Ethics *for* Health Care

fourth edition

Ethics *for* Health Care

CATHERINE BERGLUND

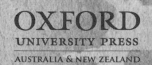

OXFORD
UNIVERSITY PRESS
AUSTRALIA & NEW ZEALAND

For my daughters, Vivienne and Ellen

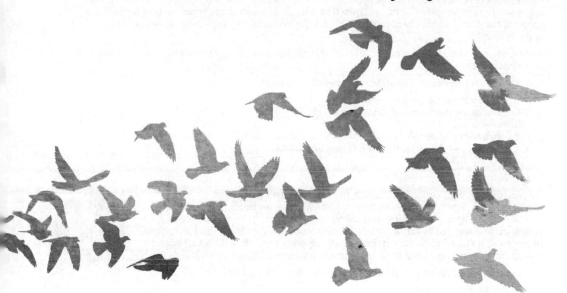

OXFORD

UNIVERSITY PRESS

Oxford University Press is a department of the University of Oxford.
It furthers the University's objective of excellence in research,
scholarship, and education by publishing worldwide. Oxford is a registered
trademark of Oxford University Press in the UK and in certain other
countries.

Published in Australia by
Oxford University Press
253 Normanby Road, South Melbourne, Victoria 3205, Australia

© Catherine Berglund 2012

The moral rights of the author have been asserted.

First edition published 1998
Second edition published 2004
Third edition published 2007
Reprinted 2007, 2008, 2010
Fourth edition published 2012

National Library of Australia Cataloguing-in-Publication entry

Author: Berglund, Catherine Anne.
Title: Ethics for health care / Catherine Berglund.
Edition: 4th ed.
ISBN: 9780195519570 (pbk.)
Notes: Includes bibliographical references and index.
Subjects: Medical ethics.

Dewey Number: 174.2

Edited by Venetia Somerset
Text design by Sardine Design
Typeset by diacriTech
Proofread by Anne Mulvaney
Indexed by Jeanne Rudd
Printed by Ligare Book Printers, Pty Ltd.

CONTENTS

List of contributions   xi
List of exercises   xiii
Abbreviations   xv
Preface   xvi
Thematic guide to text resources   xviii
Acknowledgments   xix
Contributors   xx

1   Ethics as a Process of Reflection   1

Beginning to think about ethics   2
What is ethics?   3
Absolutism/deontology   6
Consequentialism/utilitarianism   7
Libertarianism   7
Proportionism   8
Communitarianism   8
Some cases to start with   8
Principlist frameworks   11
Relativism   13
Casuistry   13
Choices to be made when reflecting on cases   13
Cases to ponder   16

2   Caring as Professionals   21

Becoming a professional carer   22
Professional goals and duties   26
Principles as fundamental propositions and summaries   29
Professional guidelines on ethics   34
Caring in multidisciplinary teams   39
Law and ethics   41

3   Caring as Service Provision   45

Accepting a job to provide service   46
Rights and interests   48
Models of justice   53
Applying the three models of justice   55

The business of provision   57
Further tools for considering fair distribution   66

4   Enter the Patient   71
Meeting the patient/client   71
The beginnings of treatment responsibility   80
A dynamic relationship   86
Negotiating treatment   89
Seeking consent   92

5   The Client and Carer Relationship   98
Expectations and responsibilities   99
Privacy and confidentiality   100
Risks facing community   110
Veracity on both sides   112
Trust in the hands of the professional   115
Risk to client or carer   117
Risk to others   120
Terminating a relationship   121

6   At the Beginning of Life   125
Personhood and beginnings   126
Genetic issues   132
Abortion   136

7   When the Patient is Young and Developing   143
Challenges to autonomy and informed decision making   144
Who decides best interests?   145
Ethically robust decisions   146
Competence   147
Information and comprehension   148
Voluntariness   149
Limiting what is asked   150

8   Mid-life and Health Care Challenges   154
Patients/clients as consumers and community members   154
Treatment in challenging situations   157
Quality-of-life choices   160
Non-compliant patients   161
Pharmaceuticals and the development of new drugs   164

9   Declining Phases of Life and End-of-life Challenges   168

Decision-making components in action   169
Declining phases and end of life   170
Suicide   175
Euthanasia   176

10   Caring in an Institutional and Social Context   182

Community input into acceptable limits   182
Institutional limits   190
Religion and health care   191

11   Monitoring and Education   197

Peer standards and implementation   197
Institutional standards and implementation   202
Legal standards and ethics   206
Self-reflection   207

12   And So to Research   209

Being a researcher and a carer   209
The patient as a research subject   211
Prominent ethics concerns in research   211
The Belmont principles   214
Research ethics committees and submitting an ethics proposal   218
Writing up   222

Glossary   *225*
A guide to further reading   *232*
Bibliography   *233*
Index   *252*

LIST OF CONTRIBUTIONS

Chapter 1 Ethics as a Process of Reflection

From Theory to Practice: Making the abstract knowable and then relevant
to clinical practice 12
Alix G. Magney

Chapter 2 Caring as Professionals

From Theory to Practice: An insight to share with students 25
Rose Leontini

From Theory to Practice: Teaching ethical behaviour in practice 29
Jenneke Foottit

Chapter 3 Caring as Service Provision

From Theory to Practice: Short supply and immediate priorities 51
Jenneke Foottit

From Theory to Practice: Staffing and care decisions 56
Jenneke Foottit

Chapter 4 Enter the Patient

From Theory to Practice: Trust and promises 76
Leanne Boase

From Theory to Practice: The doctrine of double effect 84
Leanne Boase

Chapter 5 The Client and Carer Relationship

From Theory to Practice: Tearoom chat 105
Jenneke Foottit

From Theory to Practice: Direct questions 113
Jenneke Foottit

From Theory to Practice: The client–carer relationship and fidelity 115
Leanne Boase

Chapter 6 At the Beginning of Life

From Theory to Practice: If in doubt, pair out 137
Beah Revay

Chapter 8 Mid-life and Health Care Challenges

From Theory to Practice: Consent and imbalance of power   155
Leanne Boase
From Theory to Practice: Negotiating treatment   159
Erin Godecke, Jacqui Ancliffe, and Andrew Granger
From Theory to Practice: Consent   162
Erin Godecke, Jacqui Ancliffe, and Andrew Granger

Chapter 9 Declining Phases of Life and End-of-Life Challenges

From Theory to Practice: Aged care perspective   171
Tracy Edwards
From Theory to Practice: Ethical dilemmas in health care settings   174
Jade Cartwright

Chapter 10 Caring in an Institutional and Social Context

From Theory to Practice: Ethnic perspective and ethics   184
Jenneke Foottit
From Theory to Practice: Cultural aspects of ethics and health care   193
Jade Cartwright

Chapter 11 Monitoring and Education

From Theory to Practice: Using newspapers as triggers for discussion   202
Jenneke Foottit

LIST OF EXERCISES

1.1	Multiple issues	9
1.2	Coordinating choices	10
1.3	Specific requests	14
1.4	Care and understanding	15
1.5	Worried about Mum	16
1.6	Confusion and decisions	17
2.1	Ideals and values	22
2.2	Skills and limits	24
2.3	Responsibility and accountability	28
2.4	General principles in your professional code of ethics	37
2.5	Clock on	40
2.6	Law as a basic standard	42
3.1	The sharing of resources	46
3.2	Budgets and priority decisions	58
3.3	Primary care decisions	65
3.4	Preventive testing budgets	66
3.5	Public purse and dwindling personal assets	68
4.1	People you meet	72
4.2	Preferences for privacy	73
4.3	Make a wish	75
4.4	Ideals of care	80
4.5	Duty and limits of care	82
4.6	Responsibility for harms	83
4.7	Treatment process and decisions	88
4.8	Standards of information disclosure	90
4.9	Administrative information and decisions	91
4.10	Consent forms for the everyday	93
5.1	Accuracy and records	100
5.2	Secrets and duties	101
5.3	Movement of information	105
5.4	Regulated information	106

5.5	Organisational regulation	111
5.6	Risk and assessment	112
5.7	Mandatory information gathering	117
6.1	Choices and limbo	127
6.2	Creation for others	130
6.3	Declaration—enshrined concerns	132
6.4	Genetic prediction	133
6.5	Social genetic planning	134
6.6	Personal choices and individual differences	137
6.7	Two interests and one impossible decision	140
7.1	Developing autonomy	148
7.2	Expressed wishes and capacity	149
7.3	A child's place in others' medical decisions	150
8.1	Quick decisions	159
8.2	Acceptance of advice	162
8.3	Development of a service	163
9.1	Diminishing competency	169
9.2	Tragedy and further choices	173
9.3	Final plans	175
9.4	Principles in regulations	177
9.5	Advice for professionals on assisting with final plans	179
10.1	Client and community views on practices	184
10.2	New frontiers and personal views	188
10.3	Religious conviction and actions	194
11.1	Professional concerns and trying to be heard	201
11.2	From case decisions to policy	203
12.1	Ethics analysis of research	213
12.2	A proposal for consideration	221
12.3	Monitoring and investigation	222

ABBREVIATIONS

AHPRA	Australian Health Practitioner Regulation Agency
AIDS	acquired immune deficiency syndrome
ARC	Australian Research Council
CPR	cardiopulmonary resuscitation
DNA	deoxyribonucleic acid
DNR	Do Not Resuscitate
ESRC	Economic & Social Research Council (UK)
FDA	Food and Drug Administration (US)
GDP	gross domestic product
GP	general practitioner
H5N1	strain of avian influenza
HDEC	Health and Disability Ethics Committee (NZ)
HIV	human immunodeficiency virus
HREC	human research ethics committee
IEC	institutional ethics committee
IRB	Institutional Review Board
IVF	in vitro fertilisation
NHMRC	National Health and Medical Research Council (AUS)
NHS	National Health Service (UK)
NIH	National Institutes of Health (US)
NZ	New Zealand
OECD	Organization for Economic Co-operation and Development
ORI	Office of Research Integrity (US)
QA	quality assurance
QALY	quality-adjusted life year
QI	quality improvement
REC	Research Ethics Committee
SARS	severe acute respiratory syndrome
TGA	Therapeutic Goods Administration (AUS)
UK	United Kingdom
UN	United Nations
UNESCO	United Nations Educational, Scientific and Cultural Organization
US	United States
USA	United States of America
WHO	World Health Organization
WMA	World Medical Association

PREFACE

This text meets the need to consider ethics in the routine context of health care. It follows a sequence that is familiar in health care education and practice: training, adopting a profession, becoming a team member in a health care setting, beginning to see clients, and working with clients as their treatment progresses.

The book also meets the need to learn about ethics theory. But it moves beyond the traditional theory-oriented structure of most ethics texts to a structure that is generated by practical, professional, and client needs. Key doctrines, moral distinctions, and theories are woven into the text. Principlist approaches are explored, as are frameworks such as utilitarianism and deontology. The text does not favour any one of these. Rather, it leaves the choice up to the reader. Readers are encouraged to relate the ideas presented to their own views and experiences, and to answer questions as they read.

This text takes a novel approach to teaching ethics, drawing on practical experience and contemporary issues in its exploration of ethical choices made in health care. Taking the sequence described above—training, adoption of a profession, becoming a team member, and seeing and working with clients—the book focuses on the interaction between the health provider and his or her client. This book delves into health care ethics with the workplace as the starting point. It is designed to be useful to all health care workers and students.

The author, Catherine Berglund, BSc (Psychol) PhD (Community Med), is not a practising health professional. Yet, with undergraduate psychology training, and postgraduate research and health ethics experience, she is often asked to advise on reflection processes for health professionals.

So many different health care workers offer health care: ambulance workers, specialists, speech therapists, optometrists, physiotherapists, general practitioners (GPs), dentists, rehabilitation counsellors, nurses, occupational therapists, pharmacists, radiologists, laboratory scientists, medical records and health administrators, and many others. They are all an essential part of our health system, and this book is designed to be accessible to the many and varied professions that make up a health care team.

Teachers of health care ethics can use this book as a training manual or class resource. It provides an extensive choice of tutorial triggers, and contains sufficient theory to be able to be used in an ethics curriculum, or integrated with core health care subjects. Such groups are usually led by a tutor or lecturer. This book has been written with these teachers of health care ethics in mind. Many of the exercises can be set as individual or group work, and ready-made tutorial exercises and teaching tips are a feature of the fourth edition. It is recommended that teachers work through the book first before they start a teaching program. So many of the issues are interrelated that students may raise concepts that are covered in more detail in later chapters. For those studying and teaching health ethics in a traditional thematic format, a thematic guide to recommended sections of the text is provided.

THEMATIC GUIDE TO TEXT RESOURCES

This list is to guide reading within the text if you are covering classical ethics topics in a traditional, thematic way. The chapter number, sub-headings and exercises that are most relevant to particular themes are listed as a starting point for your reading.

- Virtue and obligations to care: Chapter 1, What is ethics?; Chapter 2, Professional goals and duties, Professional guidelines on ethics
- Acting and not acting: Chapter 4, The beginnings of treatment responsibility; Chapter 9, Declining phases and end of life; Chapter 5, Privacy and confidentiality, Exercise 5.2
- Doctrine of double effect: Chapter 4, The beginnings of treatment responsibility, Exercise 4.6
- Truth telling: Chapter 4, Negotiating treatment, Exercise 4.8; Chapter 5, Veracity on both sides
- Autonomy: Chapter 1, Libertarianism, Exercise 1.1; Chapter 4, Meeting the patient, Exercise 4.3; Chapter 7, Competence
- Confidentiality: Chapter 4, Meeting the patient/client, Exercise 4.2; Chapter 5, Privacy and confidentiality, Exercise 5.3, Exercise 5.4
- Personhood: Chapter 6, Personhood and beginnings, Exercise 6.2
- Abortion: Chapter 6, Abortion, Exercise 6.6
- Genetics: Chapter 6, Genetic issues, Exercise 6.3, Exercise 6.5
- Death and dying: Chapter 9, Declining phases and end of life
- Euthanasia: Chapter 9, Suicide, Euthanasia, Exercise 9.4
- Resource allocation: Chapter 1, Exercise 1.2; Chapter 3, Exercises 3.1, 3.2, 3.3, 3.4, and 3.5.

ACKNOWLEDGMENTS

I feel privileged to have had the opportunity to learn from many people during the preparation of this book. Some are learned writers and colleagues, others are health carers and their patients, health professionals, and some are friends and family. Many have prompted me to begin this project by their writings, others by their spoken word, and others have encouraged and supported me throughout. I owe them my deepest gratitude and give my heartfelt thanks to them all.

The support of Oxford University Press in the writing and production of this book has been superb—I would particularly like to thank Jill Henry and Michele Sabto, for support during the first edition preparation, Debra James for support during the second, third and fourth edition preparation, and Shari Serjeant for support during the fourth edition preparation.

CONTRIBUTORS

Jacqueline Ancliffe is a Specialist Neurological Physiotherapist employed by Royal Perth Hospital in the Neurosciences Division. She has more than 30 years experience in the management and treatment of stroke and other neurological conditions. She is the Royal Perth Hospital trial manager for the A Very Early Rehabilitation Trial (AVERT), the largest international, multidisciplinary randomised control trial on early mobilisation post stroke in the world, a member of the Stroke Society of Australasia, the World Stroke Organisation and represents the Western Australian Nursing & Allied Health interests of the Australian Stroke Coalition. The National Stroke Foundation of Australia awarded her their Stroke Champion Award for 2011.

Leanne Boase is a Nurse Practitioner with a background in Emergency Nursing, and post-graduate qualifications in both Nursing and Education. She currently works in Victoria as a Nurse Practitioner, and lectures in a variety of nursing topics including Ethics and Law, and Patient Assessment.

Jade Cartwright is a speech pathologist with 10 years experience working in the neuroscience field in the areas of stroke rehabilitation and management of progressive neurological disorders. She is now a lecturer at Curtin University in Perth, Western Australia. Jade is completing her doctoral research in the area of Primary Progressive Aphasia.

Dr Tracy Edwards is a general practitioner working on the NSW Central Coast. After developing an interest in aged care during 14 years in family practices, she has been working exclusively in this sector for the last eight years, both in community and hospital settings. A previous Aged Care GP consultant for the Central Coast Division of General Practice, she has a special interest in dementia, palliative care and advance care planning.

Jenneke Foottit is a lecturer and nurse with many years of clinical experience in areas that present ethical dilemmas on a regular basis; caring for people with dementia who have behaviours of concern. She has a passionate interest in helping nurses live with the choices they have to make in these situations.

Dr Erin Godecke holds a Post Doctoral Research Fellowship at Edith Cowan University (Speech Pathology) which is supported by the NHMRC funded Centre for

Clinical Research Excellence in Aphasia Rehabilitation. Her PhD investigated the dose effects of early aphasia intervention, which has been included in the 2012 Cochrane Review for aphasia therapy following stroke. She has 13 years experience working as a speech pathologist in acute stroke care at Royal Perth Hospital and has a special interest in early aphasia rehabilitation and measuring stroke care outcomes.

Dr Andrew Granger is a Geriatrician and General Physician, with post-fellowship training and a special interest in stroke rehabilitation. He is currently Director of Stroke Rehabilitation Services at Osborne Park Hospital, Perth. Andrew is a representative on the Australian Stroke Coalition and on the Stroke Society of Australasia Committee. His research interests relate to stroke rehabilitation, in particular models of care including Early Supported Discharge schemes.

Dr Rose Leontini is Lecturer in Sociology and Health Ethics within the Discipline of Behavioural and Social Sciences in Health, Faculty of Health Sciences, University of Sydney. Her research interests are hereditary risk and genetic testing, health risk, youth and alcohol use, sociology of health and illness, and health ethics. She is particularly interested in exploring people's health-related experience using narrative analysis. She teaches Health Ethics and Health Sociology to undergraduate students in the health care professions.

Dr Alix G. Magney has been teaching and researching in ethics for 15 years. Her interest in the area stems from a belief that ethics is fundamental to all human inter-relations, in other words, as soon as we connect with another person we have established an ethic. Teaching ethics to health care professionals is a concrete way of valuing and respecting the intensity of the doctor/patient relationship, as well as recognising the significance of collegial relationships between all health care workers, and encouraging individual reflection on all aspects of professionalism.

Beah Revay has a background and degrees in psychology and bioethics. She has been teaching medical ethics to general studies students, nurses, and medical students at Universities in Sydney for the last 15 years. She also sits on the Macquarie University Human Research Ethics committee.

ETHICS AS A PROCESS OF REFLECTION

- Beginning to think about ethics
- What is ethics?
- Absolutism/deontology
  Consequentialism/utilitarianism
- Libertarianism
- Proportionism
- Communitarianism
- Some cases to start with
- Principlist frameworks
- Relativism
- Casuistry
- Choices to be made when reflecting on cases
- Cases to ponder

OBJECTIVES

The first chapter explains what ethics is, acknowledges the considerable theoretical tradition of ethics, and starts you on an ethical exploration of practical health care situations. The general approach in major ethics theories is explained, with a practical introduction of how theories are applied to case studies, and the arguments that might be advanced under each theory or framework. You are encouraged to reflect on your own values, and to nominate which theories you are most comfortable with. By the end of this chapter you should be able to define and

Morals
Significant lessons prompting reflection to identify virtuous, right, or acceptable course of conduct.

explain the following concepts: ethics, **morals**, bioethics, medical ethics, reflection, good, norms, ideals, and values. Note that these concepts are added to a glossary, which will grow in size as you work your way through each chapter and your understanding of ethics increases. You will also have encountered the ethics theories of deontology, absolutism, utilitarianism, consequentialism, libertarianism, proportionism, and communitarianism, and casuistry, relativism, and principlist frameworks.

BEGINNING TO THINK ABOUT ETHICS

This book is about ethics. You don't need to be an ethicist to understand ethics in the health context, and you don't need to have learnt a lot of philosophy to be able to think about ethics as you work in your health profession. This book is written so that the information it contains can be used in a practical way in your everyday work. It starts with you, the professional carer or student, and examines the way professional work and your interaction with your clients or patients is shaped by ethics.

Ethics is a tool that is meant to be used in practical situations. As more than an abstract introspective pursuit, it helps us reflect on real-life issues, and it is also a process that can be applied to real concerns and situations as they unfold.

The common theme followed in this book is that health care ethics is not only about setting acceptable standards, but is also about reflecting on what you should aim for in your work as a health care professional. It is about reflecting on optimal standards and pursuing those standards. Ethics is a reflective process of analysing and examining moral issues and problems.

The book is written in an interactive way. Dotted throughout, you will find individual and group exercises that will help you think about particular issues, standards, and styles of ethical **reflection**. Tutorial-type triggers and case studies are also included. You will encounter ethics theories and frameworks in each chapter. The way in which they may guide practical reflection is highlighted through examples and exercises. As you work through the exercises, you will become more familiar with key ways of identifying ethics issues in health care and working to resolve them. In this framework, the philosophical aspect of ethics becomes a tool that you, as a health care worker, can use to reflect on ethics as it applies in your profession and in your clinical work.

You will not be an expert in ethics after working through this book, but you will be considerably more informed. The book starts you on a path of ethical reflection and encourages you to consult with others so that you do not face ethical challenges alone. At times when you are faced with complex challenges you will naturally want to consult with colleagues who are interested in ethics. Your reading will equip you to recognise ethics issues in situations, and also recognise opportunities for discussion.

Reflection
A process of thought and analysis on past, present, or future issues, applying deep and serious consideration.

WHAT IS ETHICS?

Ethics helps you to decide what to do in routine and complex or difficult situations. It acts as a guide, a reasoned 'voice'. Thinking and reflecting is the hallmark of ethics because it is an active process.

Ethics in health contexts is sometimes simply called 'ethics'; at other times it is called 'bioethics' or 'medical ethics'. You may like to choose a definition of ethics that you understand best from the following options:

- **ethics:** 'ways of understanding and examining the moral life'.[1]
- **bioethics:** 'a popular contraction for "biomedical ethics", which is the study of moral value in the life sciences and in their clinical application'.[2]
- **medical ethics:** 'the analytical activity in which the concepts, assumptions, beliefs, attitudes, emotion, reasons, and arguments underlying medico-moral decision making are examined critically'.[3]

Some of the suggested forms of reasoning and reflecting that you will encounter in this book have a philosophical basis. In philosophical thinking, arguments are examined and analysed, underlying assumptions are tested, and arguments are carried through to extremes to test their robustness and practical application. Ethics as a discipline makes use of critical reflection processes, and also relies on practical lessons to be learnt from others. You learn from the experiences of others and you share your experiences with them, so that the collective experience of situations grows. As you gather experience, you draw on past reflections and experiences to guide you. You draw on collective ethics experience and individual ethical reflection as you decide how to act professionally and ethically.

So remember that ethics is a process of reflection. We will start with small steps, and gradually build your options for analysis and reflection. The focus of the book is to think about the health care of individuals, and that means thinking about how it is that people come to be in a position to provide care, how resources are available to allow them to fulfil that aim, and then how a process of care, with its ethics issues, unfolds. The idea of applying ethics to health care contexts is contained in the title of the book, *Ethics for Health Care*. You learn it as a tool to help with the job of health care. The idea of ethics is that an optimal standard is aimed for. There is an impetus to aim higher than the basic minimum of social responsibilities. The common process of the reflection is that moral issues are identified and examined. A moral reflection has many connotations. To some it means to reflect on a lesson that has been handed down in significant religious texts, to strive to distinguish between right and wrong, and act accordingly, given that lesson. It can also be a practical lesson learnt from past experience and reflection, again reflected on in terms of significance and importance. The term 'moral' is used in a broad sense in this book to mean a reflective examination of values and objectives, including reference to lessons, with an examination of the implications of thought and action for oneself and others.

Ethics
Reflective process of analysing and examining moral issues and problems.

Bioethics
Reflective ethics process applied to the health care context and life sciences.

Medical ethics
Specific term for ethics in the medical and biomedical context.

Ethics, as it is understood in this book, takes as its starting point the fact that, first and foremost, you are an individual. You were a unique individual before you began your training, you are an individual at work, where you are also a health care worker, and you are an individual outside work. There are very different people in this world, and one of the things that distinguishes us from each other is the way we choose to live our lives. Since you bring much of yourself to your work, it is worthwhile thinking about the sort of person you are as we begin our discussion of 'professional' ethics.

EVERYDAY ETHICS

Take a minute to think about how you live your life. Try to identify, in your own words, one fundamental value or principle in the way you live your life, and in the way you live alongside others.

Many of the philosophers whose work we draw upon in professional ethics actually wrote more about individual ethics (that is, about the ethics of decisions made by individuals) than about group standards or **norms**.

Early philosophers thought about how we should live our lives and relate to others. They thought about the structure of our society; about what we, as individuals, owe to our society; and about what we can, and should, expect in return. They also thought about our higher duties to God. Nowadays, religion is often separated from professional ethics, but if it is a large part of how you live your life it would be artificial for you to ignore it. You will see comments and exercises from many early philosophers dotted throughout the book. Try this one now.

Norms
Accepted standards, which can be used to judge conduct.

PAUSE & REFLECT

When you think about how you try to live, think about the virtue you aspire to. What is that virtue? How would you define it, and how do you know if you have achieved it?

As an important early philosopher, the key feature of Socrates' discussions was the way in which participants were encouraged to elicit and question beliefs. Some of the central values that Socrates espoused were justice, courage, and pity.[4] He tried to define them through reflection and discussion, like the reflection you just undertook for yourself. This reflection process is appropriate for our professional lives too. Justice and courage may be listed as two of the modern nurse's virtues, as nurses advance their clients' interests and attempt to maximise the autonomy of their clients.[5]

Our **values** form our ethics standards and they determine what we expect from others. In some ethics frameworks, virtue and the formation of central values is paramount. There is a sense of a moral self-development. We probably apply this notion of moral self-development, without thinking about it, in our own lives. We

Values
Concepts given worth or importance in life and interactions, making up a value-system.

do not, for instance, expect children to be rational and moral in the way in which they relate to others and the world because we know that some of this is learnt. We gradually teach them what is expected, what we value, and what we hope they will value. As they grow older, they begin to recognise, in abstract, that it is not just the fact that these values are advocated by parents and guardians that makes them desirable as guides for life. They come to value these virtues themselves.

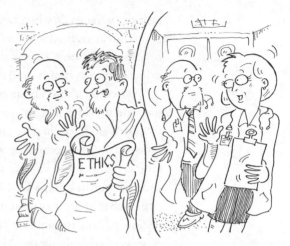

In ancient Greece and Rome there were designated forums for debating what was right and virtuous, and for reasoning about why that was so. Learned people were trained to reflect and to hold monologues or debates challenging others to refine their thoughts, actions, and reasoning. Socrates and Plato led this tradition, and there was an expectation that people who rose to prominence in society would learn to reflect and debate personal and social ethics. Plato was Socrates' student and Aristotle's teacher. Plato emphasised that winning a debate was not the purpose of the discussion. The purpose was to search for the truth.[6]

When a person becomes a member of a profession, they become one of the people who help define the ideals of the profession. They bring their own ethics to the profession, and their ethics is influenced by what others have defined as appropriate ethical standards for that profession. It is a fluid process of sharing thoughts and of learning to work together towards common goods. (Bear in mind that the word '**good**' is used as a noun here; that it is a thing or concept, not an adjective.) The process of reflecting on professional caring, identifying important aspects of caring, and debating what professionals should aim for continues the tradition of ancient debates, albeit in a different guise. You may like to consider whether you care enough about your **ideals** to defend them against others. In professional debates, we would do well to remember to keep discussion constructive, as is urged in Plato's tradition, and not simply use ethics as a tool to score points off our colleagues. The reflection process is more important than keeping score.

Good
A desirable end or object.

Ideals
A standard or concept of excellence which is aimed to be met.

What you have done so far is to start to reflect on what you value, how you live, what you strive for, and how your values are part of the way you live up to your professional responsibilities. Personal reflection on professional responsibilities has become integrated with health care, and health care ethics is generally seen as a modern phenomenon. Much has been written about the fact that technological innovation and development in health care has led to an exponential increase in ethical dilemmas, and many of those involved in health care wonder if and how we should put such advances to use.[7] Medicine and health care present such ethically stark issues that it is very useful to use ethics as a tool to unravel the issues and work out, in a reasoned fashion, what to do when faced with those issues in practice. On the other hand, even before great technological advances, the daily aspects of health care were the subject of ethics reflection. It may just be that, now that technology (including technology associated with health care) has such a high profile, ethics also has a higher profile.

You could think about ethics in health care as really being about three things: individual ethics and values, group ethics and values, and professional ethics and values. Writers on health care ethics vary in their approach. Some concentrate on individual virtue, others on group notions of ethics, or on philosophical analysis of ethical stances and values. This book gives you a wide range of exercises to do on your own or in groups so that you can experiment with these approaches. All of the approaches share a common purpose: to assist health care workers to make ethical decisions, and to monitor their own and others' practices so that the health care process is 'ethically aware'. They also potentially assist the people who plan and receive services. Ethics is becoming a joint effort, and reflection on ethics is increasingly consultative. More on this is included in Chapter 10. Throughout this book you will see examples of informed ethics debate and reflection in contemporary debates on health care, and in practical contemporary health policy and guidelines. These are the product of collaboration and joint discussion between professions and the community.

Let's start to look at what is ahead for you in learning about ethics theory and frameworks throughout the book. The emphasis for you will be on using aspects of the theories in an applied way rather than on learning them by rote.

ABSOLUTISM/DEONTOLOGY

Deontology works with the notion that there are certain absolute rules that must be followed, or upheld, regardless of the consequences. It classifies acts according to whether they must be done (because they are necessary to uphold a particular rule or rules), or are intrinsically wrong (and therefore must not be done). The rules are commonly thought to be handed down from God, such as the sanctity of life. The rules translate into duties, and an example of this is included in Chapter 2. The moral importance of acting and not acting is the subject of an exercise in Chapter 4, and you will be asked to decide which protagonist in the story, Alex or Alice, is responsible for the harm that befalls their father.

You will find the doctrine of 'double effect', a classic deontological tool which can help with this decision, in Chapter 4. The responsibility for something bad occurring, even though a good was aimed for, is a key issue for health care workers.

The question of what constitutes personhood (and life) is addressed in Chapter 6. As the discussion in that chapter shows, deontological positions are prominent in this debate on the defining characteristics of personhood and life. The discussion contrasts these deontological positions with outcome-based positions, particularly in relation to the creation, genetic manipulation, and ending of life.

Deontology is in direct opposition to relativism, in which the question of what to do is defined not with reference to strict rules but with reference to the relevant acceptable boundaries for a particular context or culture, which by definition are relative; that is, they are fluid and can change.

CONSEQUENTIALISM/UTILITARIANISM

Under consequentialist or utilitarian theories, which are teleological and focus on contributions to desirable goals, the 'right' thing to do is that which maximises the good. The outcome of an action is what is ethically important. The greatest good for the greatest number is pursued, whether that good is a specific utility, felicity, or happiness.

These utilitarian assumptions are discussed in Chapter 3. Under utilitarianism, the question of how to share a limited good is often one of how to maximise distribution. It is possible to reject such utilitarian assumptions when making ethical decisions, as you will read ethicists did when responding to the hypothetical scenario on predictive cancer testing discussed in Chapter 3.

Modern consequentialists' views on obligations to care and work, even in situations of some danger, are described in Chapter 4. This is an illustration that in some frameworks one's own interests do not necessarily receive priority if the greatest good for the greatest number is the prime consideration in the issue at hand.

To look at the effect of the manipulation of life, as is done in the case of two sisters in Chapter 6, when one sister is conceived in the hope of providing genetically compatible regenerative tissue for the other, is to acknowledge the fact that ethically problematic decisions affect not only the individuals immediately concerned and their families, but also whole communities.

LIBERTARIANISM

Libertarianism places the personal freedom of the individual at the centre of analysis. That freedom is claimed as a right, unless there is sufficient reason to limit it. Patient freedom and autonomy are explored in Chapter 4.

John Stuart Mill is referred to throughout the book as a libertarian (a philosophy closely related to liberalism) philosopher. His thesis, 'On Liberty',[8] has been used in policy debates to decide when a person's liberty can be infringed, such as in the mandatory blood testing exercise described in Chapter 5. The only acceptable reasons for limiting liberty are if a serious and imminent risk is posed to another individual, or if the fabric of society is threatened. These reasons are used, at strategic points in this book, to explore the health care worker's role in fostering self-determination and in being aware of similar rights to liberty that are held by others. The classic Mill thesis is echoed in modern libertarian writings, some of which are noted in Chapter 4.

PROPORTIONISM

Proportionism acknowledges rules and values, but does not regard them as universal. It is quite a pragmatic theory, which, without using binding principles as a guide, takes into account the human nature of the person, the situation, and the intention behind the person's actions. A broad idea of the good is aimed for.

Doing the best one can is a common pragmatic approach to ethics. The proportionist would require that the best is pursued in full knowledge of the ethics choices and practical alternatives.

Proportionism is essentially a compromise between the extremes of absolutism and relativism.

COMMUNITARIANISM

Communitarianism places the community at the centre of a value system and its corresponding ethical analysis. While the individual members are acknowledged, it is the good of the community, its goals, and the threats it faces that are the key considerations. Communal and public goods are emphasised, and community views must be sought to unravel difficult issues.

The process of seeking and acknowledging community views is discussed throughout this book. In Chapter 2, a comment by a former Director-General of the World Health Organization (WHO) is included to show that professional ethics takes place within a community context, and an expectation that the values of the community should be respected.

The fact that there are many different community values in relation to informed consent is noted in Chapter 4, so it is important to be able to check what the relevant values are. The processes that make community views on ethics known are outlined in Chapter 10.

SOME CASES TO START WITH

The reflective exercises that you will be asked to do throughout this book are intended to galvanise you towards your own preferred ethics theory. Your own reflection on ethics is a continuing process that is only just beginning. As it develops, it will be moulded and tested by the challenges you will face in your work as a health care practitioner.

A number of cases are provided in this chapter as a starting point for your practical ethics reflection. As you reflect on your first reaction to each case, think about the values and concerns that are prominent for you. Later, when you use the cases for revision and you read back over your notes in the book, you should be well on the way to recognising which ethics theories you favour and identifying the ethics tools that are useful in your ethical reflection on your health care work. This process of reflection is the start of routinely integrating ethics in your own health care work.

The process of reflection is well suited to groups. If you have finished your training and are working, you may like to do a few of the exercises with some colleagues in an informal group, or as part of a professional development program. If you are training, you may have a group of colleagues and students around you, in which case you are fortunate enough to have a ready-made group for ethical reflection.

Now you might like to consider the following case studies. After each case study is set out, the aspects that might be focused on under different theories are explained. It is up to you to ponder the key elements and think about how a solution to each problem might be arrived at. As you think, be reassured that you will learn more about how to analyse the cases in detail as you work through the book. If you return to these cases as a revision exercise, you might also reread sections of the book to bolster your analysis, your argument, and ultimately the ethics position that you recommend.

EXERCISE 1.1 MULTIPLE ISSUES

CASE ONE

When you first met Ms Tan, she was 14. She has a slight mobility disability, from a congenital spinal problem, and a mild intellectual disability. With the aid of an interpreter (English is her second language), you arrived at a course of treatment and management for her recently diagnosed asthma in close consultation with her other health care workers and her parents. Now, three years later, Ms Tan returns. She has left school, is working part-time, and has more ambitious life priorities, in keeping with a young adult. She asks for your help in continued treatment, but also in gaining more independence from her family. She feels that they closet her because of her medical problems.

Patients rarely have just one medical or health concern. Their social context is also complex. How you define 'health' will lay the foundation for your reaction to this case with Ms Tan. You should first consider whether your definition of health is as broad as the WHO's, which includes the physical, social, and mental aspects of life. The definition of health, and the good to aim for as a health care worker, is a central focus of Chapters 3 and 4.

Deontological theory would emphasise the duties owed to Ms Tan as an individual, especially the duty to further good for her and limit harm coming to her, particularly intentional harm. There may be some rules that would preclude doing what she wants—for example, you might think that the process she has asked for is fundamentally wrong.

If you adhere to the ethics theories that place the most weight on patient autonomy, such as libertarianism, upholding Ms Tan's choices will be important to you, even if you do not agree with the choices she makes. You will be concerned with establishing that Ms Tan is competent to make certain relevant decisions and life choices. The issue of competence is covered in Chapter 7.

Ms Tan's cultural and family contexts are especially relevant with regard to proportionism and communitarianism. Both theories balance goals, such as life and health goals, with individual variation and choice in relation to these goals, according to cultural and societal limits.

The question of whether allowing the choices she wants to make will result in good for her, her family, and society is a key factor in utilitarianism. This is because the good that is aimed for also has a societal context—that is, it has ramifications beyond Ms Tan as an individual.

So while all theories rely on an obligation to care on the part of the health worker, they give startlingly different reasons for the existence of that obligation.

EXERCISE 1.2 COORDINATING CHOICES

CASE TWO

You are involved in a coordinated-care program, in conjunction with many different health care providers in your local area. The money available for care is controlled by a central coordinator, in this case a nurse, and the money is hypothetically capped for each chronic health problem. Your client, Mr Helm, is in his mid-forties and has many complex medical problems resulting from a car accident that happened five years previously. This accident left him with internal injuries. A new drug has just finished being tested and has been registered. There is a possibility that the drug could significantly help your client, but it is not known if the results, as published in your professional journal, apply to him. The drug is also very expensive. Mr Helm does not know about the new drug. He comes to see you as part of ongoing rehabilitation, and expresses dissatisfaction with the current treatment plan. He wistfully says that he wishes there was something else he could try.

Coordinated care places emphasis on working as a team. In relation to any particular client, the objectives of care, arrived at by the team, are crucial. Discussing what each member of the team is aiming for is important, as is discussed in Chapters 2 and 3 (coordinated care is discussed in Chapter 3).

Libertarian theories, in particular, would allow as much choice as possible to be made by the individual patient. The professional may be obliged to promote such a choice if they adhere to libertarian or other autonomy-based theories. Apart from questions of ability to make treatment and life decisions, apparent in case one, there is an issue of information disclosure here. The professional holds information that may be relevant to the patient's choice. The importance of the patient knowing the relevant information before treatment decisions are made is discussed in Chapter 4. Paternalism, which contrasts sharply with libertarianism, may be at work if the practitioner is withholding so much information that it effectively nullifies patient choice.

Deontology would ask whether the possible treatment really is better for this client. Research is essentially a balance of risks and benefits, as discussed in Chapter 12. This is the case in drug development and research too, as outlined in the section on drugs in Chapter 8. Is a new untried treatment better than the myriad treatments and side effects currently available to Mr Helm? This value judgment clearly needs to be made with professional clinical expertise and with the relevant medical facts available.

In the case study of Mr Helm, the facts given are scant. If the risks include significant harm, the ethical obligation to care may translate into an obligation to protect rather than chance further injury. The chance of further injury can be hard to predict in situations where complex conditions are treated with multiple powerful drugs. You may like to consider whether you are sufficiently knowledgeable or skilled to deal with that drug, or with the combination of it and other medications that Mr Helm is currently taking (and will, no doubt, continue to take). The limits of skill are a central issue in caring, and this is the subject of a reflective exercise in Chapter 2.

The obligation to provide the best available treatment is double-edged. You may have an idea of what is best, but is it 'available'? Certain utilitarian theories hold that a good should be available to the greatest number, giving society the ethical authority to limit the availability of resources. Under these theories, limiting the access that certain individuals have to certain resources is justifiable if those individuals consume 'too much' of the health care budget.

PRINCIPLIST FRAMEWORKS

Principlist frameworks for decision making are a modern phenomenon. They are tools for summarising, in shorthand and in a thematic way, the obligations and aspirations of health care workers. These frameworks are a facilitative naming of principles, and rather than providing an answer or sole principle to follow, they foster exploration of various aspects of a health care role.

The principles themselves are ideals that guide health carers in their work: to care, to do no harm, to respect integrity and autonomy, and to share resources fairly. Different principlist frameworks are described in Chapter 2, together with the different principles that are named, including those of Beauchamp and Childress—beneficence, non-maleficence, autonomy, and justice—and Gillon—respect for autonomy, beneficence, non-maleficence, and justice.[9] Chapter 2 uses the principles of Beauchamp and Childress as a tool to summarise issues in a vignette on general practice. They are also an essential part of the exercise requiring you to summarise your code of ethics. In Chapter 12, the similarly constructed principles of beneficence, respect for persons, and justice are also used to highlight key ethics concerns in health care research.

These principles can be shown to be compatible with diverse ethical theories, as is shown in Chapter 2. Some thought needs to be applied in situations in which the principles conflict though, as different theories would prioritise the principles quite differently. For instance, while libertarianism's central value—individual freedom—emphasises autonomy, communitarianism's concern with achieving good for all (in a fair manner) emphasises justice. Drawing the line at harm that is unacceptable (even when the patient has indicated a willingness to be harmed, or there is a good that must be promoted) emphasises beneficence. Because the principles used in principlist frameworks are summarising principles, they should not be used alone. You can use a principlist approach in combination with any of the ethics theories outlined above.

FROM THEORY TO PRACTICE

Making the abstract knowable and then relevant to clinical practice

Contributor: *Alix G. Magney*

At face value clinical ethics seems intuitive: be kind to patients, make good decisions. But each of the terms 'kind' and 'good' are value-laden and unspecific in their meaning. Beginner students don't understand why they need to 'learn' ethics. In essence the problem is that students don't know enough to know that they really need ethics. As one medical student said, 'Ethics is abstract; shades of grey, not like a list of things you have to learn'.

The challenge of teaching ethics is making the abstract knowable and then relevant to clinical practice.

I firmly believe in learning the theory first and immediately applying it. For example, when teaching the Principle Approach—autonomy, beneficence, non-maleficence and justice—I ensure that the students have a clear and plain understanding of the terms. In small groups they are asked to analyse a public health scenario with at least five stakeholders using the four principles. They are asked to adopt a role and debate the issues that have arisen. In a large class discussion we evaluate the concerns of the various stakeholder groups.

The value of this exercise is that the students learn that the Principle Approach is more than a list of abstract terms. It is a valuable tool for drawing out the ethics concerns of any situation.

Using the Principle Approach students elicit issues and examine a range of perspectives from each of the stakeholders. It is imperative that they apply all the principles to every stakeholder because in doing so they come to recognise the entirety of the stakeholder position. Furthermore, the inherent efficacy of the approach becomes apparent to the user.

Through the application of the Principles, students appreciate the significance of each of the terms. It is one thing to say autonomy is 'an individual's freedom to choose'. In reality, valuing individual choice can be confronting, particularly when you don't agree. Autonomy is a weighty term and comprehending and truly respecting someone else's autonomy requires you to have tolerance, empathy, and grace.

Quite often students are scared of using words if they think they are going to pronounce them incorrectly. I get the entire group to chant the terms out loud, so that they get used to saying the words. I also insist the students use the terms when they are explaining their positions to the class.

Learning needs to cement the words and their meaning in the minds of the learners.

RELATIVISM

Relativism is mentioned in Chapter 2. It is an example of an approach to the search for minimum acceptable standards that is often conducted when two groups differ on the appropriate course of action in treatment.

Relativism is not compatible with deontology, in which rules are universally applied, but it can be used in combination with other moral theories, such as utilitarianism or communitarianism. Relativism takes note of the rules or values that are appropriate for the context in which decisions are made.

CASUISTRY

Casuistry is also a pragmatic addition to ethics. It emphasises the importance of understanding value-laden decisions in their appropriate factual context and culture.[10] Legal reasoning, such as is discussed in the context of informed consent in Chapter 4, is very close to casuistry. It starts with the facts and context, and relates them to precedent. Precedent is law derived from previous decisions in cases involving the same or similar circumstances. To apply precedent in a legal context is to use a type of case-based legal decision making that applies certain legal principles derived from an accumulated history of case law to the particular facts of the dispute. Each new case tests whether the same precedent applies, given the slightly varied facts and circumstances.

CHOICES TO BE MADE WHEN REFLECTING ON CASES

The next two cases highlight the different approaches you can use to begin your analysis if you make use of the various models of ethics analysis.

CASE THREE

A 15-year-old girl, Karen, who is doing her Year 10 exams soon, comes to see a general practitioner. She says she feels tired but can't sleep, and is very worried that she won't do well in her exams. Karen asks for sleeping tablets. She does not want her parents or her normal doctor to know that she is seeking medical treatment.

The most common starting point for ethics analysis is the principlist model suggested by Beauchamp and Childress, which uses the principles of beneficence, non-maleficence, autonomy, and justice. Once you separate out the issues into these four categories, or try to brainstorm what might be a concern in each of the four, you will have made a good start to recognising the complexity of the case. For Karen, autonomy and the decision-making process will loom large. Once you have the issue tagged under autonomy, you can start to identify what is problematic about it. You might look to the sections on competency and decision making, as in Chapters 4 and 7, or to those of confidentiality in Chapter 5. The purpose of care might be discussed, and you could consider the options that may be open to the professionals who see Karen. Just stating the existence of an issue does not solve it. You will need to explore each issue and discuss if the issues are in conflict: such as if a patient's choice (autonomy) conflicts with the needs and resources available to others (justice).

The ethics theories and frameworks are very helpful in deciding how to resolve conflicts between the shorthand principles.

The Beauchamp and Childress model has appeal partly because of its simplicity, and partly because it can be realistically undertaken by any interested party. Professionals can readily use it. So can patients themselves, if they wish, or their family. It is useful for policy makers and administrators too, as it includes big-picture issues of resources alongside the potential complexities of individual circumstances and situations. It is quite useful in 'macro' community-type decisions, as well as 'micro' individual issues.

Thinking about the practical casuistry approach in the case above, given this situation of a teenager asking to be treated, independent of her family or guardian, and seeking a specific short-term 'fix' to what may be a larger complex problem, the usual approach of the clinic may well largely determine how her request is handled. An 'acceptable' course of action may already be defined by other experienced team members, and even if the ethical reasons remain unarticulated, actions by team members in the past in similar situations could guide the person treating the 'Karen' who presents as a patient this time. Tea room chats and team meetings provide a wealth of lessons learnt from past cases, and these stories are the material of casuistry.

EXERCISE 1.4 CARE AND UNDERSTANDING

CASE FOUR

An 87-year-old man, Mr M, is in a nursing home, in reasonable health for his age apart from forgetfulness of recent events and chronic hip pain. He was admitted after the death of his wife from cancer. The local GP said Mr M had been about to have hip surgery but postponed it to a few weeks after the funeral. The nursing home is preparing Mr M for the trip to hospital for a hip replacement. Each time the process is explained to him, he forgets by the next day. The operation is booked for one week's time.

What should the nursing home staff do, and why?

Two models that summarise issues into meaningful clusters that will be presented for you are those by Jonsen, Siegler, and Winslade,[11] and the rules of thumb by Jennett,[12] both included in Chapter 4. These are clinically focused, and seem to be compatible with an analysis undertaken primarily by the clinician. If you were to start with Jonsen, Siegler, and Winslade's model in your analysis, you would first try to understand the 'medical indications', or what the medical situation facing the patient is. Then you would look for evidence of client preferences, consider quality of life, and finally contemplate contextual features like the resources and so on. Note that you would summarise the issues in a different sequence from that if you were using Beauchamp and Childress's model. Some of the same issues would appear of course. The primary starting point is the health or medical issue to be dealt with, so the process is driven by the health carer, and seems in that sense to be favouring a carer's view of the important features to consider. This is similar to the 'enhanced autonomy' model you will read about in relation to decision making (Chapter 4), in which the decisions to be made are limited to those judged to be appropriate by the clinician. This seems a sensible emphasis, given that the health professionals are making themselves available to offer benefit to their patients.

If you were to apply Jennett's rules of thumb, which are explained in Chapter 4, you would explicitly consider whether to apply a specific action or treatment option. So it is important to identify the likely treatment options, and then analyse each one. You would consider whether the proposed treatment is appropriate, or rule it out if it is unnecessary, or likely to be unsuccessful, unsafe, unkind, or unwise. Some of these models emphasise judgments of care and likely benefit, some emphasise likely harm, and some emphasise questions of resources and justice. So, again, the elements that you would discuss if you used Beauchamp and Childress's principles appear in your analysis. Notice again, though, the emphasis on care issues, and a clinician's interpretation of those issues. There is little explicitly on autonomy built in to this rule-of-thumb analysis, except that each treatment is an option or choice potentially to be offered to the patient.

A relativistic approach would cast your net for gathering up issues to ponder a little bit wider than either of these models, or at least, it would emphasise the personal, cultural, and community context of the issue, and acknowledge diverse perspectives on the definition of the ethically tricky issues and their resolution. Given his view of the facts, Mr M's own preferences are important, but not more so than those of the health carers or indeed the community that is effectively providing the health care options under contemplation.

CASES TO PONDER

The following cases invite you to think through developing scenarios. It is quite routine in health care for situations to develop over time, and for different ethical challenges to emerge at different points of the process of care. Make your preliminary notes on these cases now, then, as you work through the book, look back here occasionally to add your suggestions for how to analyse the emerging ethical issues.

Remember that when making your decisions in the future, you can rely on a rich tradition of reflection and analysis that can be found in the ethics writings of others. Listen well to learn from the thoughtful decisions that have been made by those who have worked in health care before you or who work alongside you, and actively reflect on your practice. The wisdom that you will build will serve you well in making robust decisions in your everyday practice.

EXERCISE 1.5 WORRIED ABOUT MUM

CASE FIVE

Ms B has recently moved from the country to an outer suburb of a large city, to take up a student place at a college. She has two small children, and is receiving a government study subsidy and family support benefits. She is enrolled in a diploma course, and hopes eventually to be able to support herself and her children, for whom she is the sole carer. Ms B wants to arrange routine immunisation for her children and visits a local GP. She takes their previous record of immunisation with her, which is entered in the back of the children's 'child health book'. This book, kept by Ms B, contains entries of the child health nurse visits from when they were babies, and the immunisations they had received. The children are examined, and a history of their health and previous illnesses is taken by the GP and noted in their new medical records. Both children appear to be well, and are given the vaccines that are due for them according to the government-recommended immunisation schedule. This is only done after checking that they didn't appear to have been given any of them previously, both by asking Ms B and by reading the entries in the immunisation record page of the book.

Ms B is advised when to bring the children back for their next booster. A record of immunisation is entered into the 'child health book', and also in the GP's own records. The GP bulk-bills for the children's consultation, asking for no money from Ms B directly for either the consultation or vaccines, noting the Medicare and pension card that Ms B has produced to the reception desk earlier. The GP also asks Ms B whether she already has a GP for her own health needs since she has moved. The GP has noticed that Ms B appears to be thin, tired, and withdrawn, and that her teeth look chipped and damaged and her gums look swollen. She doesn't appear to be well. Ms B replies that she hasn't been to a GP as yet because she hasn't been sick. Then she volunteers that she was in an 'accident' in the country and is waiting for dental care. She says she can't afford to go to a private dentist, and had been on a public waiting list a while back, but hadn't heard yet that an appointment was available. The GP offers the number for a more local public dental clinic, and suggests that if Ms B rings, she may be able to have her appointment moved to that clinic.

Ms B returns at the next scheduled time. The children have a cold and can't be immunised that day. The GP examines them and rules out more serious febrile illnesses, but explains that the process of immunisation can have more serious side effects if a child is unwell, so it is safer to return the next week.

A week later, when Ms B returns with the children, she apologises that she has forgotten to bring their health books. The GP suggests that Ms B drops the book in to reception some time, or just to bring it along at a subsequent visit, so the details can be updated from the GP records. Both children have recovered, and receive their next booster. Ms B volunteers that a date for her dentist appointment hasn't been set yet, but that it seems possible to move it. She seems resigned to wait her turn. The GP worries that there may be more gum deterioration in the meantime, but feels that public dental care is really outside her control. She suggests that Ms B come for a check if she feels she has unusual tooth, mouth, or jaw pain, or for other health issues.

Ms B continues to return at the relevant times for the children, but does not present as a patient herself. The GP continues to worry about Ms B's overall health, particularly given Ms B's heavy study workload and sole caring responsibilities.

EXERCISE 1.6 CONFUSION AND DECISIONS

CASE SIX

Lian is a new graduate in nursing and Dr S (Phil) has just finished his specialist physician medical training. They will be working together in a public hospital inpatient ward. It is a new posting for both Lian and Phil. Lian is quite young, having gone straight from school to uni, and is just 21. Phil is older, with six years of undergraduate medicine training, a year as intern, then two as registrar before starting his postgraduate training. He is 32.

(continued)

Jan, an experienced social worker, is part of the ward team, but is also on call to three other wards with elderly patients. She has been in her position for almost 15 years. On a break in the tea room they cross paths, and Jan takes the initiative to welcome the newcomers. They chat easily about new developments in the field, and Jan comments on not only how the changes have improved patient outcomes and potential quality of life, but also on how families bear a large carer responsibility. Phil mentions a new technology he heard about at a conference the previous month that is being developed and trialled as an alternative to a particular operation. He is hoping it might become available for trial at the hospital. Lian mostly listens, but feels lucky to be part of such a pleasant ward dynamic. She has heard that some places aren't as ideal. She lets Phil and Jan know she is a new graduate, and might have to ask lots of questions. The others encourage her to let them know if she's not sure of anything and hasn't had a chance to ask her supervising nurse. She thanks them.

The public hospital budget is stretched. Three of the beds are effectively closed, and there is pressure to discharge patients in a timely manner so that other more seriously ill patients can be admitted. Jan is worried that the time needed to check that home care arrangements are in place is being curtailed, and that sending sick people home in that circumstance is potentially dangerous and stressful for family members. Lian is just run off her feet, doing a few double shifts to cover for other staff when they are sick. Fewer casual staff are being called on to help given the budget situation. She feels like she is on a steep learning curve. Dr S is busy, in clinics, operating, on ward rounds, testing procedures, and some private consulting, but enjoys the pace.

Mr I has been admitted overnight, dazed, confused, and ill. He will be having a series of tests and has been given a bed on the ward. Lian introduces herself when she comes on shift. Mr I says he just wants to sleep. Lian checks the tests that he is booked in for, and explains to Mr I that he will be coming and going from the ward, with the orderlies and a nurse if necessary, for the tests the doctors want done. She tries to disturb him as little as possible, but makes sure that he is ready and gowned when the orderlies are expected. He seems a bit confused to her, calling her Nina repeatedly. He doesn't refuse to go for the tests, but he doesn't seem happy. From her reading of the notes, Lian can see that Nina is one of his daughters. Lian puts her observation of confusion in the nursing notes as well as the routine observations (temperature, blood pressure, and so on) she records. Some of the family visit, including Mr I's elderly wife and his son. They comment that 'Dad seems a bit out of sorts'.

Throughout the day, there is some progress in identifying the cause of Mr I's current illness, with test results ruling out some of the more serious possibilities, but still identifying a condition likely to become very serious if not eventually corrected surgically. Some stabilising medication is discussed among the doctors, then Dr S meets with Mr I and family members who are present in the ward at the time of his ward round. This time, it is a daughter, Kim. The medication is discussed, and orders for it are written into the notes. Lian starts the medication regime straight away in conjunction with the supervising nurse.

The possibility of Mr I undergoing an operation, as soon as he is sufficiently stabilised, is discussed with Mr I, who is advised to think about this.

The next day, Dr S returns on his ward round to see some further progress in Mr I's condition. He seems to be almost stable enough for the operation. However, Mr I seemingly has no recollection of his discussion about an operation. Dr S was hopeful about scheduling it for the more urgent list, to be done any time within a month, but feels uneasy that Mr I is not retaining or understanding what was said yesterday in their consultation. No family member is present. Phil puts a call in to Jan for a social/competency assessment as part of the consent process. He wonders if it is a temporary problem or a more long-standing one, and plans to seek more structured family input if need be, after the competency assessment. When an operation is raised, Mr I objects.

Mr I seems more lucid as the next day approaches. He tells Lian he doesn't want an operation, and he also doesn't want to be resuscitated if 'anything should happen'. Lian lets Phil and Jan know and the request is entered into the notes. A process is put in place to double-check that this is what he has decided, having understood current treatment plans, management options, and the implications of not pursuing active treatment, and that he is competent to make such a decision. Dr S is then confident that Mr I understood the relevant information and is competent to make such a decision, concluding that his earlier confusion was temporary, and related to having been quite ill. He records the clarification of Mr I's decision not to pursue invasive treatment and his 'do not resuscitate' request.

The family asks Lian why nothing is happening, and if an operation is still likely. A meeting is arranged for the family and Dr S, who discusses the options, but also Mr I's request to refuse further invasive procedures and resuscitation. They are distraught, and ask to be the decision makers. They say 'He doesn't know what he is doing. He wouldn't do it, just give up. It is against our culture and religion.' Jan spends some time with them, assuring them that if he changed his mind it would be different, but that respecting his views and wishes is the utmost priority. They are assured that the medication will keep him fairly stable for as long as possible, and he will be reviewed in the outpatient clinic periodically by the doctor. Plans are made to discharge Mr I into his family's care.

Phil comments in the tea room that Mr I would be a candidate for the new procedure he had been talking about a few days earlier, if the research trial was under way as an alternative to the operation that was standard now. Of course, he would have to consent, he says, with a shrug of his shoulders and two raised hands.

SUMMARY OF KEY ISSUES

- Theoretical traditions
- Reflection on practice
- Joint responsibilities in professional life.

SHORT NOTES

1   Gillon, *Philosophical medical ethics*, p. 2.

2   Moreno, *Deciding together*, p. 4.

3   Gillon, *Philosophical medical ethics*, p. 2.

4   Collinson, *Fifty major philosophers*, p. 16.

5   Beauchamp and Childress, *Principles of biomedical ethics*, 4th edn, p. 465.

6   Collinson, *Fifty major philosophers*, p. 21.

7   Spicker et al., *The use of human beings in research*.

8   Mill, 'On liberty'.

9   Beauchamp and Childress, *Principles of biomedical ethics*, 4th edn; Gillon, *Philosophical medical ethics*.

10   See Brody, 'The four principles and narrative ethics', p. 211.

11   Jonsen et al., *Clinical ethics*.

12   Jennett, 'Quality of care and cost containment in the U.S. and the U.K.'.

2

CARING AS PROFESSIONALS

- Becoming a professional carer
- Professional goals and duties
- Principles as fundamental propositions and summaries
- Professional guidelines on ethics
- Caring in multidisciplinary teams
- Law and ethics

OBJECTIVES

This chapter identifies ethics in practice, for individual carers and groups of carers. Personal and professional bounds and ideals are explored. Ethics is explained as an optimal standard of thought and action. Training and role boundaries are discussed, and broad beneficence issues are canvassed. The difference between law and ethics is explained and their complementary nature is discussed.

By the end of this chapter you should be able to define and explain the following concepts: health care, health care professionals, patient, client, skill, goals, duties, obligation, rules, responsibility, accountability, professional codes of ethics, and law. You will have learnt more about the principles of beneficence, non-maleficence, autonomy, and justice, and the ethics theories of utilitarianism, consequentialism, deontology, absolutism, and relativism.

BECOMING A PROFESSIONAL CARER

Becoming a professional carer is not an easy decision. It can take years to decide which profession to choose. People are often asked, as they approach their final years of school, 'What do you want to do?' Think back to when you started your training. This might be when you left school, or it might be later. Why did you choose to train in your health profession? Did you hold certain values and ideals of caring, or was it something else that prompted you to choose your profession?

Education selection specialists are people who advise students on careers and courses, or who advise institutions on which students to accept. They know that there is more to being a successful and productive professional **health care** worker than academic marks. Increasingly, selection panels are searching for those with the capacity to work with others, to reflect on difficult problems, to make a virtue of wanting to care, to serve, and to go beyond self-needs to meet the needs of others. They are interested in why people want to become **health care professionals**, beyond any superior intellectual capability of remembering facts and performing certain procedural skills. In other words, they are looking at the person who will be carrying out the work, not just at their narrowly defined 'technical' ability to do the work.

The following exercise asks you to think about the values and ideals that you held at an early stage of your health care training. It has been adapted from a reflective exercise written by Ken Cox, a surgeon and medical educator, for a jointly authored distance-education course on clinical ethics.[1] Think about when you were just beginning training, when you were just beginning to learn to be a health care professional. You might like to look back to photos of yourself when you were beginning training to jog your memory.

Health care
The provision of care with the objective of maintaining, restoring, or improving health or comfort.

Health care professionals
Those trained in recognised and registered professions to be providers of health care.

EXERCISE 2.1 IDEALS AND VALUES

Write down the words that spring to mind about your images of yourself and your ideals and values as a beginning clinical student.

It is part of reality that ideals, values, and circumstances can conflict. From your list, strike out the ideals that you no longer hold; write down what changed your values and add some new ones. More importantly, think about what might have reinforced or changed your values.

Looking at your list of current ideals and values, do you think you are ethical? Do you have the potential to act ethically as a health care professional if you implement those ideals?

Ethics is more than an expression of what might be. It is more than writing down what we agree with, or what we think we should aim for. Learning to be a professional is also about learning skills, and about becoming able to put those **skills** into action. We learn to put our ethics or ideals into action too. The skills aspect of professional work is inextricably linked to professional ethics. As Pellegrino has stated, the ethics of a profession are not 'the norms actually followed by professionals, or the professional codes they espouse, but rather the moral obligations deductible from the kinds of activity in which they are engaged'.[2] So your individual natures, and the skills you learn, are intertwined with your sense of professional ethics.

This is just starting to be recognised by teachers of health care ethics around the world. They are increasingly stepping away from the dramatic bioethics dilemmas, and the purely philosophical discussion, and are beginning instead to bring ethics back into our everyday lives, helping us to acknowledge its existence in everyday health situations.[3] That is the approach of this book. You need to be constantly re-examining your list of ideals and values, and as your list of professional skills and types of professional activities grows, you should be thinking about how you should act. You need, in other words, to think about ethics in your everyday work.

While wanting to care for others is a common reason for becoming a health care worker, the decision about what type of health profession to join is much more complex. What skills you might be good at should be considered. If you are making this decision, you need to ask yourself what sort of work do health care workers in a particular field really do, and what sort of work would you enjoy? Talking this over with career counsellors, or seeing health care in action, will help you to decide.

Work experience can help too. Many budding health professionals take on part-time work in health contexts, and this exposes them to a variety of health care work, and to the reality of the day-to-day aspects of health care. When I was at university, doing an undergraduate psychology degree, I worked in the kitchen of a large private hospital. I learnt a lot, saw a range of health professionals in action, and I got a feel for how health care was being practised in that hospital. I learnt that the ethic of caring extends not only to medical staff and other health professionals, but also to the auxiliary staff. They are all part of a health team. The ethic of caring is warmer in an institution in which that is acknowledged at all levels. We regularly took the time to stop and chat to patients as we delivered their meals, if they initiated conversation. Some patients became very friendly; they and we looked forward to us popping in for a hello or a chat. If patients obviously needed privacy we respected that, and we learnt to be as discreet as possible in delivering and collecting trays. When people felt more ill than usual, we would try to substitute more easily eaten food (after checking with the dietician and ward staff of course), and if they just had an appetite for something else, we tried to accommodate that. We learnt to respond to needs and wishes, behave with respect and courtesy, and work smoothly as a team so that there was maximum

Skill
Level of competence in a specific task or series of tasks.

service and caring. 'Providing care' and 'providing it caringly' may be subtly different. The ethic of caring is not just about technical application of skill; it is also about how that skill is applied.

PAUSE & REFLECT Think about the first time you felt the ethic of caring, and make a note of it. Also, think about how non-health care professionals show this ethic where you work.

The process of learning, and the awareness of the culture of caring, continues throughout professional life. It starts very early. Your own early learning should be recognised, even if it appears to be less glamorous than 'real' health care or 'real' professional work. You perhaps learn as fast in your early work as you do in your later years as a senior, or more qualified, health care worker.

The professional training system is openly acknowledged to be a slow process. It takes time to accumulate knowledge and skill. And it takes time to gather insight into proper standards. Our society acknowledges that it is necessary to fund training through public taxes. We have teaching hospitals, which are centres of excellence and strive to train others in that excellence. Teaching hospitals work in partnership with colleges and universities to train a skilled and experienced workforce. Our system lets students and juniors 'do' health work under supervision, and, by applying less rigorous skill standards to them (in the presence of a trained person to support, supervise, and back the student up), it allows them the freedom to learn. As their skill and knowledge level increases, students do increasingly difficult tasks under decreasing supervision. The professional skill is slowly transferred from supervisor to student. The professional power and discretion to decide the 'right' manner in achieving that work is also slowly transferred. This happens in professional ethics too. Through mentoring, academic instruction, role modelling, group discussion, and other systems, we gradually form the 'moral professional', and we trust that by the time students graduate they have sufficient understanding of standards in the profession.

EXERCISE 2.2 SKILLS AND LIMITS

Think about one professional standard that you have learnt. Make a note of how and when you learnt it, and when you first put it into action.

You may have chosen a level of knowledge (or practical skill), or you may have chosen a standard that is more about the way that skill is delivered. Learning increasingly difficult and finely tuned professional standards is part of becoming a professional carer. You learn, in fine detail, what the job is, and how you are expected to do it.

When you are trained as a professional, you acquire the privileged knowledge of that profession. You will continue to learn throughout your professional life, constantly updating or extending your knowledge and skill base. Part of being a professional is this commitment to keep learning, to strive continually to be able to deliver the best possible care for your clients. The flip side of this is that there are limits to your knowledge and skill. You need to have insight into how knowledgeable and capable you are. There is a danger for others if you think you are much more skilled than you actually are, and you go beyond your safe limits in dealing with people. This reflection on skill and knowledge is essential. Practising insight into your skill level actually gives you a model for reflecting on your ethical limits.

PAUSE & REFLECT

Think of a skill that you are still learning, and try the following reflection.

My safe limits in performing the skill are:

My judgment of my safe limit is based on:

The consequences of exceeding this limit for the client are:

Recognising your limits in skill is very helpful because it starts you on a process of self-reflection, and on reflecting on all aspects of health care. Reflection is a key part of ethics. It should continue throughout your career.

Lifelong commitment is not uncommon in professions. Historically, people entered the equivalent of holy orders to receive the depth of training that was required, and they often pledged themselves to the ideals of learning and service. To have a profession was, literally, to have professed oaths, such as obedience to church values, honesty, and high standards of service.[4] This is similar to the intensity of devotion and long apprenticeship that a successful professional still needs today. There are still professional ideals that are avowed by particular health care professions. These ideals go beyond a particular duty to an employer or contract of employment. Once professed, they apply wherever that professional works. Professionals have an ongoing duty to consider appropriate moral or ethical standards, and to reflect on their own behaviour.

FROM THEORY TO PRACTICE

An insight to share with students

Contributor: *Rose Leontini*

One topic I teach in my unit, Health Ethics and the Law, is the ethics of the care of the self. This is about health care professionals practising an ethos of self-care, in view of the large volume of stressful work they often engage in.

As a researcher (using qualitative methods) I like to share with students my own experiences as a researcher in areas of interest that can be emotionally and psychologically demanding. For example, investigating people's experiences of losing loved ones, of physical and mental health, of child or other forms of abuse, pain, loss, etc.

(Continued)

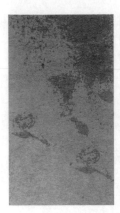

In anthropological and sociological studies (my background) there has been a lot of research into the sociology of the emotions (and emotion work performed by health care professionals) and of the toll this can take.

In my lectures and tutorials on the subject I raise examples of my own experience, as well as the experiences of colleagues and PhD (Doctorate of Philosophy) students. This resonates with many of the students who are placed on clinical appointments, and in particular with the nursing students.

I think this is a topic that is underdeveloped in conventional ethics, which focuses primarily on how to treat others.

PROFESSIONAL GOALS AND DUTIES

By definition, professional work is skilled, and is done to benefit others. The community trusts that proper standards are applied in carrying out that work. You need to be familiar with the extent of your skills, and by carrying out that skill properly, which includes doing it competently and ethically, you fulfil the trust placed in you. Just as the community places its trust in you, so too you trust others to carry out work involving skills different from your own.

Proper standards, of course, need definition. Professions, by their very nature, have a responsibility to define what their goals are; the expected role, and corresponding duties, of practitioners; and the limits of the service they can be expected to provide.

Goals are something to aspire to; they are the ethically optimal position. In contrast, **duties** are something we are obliged to fulfil. It is a minimal position to only fulfil strict duties without aspiring to higher goals. The idea of virtue is receiving renewed attention in modern ethics texts, incorporating the Aristotelian notion of ideals. The motivation towards ethical action, as well as achievement of ethical actions, is reflected upon. Some people who accept special roles, like health care professionals, can assume certain higher responsibilities than others. They are expected to exceed normal moral requirements towards what would be regarded as moral ideals and excellence in others.[5] Basic duties can translate into lists of duties, or **obligations**, and prohibitions, all of which are outlined for you before you start working in your profession. The first documentation you might see when starting a new job is a 'statement of duties', or a general job description that implies duties. These vary widely between professions because of the different skills and corresponding responsibilities involved in that profession. They also vary between different units or specialisations within that profession because of the different services those units provide.

Goals
Ideals and objectives aimed towards.

Duties
Obligations and specific tasks that one is bound to fulfil, or actions from which one is bound to refrain.

Obligation
Something one is bound to fulfil or perform.

Do either of the following sets of tasks, associated with the jobs of occupational
therapist and registered nurse respectively, come close to the basic duties of your job?

• An occupational therapist helps 'mentally, physically, developmentally, or
  emotionally disabled individuals develop, recover, or maintain daily living and work
  skills'. Occupational therapists will often be assigned, in their duties, to individuals
  in one particular age group or disability, and will be required to design programs that
  assist with day-to-day life skills.

• A registered nurse is required to 'observe, assess, and record symptoms, reactions,
  and progress; administer medications; assist in convalescence and rehabilitation;
  instruct patients and their families in proper care; and help individuals and groups
  take steps to improve and maintain their health'. The level of responsibility varies
  with experience.[6]

Care to self is also a responsibility: to keep oneself safe and well, and then set about
the duties of helping others. Codes of practice, and the ideals they profess, are there
to encourage optimal behaviour, and serve as a safeguard to ensure that certain basic
standards of behaviour are adhered to and that professionals are committed to offering
a proper quality of care. Registration bodies are established to make sure that only those
people who are trained and are currently competent to practise in health care do so. When
you enter your profession, you effectively agree to meet the standards of professional
behaviour expected of you. Formal registration makes this clearer. Your professional
body then fully expects your approach and conduct to be competent and ethical. Your
peers, in effect, expect you to uphold professional standards. If standards are breached to
a significant extent, professional bodies may take the step of deregistering professionals.
This is effectively a statement that the standard of care offered by that professional is
deficient. This assessment of the standard of care can be made in relation to ethics
as well as practical skill. These professional regulatory mechanisms are discussed in
Chapter 11. If people who purport to be professionally trained are not, then we become
worried. Consider the report from South America of a man with no medical degree who
worked as a neurologist in a major hospital for 16 years, chaired a specialist conference,
and co-wrote a book on medicine. Described as 'a great seducer with the gift of the gab',
and both brilliant and a psychopath, he was subsequently charged with forgery, false
exercise of a profession, and causing serious injury after a woman told police she had
suffered brain damage in an operation he recommended.[7]

We are worried about such people because they have not gone through the training
of the profession, nor are they subject to the same degree of rigorous peer review and
sanction as member professionals are.

Similarly, an American doctor who promoted his 'suicide machine' as an option
for terminally ill patients also troubled professional medical practitioners. Even apart
from the arguments of whether suicide, professionally assisted or not, was ethical

(and this will be discussed in Chapter 9), he was retired from medical practice. He was, in effect, beyond professional sanction, but was still using his title of doctor.[8] His actions attracted significant media attention; he was tried in a number of criminal courts, and certainly succeeded in prompting debates and discussions on how to end life with dignity. You may like to consider further the border between ethics and law, and read ahead to Chapter 11 if you want to do so now.

Similarly, practitioners who work alone for an extended period of time are disproportionately the focus of disciplinary and remedial practice programs. An extreme example is that of the British GP Dr Harold Shipman, who was convicted in 2000 of murdering 15 patients. Shipman had a long-term pattern of working alone and making unannounced home visits. The fact that many of his patients were dressed in their day clothes was noticed by a local undertaker and thought to be unusual, as people who feel ill are normally lying in bed in pyjamas. The patients were also sometimes found in a seated position in their lounge rooms. Then a local GP expressed concern about the rate of death certificates she was being asked to countersign, prompting an initial police investigation, which was completed without specific conclusion. The possibly fraudulent inclusion of Shipman's name as a beneficiary in a will prompted the eventual successful criminal investigation, and subsequent commission of inquiry.[9] Audits of his patient files and deaths of other patients led to calls for further charges.[10] Commentary from the UK focused on concern that the activities were not detected sooner, and restoring public trust in the quality, appropriateness, and accountability of professional medical services.[11] Opportunities for detection are highest when individual actions and judgments are accountable to others. This was emphasised by the Shipman Inquiry chairman, Dame Janet Smith, in her lengthy findings into the practice and death certification process. In the Inquiry, Dame Smith estimated that over 200 patients had been killed.

EXERCISE 2.3 RESPONSIBILITY AND ACCOUNTABILITY

Responsibility
Obligation and duty to fulfil certain tasks or series of tasks.

Accountability
Process of being open to scrutiny for assessment of conduct of responsibilities.

Try the following exercise. Look through the suggested process for certification of a death in England, as in the Shipman Inquiry Report (in Third Report, at pp. 496–510), and write them out again as a series of steps. Then circle the steps in the process that set out who are the appropriate people to undertake responsibilities in certifying and checking the circumstances of each person's death, and those that link the opinion of individuals to the scrutiny of others. This is to build in accountability. Consider who is undertaking each **responsibility** and who their **accountability** is to.

Form 1 is to be completed by a health professional (doctor, nurse, or paramedic) to confirm the fact of death, the circumstances of death, those present, and their contact details. An external examination of the body is undertaken, and findings recorded. This form is transmitted to the coroner's office.

Form 2 is to be completed by the doctor treating the last illness, confirming the medical history, and attaching relevant extracts from the medical records. In a hospital setting, it could be the same person as that completing Form 1, but this person must be a senior doctor. In a community setting, the general practice with which the patient is registered has responsibility for completing the form. The Form 2 doctor has an option to express an opinion on the cause of death. Full coronial investigation is possible in either case, but is more likely when no expected cause of death is probable. This form is transmitted to the coroner's office.

Coronial certification is a process of analysis. The family of the deceased is consulted by a trained coronial investigator. Considering the **information** in Forms 1 and 2, the coroner can certify the death, after consultation with the deceased's family, or proceed to full coronial examination and inquiry. Random checks should be conducted on a portion of the cases certified.

Information
Details specific to issue under consideration.

FROM THEORY TO PRACTICE

Teaching ethical behaviour in practice

Contributor: *Jenneke Foottit*

Ask students to debate issues that may arise in practice:

- Resuscitating a patient with a DNR order
- How medication errors should be dealt with
- Dealing with an impaired staff member for 'ordinary' reasons: coming onto night duty without sleep; coming to work smelling of stale alcohol and may or may not be under 0.05
- Staff member who does not do a fair share of the workload.

These issues often get argued from an emotional point of view. The challenge for the student is to argue them from an *ethical* perspective.

PRINCIPLES AS FUNDAMENTAL PROPOSITIONS AND SUMMARIES

Expressing professional goals and duties is quite complex. Some are broad notions; others are more specific. There has been a move in recent times to simplify the ethical goals and duties for health care into broad principles, such as the following, espoused by the American ethicists Beauchamp and Childress: beneficence, non-maleficence, autonomy, and justice.

Beneficence
The principle
of doing good
and providing care
for others.

Autonomy
The principle
of allowing and
promoting self-rule,
of people making
decisions about
their lives.

Principle
A fundamental
proposition, from
which specific goals
or duties can
be derived.

Justice
The principle of
fair allocation
of community
resources and
burdens.

Non-maleficence
The principle of not
harming others, and
of minimising harm
to them.

Respect for persons
Principle of
upholding
autonomy, generally
used for research
participants.

Beneficence encompasses the obligation to do good, to care for people, and non-maleficence is the paired obligation to do no harm to them. **Autonomy** is the **principle** of self-rule, of clients making decisions about their own lives. **Justice** is about fair distribution of resources, particularly when the pool of resources is limited.[12] A British ethicist, Gillon, proposes similar principles of respect for autonomy, beneficence, **non-maleficence**, and justice, but provides a slightly different definition of 'respect for autonomy', which he defines as 'the moral obligation to respect the autonomy of others in so far as such respect is compatible with equal respect for the autonomy of all potentially affected'.[13] In essence, this definition builds a social context into autonomy.

Slightly different principles have also been used to think about ethical duties and proper behaviour in health research practice. These research principles—beneficence, **respect for persons**, and justice—have been termed the Belmont principles because they were coined by the US National Commission for the Protection of Human Subjects of Biomedical and Behavioural Research, in the Commission's Belmont Report. Beneficence, in the Commission's terms, concerns a dual obligation to, on the one hand, do no harm and promote the well-being of individuals, and, on the other, to maximise the potential benefit to society. 'Respect for persons' refers to an obligation to uphold the autonomy of individuals. The principle of justice relates to an obligation to share the benefits or burdens of research fairly in society.[14]

The principles suggested by Beauchamp and Childress (beneficence, non-maleficence, autonomy, and justice), and Gillon (respect for autonomy, beneficence, non-maleficence, and justice), and the Belmont principles (beneficence, respect for persons, and justice) have gained support because they provide a shorthand for thinking about ethics issues. The principles are used as tools to collect and summarise issues expressed by professionals, clients, and the community as being of concern. They are tools for ethical analysis and comparison. They do not, in themselves, give ultimate guidance on 'right' or 'wrong' behaviour.

The following dilemma is an exercise in using the principles to aid ethical reflection. The vignette is drawn from a study on ethics in the general practice setting in the mid-1990s: a group of multidisciplinary researchers and I asked general practitioners and consumers of the services of GPs to nominate their ethics concerns. Vignettes were written to reflect these concerns, and the GPs and consumers were then convened to discuss possible solutions to the dilemmas contained in the vignettes.[15]

A 22-year-old man, Mr Y, had been very active until experiencing some unsettling symptoms. He saw his GP, had a lot of tests, and was eventually diagnosed with early-stage multiple sclerosis. His GP said nothing much could be done at this stage, but advised Mr Y to stay active, and gave him something to help with that. The GP explained that this medication was called 'dexamethasone', and explained the dosage required, without giving further instructions. Mr Y was worried about the medication and was surprised to find out six months later, when he read the pharmacist's instructions, that he had been taking steroids.

In discussing the dilemma, many consumers focused on the responsibility they thought each patient should take to inform themselves about the treatment being offered—this translates, in terms of the ethical principles discussed above, into the principle of autonomy. Consequently, they focused on the fact that Mr Y did not seek more information about the medication and did not read the pharmacy details until six months after purchasing the drug. The general practitioners, however, wondered at the apparent **paternalism** of the doctor, who had decided that acting beneficently did not include allowing the patient to make an informed decision.

The balance between the possible long-term effects of steroids and the benefit in prescribing something to stave off early degeneration in multiple sclerosis could also be raised. If these steroids are thought to be beneficial, then under the principle of justice such drugs should be made equitably available to all those who might benefit. You could apply the same discussion to more recent drug treatments for multiple sclerosis. How, then, should the care be delivered? There is a caution to be made here: justice is about the distribution of a good. This is different from the legal sense of justice. In other words, in ethics, justice is a question of resources, as is explained further in Chapter 3. A further caution is that the autonomy at issue is the client's autonomy, not the professional's. Autonomy is discussed in some detail in Chapter 4. It is clear that, when possible concerns have been summarised, and the principles used as an aid, further discussion needs to take place on the issues raised in the vignette. Neither the principles nor the summarising process alone solve the dilemma.

The Belmont principles—beneficence, respect for persons, and justice—were formulated to provide an 'analytical framework' to 'guide the resolutions of ethical problems' in research.[16] They may have been attractive to the Commission because of their practical application.[17] The principles represent a minimal position because they capture what are regarded as key issues in diverse ethics frameworks. Beauchamp and Childress have also stated that they came up with their principles of beneficence, non-maleficence, autonomy, and justice despite a fundamental difference between their theoretical positions: Beauchamp's stance can be broadly described as utilitarian, whereas Childress's is, again generally speaking, deontological. A utilitarian concentrates on the outcome of behaviour for the greatest number, and aims for the happiness, or utility, of the greatest number in society. A deontologist, on the other hand, looks at the fundamental rule (the Greek *deon* means obligation or duty, from which laws or rules arise) that should be applied, in all situations, to ensure an ethical process. In general, **consequentialism**, an ethics theory that focuses on consequences, is incompatible with **absolutism**, in which a rule-driven process is the focus of analysis. **Utilitarianism** is a theory that is compatible with consequentialism, and nominates utility or usefulness as the outcome that should be assessed. **Deontology** is an ethics theory that is compatible with absolutism, describing the process of identifying rules and the derivation of those rules for use

Paternalism
Decision-making framework in which care and control of another is undertaken.

Consequentialism
An ethics theory in which the consequences of actions are the focus, both on the actor and on others affected by the action.

Absolutism
An ethics theory in which a rule or rules are identified as fundamentally important, and of unvarying significance.

Utilitarianism
An ethics theory in which the outcome of actual or proposed action is the focus, and the acceptable course of action is that in which the greatest good for the greatest number is achieved.

Deontology
An ethics theory in which the process and components of actual or proposed action is the focus, with reference to agreed values and rules.

in guiding ethically acceptable processes. These theories were initially described in Chapter 1. Beauchamp and Childress acknowledge that many different ethics theories can legitimately claim to have advanced health care ethics.[18]

The next two paragraphs discuss some of the support, advanced by different ethics theories and frameworks, for the principles of beneficence, non-maleficence, autonomy, and justice. The key idea is that each principle has its merits, even though different ethics theories and frameworks provide different supporting arguments. How much you emphasise each principle may shed some light on your overall ethical framework. This is discussed further in Chapter 4, in the section headed 'A dynamic relationship'. (You may decide to skip over the next two paragraphs now and return to them later when you feel ready to delve into ethics theory.)

Immanuel Kant was the founder of deontological theory. The central issue in Kant's deontological theory is the individual pursuit of morality. Freedom underpins this theory because it is needed for individuals to develop and act on their moral laws. A duty to uphold freedom entails respect for oneself and respect for others. Although Kant rejects a perfect duty to benefit others and not to harm them, he maintains that a duty to benefit oneself and to refrain from harming oneself is part of the fundamental duty of respect. As respect for others is also fundamental, duties to benefit others and refrain from harming others stem from allowing them freedom to safeguard their own well-being. Justice implies that we fairly respect everyone's need to develop their own moral selves. It also implies the ultimate good of 'moral perfection'. The way of achieving moral perfection, according to Kant's theory, is to treat individuals with respect, and to extend that respect to all people equally under a framework of justice as fairness. In other words, it stems from treating individuals with respect, and not as a means to an end.[19]

Utilitarian theory aims for the smallest possible amount of harm and the greatest possible amount of benefit. For utilitarians, beneficence involves maximising benefit and minimising harm. This is best achieved by allowing autonomy, because it is assumed that each person acts to pursue their own well-being and happiness. John Stuart Mill was a founder of utilitarianism. Under Mill's utilitarianism, liberty should be limited to a certain extent to allow for justice and the fair distribution of burden and benefit. Individual liberty is limited when exercising liberty may unreasonably infringe on others; liberty would be denied in circumstances in which other individuals were severely harmed or their similar liberties were threatened.[20]

The shorthand principles of beneficence, non-maleficence, autonomy, and justice make little sense on their own. They are simply tools, expressions of key ethical obligations that health care workers should fulfil, and goals to aim for. At best, the principles are a shorthand expression for drawing together concerns, and for referring to a considerable body of thought and literature about health care ethics. They extend the context for considering key issues in health care to the community and social contexts in which we live. At worst, the principles are used as a narrow and prescriptive decision-binding tool. It is not enough to think that summarising concerns under these or similar principles will lead to a solution. In addition to knowing the ethics principles, we have to apply them constantly within an ethical framework. We need to know our obligations, and we must live up to them.

In applying principles and meeting our obligations, the particular values and beliefs of the individuals and groups we care for, and the specific situations to which the principles are applied, must also be taken into account.[21] Professional standards, which reflect a shared sense of obligation, must be able to be communicated to relevant groups, and the ethics of relevant groups must be heard by the professions. In essence, it is the issues themselves, not the principles that summarise them, that should have prominence in ethics discussion and analysis.

As simple, shorthand points, the principles of beneficence, non-maleficence, autonomy, and justice have the potential to be very useful. Many students and health professionals use them precisely because they are easily grasped and applied. They do not in themselves provide answers for ethical dilemmas that you might face, but they do provide a starting place for reflection on ethics in your work as a health care worker. The lack of ready answers or solutions is perhaps a strength of the principles. The reality is that ethics is dynamic: times change, people change, medical problems and health issues change, and social contexts change. The principles will continue to be useful tools precisely because they do not lay down strict rules to be applied whatever the situation, culture, client, or professional involved.

In a concise historical review of approaches to medical ethics, Edmund Pellegrino argues that some dissatisfaction with principles as they apply to specific cases led to a sceptical and chaotic chapter in ethics in the late part of the 20th century. Yet difficult decisions and clinical realities remain, so ethics reflection continues.[22]

This consideration of cases is how health care has been taught over generations. It is not incompatible with understanding important links and theories. In clinical case description, the story about an individual demonstrates 'what can happen' and serves as a guide on 'what to do'.[23] Teachers develop students' case-based reasoning and ensure they are exposed to enough diverse case situations to gain a broad and complex understanding of case management in clinical practice. This book is structured so that the focus is on the individual and their story. You are encouraged to think about the ethics implications of health as each individual travels through the sequence of treatment with you. The stories you reflect on will challenge you ethically in the same way as your clinical reasoning is challenged as you develop it.

Two longer cases were included in Chapter 1 as review cases, and can be returned to after you complete the new work in each chapter. You might like to reread them now. They are case five, 'Worried about Mum', and case six, 'Confusion and decisions'.

PROFESSIONAL GUIDELINES ON ETHICS

Individual reflection on standards, skill, and ethics is vital, yet individual reflection alone is problematic. It is difficult to act ethically without some guidance. Some of that guidance is found in discussion with fellow professionals, and some is found in written form, in professional codes of ethics. A profession is an occupation that

- is skilled
- requires training to a high level (to which considerable time is devoted, leading to the expectation of relatively high remuneration)
- gives rise to expectations of a high standard of proficiency
- is bound by a code of ethics of ideals of service to society.[24]

Rules
Derived and specific expressions of fundamental principles or ideals that are agreed to have moral force, so as to obligate subscribers to that moral stance to abide by them.

In professional life, there is some sense of setting moral rules and moral ideals. Moral **rules** may not be left to individual discretion as much as moral ideals. A moral *rule* is something that must be obeyed, and can therefore form the basis of a list of prohibitions, such as 'Thou shalt not kill'. In contrast, a moral *ideal* is something that should be strived for; it requires some positive action.[25] So there is a sense that 'lower' limits of behaviour exist and that we should strive for 'upper' ideals. Since we should abide by moral rules, we would regard behaviour that breaks these rules with disfavour. We might be forgiving when ideals are not upheld, as long as the person strives for them in the future with a moral imperative to strive towards the aspirational goods.[26] A written code makes this more explicit, and provides members, as well as outsiders, with clear expectations of the rules and ideals that are central to the profession.

Philosophically, the principles that the professions seek to uphold translate into moral rules that guide behaviour.[27] Many different ethical frameworks support, to some extent, the notion of practical rules. Moral rules are especially important in rule forms of deontology and utilitarianism, which regard rules as ethically necessary.[28] Rules can be formed and adopted so that moral goals may be achieved. While the rules can be formed by individuals, according to Kant the collective notion of shared rationality implies that rules formed by rational individuals will be shared and will have commonalities.[29] As a professional working in a community of other member professionals, you are expected to share some common 'professional ethics' rules, to have a sense of purpose in expressing those rules, and to strive to abide by them. Your strict professional duties can be defined with reference to the rules that your profession adopts. Your goals go further than that: you have a general duty to aspire to the optimal goals; to go, in other words, beyond minimum duties. Thus goals and duties go hand in hand.

So codes of ethics can be thought of as 'general action guides' for professionals.[30] As a health care professional, you are required to abide by your association's code of ethics in carrying out your work. Your code is a potential influence on your conduct, because it can define how you should act, and mould you to conform with your profession's standards. The code is a collective responsibility in the ethical conduct of health care by you and your fellow professionals.[31] The codes may be evidence of existing ethics standards, rather than creating obligations in themselves. According to Knultgen, the purposes of professional codes are to promote a sense of community among members, to discipline the behaviour of members, and to ensure public trust in professional actions.[32] Guidance on proper behaviour by those with relevant expertise is crucial. As Hans Jonas has said, it is especially difficult to define ethical conduct in a technologically complex situation, which modern health care inevitably is. People who have the relevant technological expertise can help to predict the consequences of actions. Without their help, actions, even if done with good intentions, could easily result in harm to others.[33]

This has particular relevance for health care teams that combine different sorts of expertise. You should get used to checking ethics limits with the whole team. The minimum is to check with your own peers. The importance of relying on others for guidance is evident even in Kant's otherwise individualist writings, which stress virtue in relation to one's own moral laws. According to Kant, the acceptability of actions to others is important because the praise of others is essential in reinforcing virtuous actions.[34] In simple terms, you check and discuss matters with your colleagues to see if you have acted properly or if your planned action is ethical. It seems appropriate that the group of people who best understand the professional skill and actions involved are ethically active, in effect setting their own goals and limits. It is worrying if outsiders have too much control over the ethics of a profession. As one commentator has stated, 'a morality of those whose hands are clean only because they have the position of an observer, charging others with the responsibility, seems doubtful'.[35]

But if professions fail to set their standards, and outsiders are worried about standards, outsiders may well step in and set the limits of acceptable professional conduct. Professions have sometimes refined and discussed their standards precisely because of the threat of such an external imposition of standards. They should be wary of thinking that the community trusts them entirely. A growing distrust of professions on the part of the general public has been reported periodically from the early 1990s. The public fear is that professionals enter into their chosen field solely, or primarily, to gain money and prestige, and that professionals can be held captive by business interests rather than being bound by the traditional values of service.[36] Sociological studies about the integrity of professionals have routinely included concerns that professional ethics is a product of powerful institutions, merely a tool of monopolisation, such that the 'values' of any profession are constructed to serve the interests of the profession, and that group ethics is imperfectly internalised, and ultimately is neither shared nor acted on by individual professionals.[37]

The community trust in professional standards is premised on the expectation that the community as a whole will ultimately be served by the profession. The view of authority and power is not so stark in modern sociological theory, but the consistent message is that the community response to continued distrust is that society may judge that more outside regulation is needed, effectively limiting the power and discretion of professionals. The public and social interpretation of health, science, medicine, and health care is part of the modern critique.

As **professional codes of ethics** provide guidance on the values and aspirations of a profession, there is little doubt that codes are looked to by the profession and the public as a measure of professional approach and standards. The formation of the code is itself a valuable ethical process, and, as is explained by business ethicists Stephen Cohen and Damian Grace, the process of reflection is perhaps ethically more important than eventually enshrining a code.[38] In other words, the existence of an ethical code should not replace individual conscience and reflection; we need to distinguish between the teaching of custom (or group norms) and what is moral.[39] Continual assessment of the existing standards in the codes of ethics is needed as part of ethical reflection.

From time to time guidelines are updated. As a profession develops, and the context in which it is called to practise changes, so codes become increasingly defined. You must be ready to be part of the discussion and be alert to changes in context and professional limits. Different professions applying their own particular codes of ethics can make different assessments of the same situation. Nursing codes and medical codes are frequently compared, and it has been noted that they differ in their emphasis on autonomy, with nursing roles aligned more explicitly with patient advocacy.[40] How professionals view their code is also important. When practising physicians in the USA were surveyed and asked to rate the influence of codes, religion, and other moral guidance, a 'personal sense of right and wrong' was reported as a significant influence on their professional practice by the vast majority, and to a lesser extent, 'great moral teachers'; student or professional codes themselves were not explicitly nominated as influential.[41] So the codes of ethics may not be routinely sourced, but in times of reflective need they are there as a guidance document that is readily available.

Codes of ethics need to be more than window dressing, and there is a strong potential for criticism if the values enshrined in them are thought to be either rarely enforced or applied by practitioners.[42] At the heart of the potential criticism is that, having established professional codes of ethics and justified them if need be, professionals also need some mechanism for giving effect to those ethics, beyond that of the virtue of the individual health care worker. More on mechanisms that give effect to codes and standards of behaviour is included in Chapter 11.

There is a move by some professions to assemble performance standards and ethics in the one professional code, and this means there will be little excuse for professionals not to be familiar with their latest standards, including their ethics obligations. You are asked to access your latest code in the following exercise.

Professional code of ethics
Expression of principles, rules, ideals, and values of specific professional group, creating responsibility to strive for states, ideals, and goals, and to uphold certain rules, in each member professional's conduct.

EXERCISE 2.4 GENERAL PRINCIPLES IN YOUR PROFESSIONAL CODE OF ETHICS

You should have at hand your professional code of ethics. If you do not already have it, you could try looking up the association website, ringing your association to have one mailed to you, or visiting a library where it may be held. Examples of the latest codes of ethics for your profession can also be available through relevant registration authority websites. The Australian Health Practitioner Regulation Agency (AHPRA) has been the relevant authority to register practitioners and students from the health professions of dentistry, optometry, pharmacy, physiotherapy, psychology, nursing, medicine, osteopathy, podiatry, and chiropractic since July 2010. The relevant national boards and state councils produce professional standards and guideline documents, which can be sourced directly from the AHPRA website (www.ahpra.gov.au). The latest codes outline duties to patients, the community, and the profession. You should remember to check with your association and obtain updates whenever your code is altered.

Using your own code, try the following exercise.

Place the principles and comments of guidance in your code of ethics under the broad headings listed below of beneficence, non-maleficence, autonomy, and justice. You may like to refresh your memory on the definition of these principles, according to Beauchamp and Childress. The definitions were given earlier in this chapter.

CODE OF ETHICS
My profession is:

PRINCIPLES OF NOTE IN MY CODE OF ETHICS
Beneficence
Non-maleficence
Autonomy
Justice

To follow group-defined ethics standards, without making an input into the evolving standards, would be a minimal position to take. It is preferable that all professional members actively consider their ethical stance and be ready to explain it or pursue further discussion on it. Opportunities for discussion and explanation often arise casually—for example, in the tea room, at handover, at professional conferences over lunch, or as you talk about what happened during the day with your flatmates or partner. Professional discussions can also be scheduled if there is an issue that seems to be arising consistently or is of some moment. These meetings and discussions are of utmost importance to the dynamic nature of health care ethics.

The philosopher John Rawls thought that principles of conduct, such as we find in some codes of ethics, were important. He also thought that we need more than principles to bring ethics into action. Rawls distinguished between the principles and the subsequent judgments of value in relation to those principles.[43] We need to make individual and collective judgments before principles are put into practice.

PAUSE &
REFLECT
Think about one of the basic principles that you might find in your professional association's code of ethics (or you might like to look to another profession's code for this exercise). Think of situations in which you have applied this principle and make a note of how you have seen others apply it.

You may apply it slightly differently from another health care worker, or someone else in your own profession. Part of that difference may be the values that you use when you interpret and apply the principle. One of Rawls's points is that the judgments we make may depend on the contractual situation to which the principles and values are applied (the word 'contractual' here is being used to refer to any agreement, whether implied or explicit, between people). We can expect some differences in 'ethical behaviour'. Just because someone behaves differently does not necessarily mean that they are unethical, but it does give us pause for reflection and discussion. The next time you see something quite different in the application of a principle, take a moment to think about the values that may have influenced that professional's behaviour, and the contractual situation in which it was applied. You may be witness to extreme values or a contractual situation that puts considerable constraints on professional behaviour.

An editorial written by a former Director-General of the World Health Organization reinforced the need for, and the value of, both professional expressions of ethics in professional codes and the recognition of the diversity of values in the community when offering health care:

> To be ethical, our responses must be both honest and humane: first, they must
> be applicable to people's concrete circumstances and meaningful to them; and
> second, they must be respectful of their rights, values, and personal dilemmas,
> as lived within their own communities. In other words, ethical issues must be
> worked out with the people concerned.[44]

An international commitment to basic goals and duties such as promoting human dignity and human rights and freedom is also found in the United Nations Educational, Scientific and Cultural Organization (UNESCO) Universal Declaration on Bioethics and Human Rights, which aims to promote human dignity and human rights and freedom. The Declaration provides useful reference to fundamental notions of collective responsibility to promote health and social development, respect and integrity of individuals, and protection of the vulnerable in health care and research contexts.

More on community input is included in Chapter 10. The issue of individual client autonomy and input is discussed throughout this book.

CARING IN MULTIDISCIPLINARY TEAMS

We live and work with the reality of different professions in health care. Different professions train their members in different skills, and these differently skilled workers all tackle health care together. The basic aim of all health professions is to care for **clients** or **patients**, to be beneficent towards them and the community that is served. Yet sometimes there seem to be differences in attitude among health professionals. You may seem to be at loggerheads over health-system priorities, or decisions over individual client care. Despite your differences, you must learn to work together, because you need each other's skills to provide proper health care. Some professionals prefer the term client to patient, and vice versa. Both will be used in this book. Their common meaning is a person who receives something: care or services.

One step towards professionals working well together is to understand each other's different skills and objectives in providing care. A common example of two professions working together is that of doctors and nurses. Nurses acknowledge both the difficulty and the importance of working with doctors, who have different skills and objectives. Working as a team does not mean always working 'under' another profession. It means being aware of and working towards goals, and on occasions being 'guided by others who possess greater knowledge and expertise'.[45] Of course, establishing team leadership will depend on what goals are aimed for and who has the skills to lead the team towards that goal. Junior residents find themselves learning a great deal from senior charge nurses. Experienced nurses and their favourite doctors appear to work together effortlessly. Perhaps they have come to a common understanding of the goals of care in their own context and appreciate each other's skills so much that there is true team harmony in providing that care. You could apply the same assessment of successful teamwork in other professional combinations.

Discussing basic values and objectives in health care with the multidisciplinary teams with which you work can be useful in establishing common ground and acceptable aims. There are philosophical processes that can help us to achieve this, such as those that rely on relativism and the understanding of different cultural stances and beliefs. Yet there is also a danger, as noted by Moreno, that aiming for consensus too early, and sacrificing differences of opinion to achieve that consensus, can hide the difficulty of an issue, or even hide divergent views on an issue.[46]

Harman is a philosopher who has defended **relativism**, a theory that suggests that there are no hard-and-fast rules in ethics. Rather, ethics can change depending on the perspectives of key participants in a dilemma and the stance of the group to which they belong. Not all people agree with relativism. It is useful to think about it here though, because it stresses how an agreement can be reached between people with different perspectives on what might be best or right. Harman claims that a judgment of proper conduct by one party towards another depends on the agreement between the two parties.[47] In a practitioner–client relationship, both parties should

Client
Person or organisation investigating or receiving service.

Patient
Person receiving care.

Relativism
An ethics theory in which divergent perspectives are canvassed, with a view to establishing courses of action that are acceptable to those perspectives in their given context.

agree that what is being undertaken is proper. In the context of a health care team, the team should also agree that it is proper. Remember that they might agree for different reasons. Reaching this agreement does not necessarily mean minimal standards. In any contractual situation, an upper level, beyond a bare minimum, can be negotiated. The discussion in this book is based on the assumption that an optimal level of ethics behaviour is what should be sought—that is, it assumes that we should strive to go beyond the minimum and aim for an outcome that will raise and uphold standards.

Recognising when important values are being threatened is a challenge in the hectic pace of health care practice. Try to identify what is being threatened in the situation in Exercise 2.5.

EXERCISE 2.5 CLOCK ON

A health care professional, let's say a medical resident, who is new to a training position in a major public hospital, is rostered on to work a double shift. At the end of that shift, the next person phones in sick. The resident is asked to stay on duty until alternative staff can be found.

How long should that person be asked to work in one stretch? What is threatened by breaching this limit?

Does your estimate vary if you consider 'safe' or 'optimal' work capacity?

Does this vary depending on what work the staff member is performing? That is, would your estimate of acceptable shift extension be different for doctors, nurses, laboratory technicians, administrative staff such as medical records staff, or cleaners?

So what about moonlighting? That is, what if the person has held on to a second job, and is also working elsewhere on their time off?

This exercise will lead you back to a consideration of skill and limits, which is what we started with at the beginning of this chapter. The environment also needs to be conducive to safe and effective practice for your professional responsibilities to be met.

When tasks and responsibilities are divided in a health care team, it is easy to lose sight of the fact that the team, as a whole, is responsible for the care of the individual patient. You routinely work in teams that share skills and responsibility for client care. When you are part of that system, the standards of care from each of the health care professions apply. Everyone would do well to acknowledge a team ethic of caring. It is worth spending time with one's own team, discussing and defining team goals, and minimum rules and optimal ideals, so that compatibilities are recognised and potential problem areas are identified before they occur in practice. In an interdisciplinary approach to ethics education at a US university health centre, one benefit was thought to be a complexity of issues that different training professionals brought to the ethics discussion. The lecturers felt that when students understood each of the team members' roles and responsibilities, they had the prerequisite for discharging their ethical obligations to their patients.[48] So the ethics discussion and decision cannot be in isolation from other members if it is to be realistic. The development of both professional team responsibility and team ethics that are specific to your work practices are valuable and practical additions to your implementation of professional ethics. Think about where you can find up-to-date versions of different stances of professionals that you are likely to work with, and keep a note for yourself to stay in touch with updates from time to time. Also, think about opportunities for your team to talk about ethics concerns and expectations.

LAW AND ETHICS

When you learn about ethics, you also encounter the **law**. The law represents the basic duties of citizens and the accepted lower limits to their behaviour in their given social and professional context. It is a contemporary statement of the standards that you are expected to maintain in your dealings with the social institutions of your state and country, and with others in personal interactions. It can be different therefore in different countries and states, as each 'jurisdiction' may define different duties and limits.

Law
System of basic rules and regulations of interactions in a specific community, binding on members as expressed in that community's government-enacted rules, or derived from its judicial decisions.

Law is represented in statute law and subsequently developed regulatory guidelines, case law, and criminal law. There are special requirements made of professionals under law, and these are contained in different areas of law.

Statute law is legislation that has force because it has been passed into law by the governments of states or countries. You can look up statutes and read the exact wording of what the expected standard is. For instance, you could look up the statute that provides for your registration and the expected standards of registered health care professionals. The statute is also likely to set out the process for dealing with potentially incompetent or unsatisfactory professional conduct.

Civil case law is the body of determinations and reasoning from tribunals and courts. Decisions stem from disputes between parties; they capture the essence of what was in dispute and the judicial decision on why certain action or behaviour was acceptable or not in a particular context. This is the area of law in which negligence and, particularly relevant for you, professional negligence are tested.

Criminal case law represents the application of criminal statute law to an alleged crime, which is conduct that is so reprehensible it is deemed by society to be punishable by a criminal law penalty. The judge, or in some cases judge and jury, decide if the facts as tested in court amount to a certain 'crime'. The judge then decides on an appropriate punishment, in accordance with expected punishments as provided for in the relevant statute.

You can extrapolate from case law to work out what the accepted standard likely to be held up would be if tested in a court, by comparing the circumstances, context, and facts of any new situation that arises. Therefore, if you had a hypothetical situation, you could then look up case law to see what, if any, decisions could help you to decide what should or should not be done.

Ethics is about both basic standards and optimum aims or objectives of thoughts and actions, standards, and behaviour. It is more esoteric and arguably far less simple to capture than law, largely because it is in essence a process of debate and thought and reflection, by an individual or a group. So it is the process of analysis as much as the position that is argued, and that is the subject of ethics writings and discussions.

Law and ethics complement each other, and the process of debating new laws, in particular, exposes the thoughts behind the way standards are set as community givens and enshrined in law. The opportunity to view this is often available in parliamentary debates or law reform discussion documents. Throughout this text, you will notice examples of discussions from law reform processes. You will also notice examples of statute law, in terms of acceptable lower limits of behaviour, and, of course, professional guidelines and regulations, which have force because of statute law. The complex interplay of law with ethics is that lower limits are defined, and debated, and optimal standards are more readily defined as a result. The interplay is a social process, and to treat law and ethics as totally separate would be artificial.

EXERCISE 2.6 LAW AS A BASIC STANDARD

As a start in examining what the law could mean for you in a practical sense of identifying basic standards, try the following exercise.

Find one example relating to your profession in each of the areas of legislation, civil case law, and criminal case law. Your library may have search systems to help you, or you may be able to conduct your search through a library facility on the web.

Summarise what you could deduce as acceptable or unacceptable behaviour from each of your chosen examples.

Share these with a group, if possible, and see if you can find a pattern in terms of the basic setting of minimum standards and safeguards, protection of the public, compensation apportioned for unfortunate mistakes, and punishment for grave and intentionally disruptive or destructive behaviour.

Reflect on how such standards would have come to be accepted as community expectations and standards.

Remember, though, that a professional is open to a 'higher' moral aim than that required by law. It is also possible for individuals to behave differently and, in effect, never really have their behaviours tested by the legal limit, because they rise well above that level. Personal ethics and professional ethics are evident in the objectives chosen by them, and the efforts to which they go in striving to meet those optimal standards.

As in any process of social negotiation, agreement on ethical conduct may change. Appropriate standards are, therefore, dynamic rather than static, fluid rather than absolute. They may be different in different situations and at different times. This book highlights what would be acceptable as you begin to work in health care and in treatment relationships with clients. The word 'acceptable' is used to mean acceptable to you as a professional, to the professions, to the patients or clients, and to the community in which you work and belong as a member.

SUMMARY OF KEY ISSUES

- Fundamental values

- Debate and reflection

- Skill and limits

- Caring and commitment

- Goals and duties

- Codes of practice

- Principles: beneficence, non-maleficence, autonomy, and justice

- Judging the importance of principles, and applying principles

- Understanding the difference between law and ethics.

As a way of revising this chapter, look back to the introductory paragraphs. Can you define all of the glossary terms?

SHORT NOTES

1   Berglund et al., *Exploring clinical ethics*, 2nd edn, p. 4.

2   Pellegrino, 'Character, virtue and self-interest', p. 56.

3   See, for example, Hubert et al., 'Context in medical education'.

4   Barker, 'What is a profession?', p. 86.

5   Beauchamp and Childress, *Principles of biomedical ethics*, 5th edn, p. 45.

6   Marino, *Resumes for the health care professional*, pp. 36, 37, 39.

7   'Hospital faker ends in doc', *Sydney Morning Herald*, 30 December 1995, p. 10.

8   'Doctor helped woman commit suicide', *Sydney Morning Herald*, 7 June 1990, p. 12.

9   Smith, *The Shipman Inquiry*.

10   Ramsay, 'Audit further exposes UK's worst serial killer'.

11   Horton, 'The real lessons from Harold Frederick Shipman'.

12   Beauchamp and Childress, *Principles of biomedical ethics*, 4th edn, p. 38.

13   Gillon (ed.), *Principles of health care ethics*, p. xxii.

14   US Department of Health, Education, and Welfare, *Ethical principles and guidelines for the protection of human subjects of research* (the Belmont Report), pp. 4–10.

15   Berglund et al., 'The formation of professional and consumer solutions'.

16   The Belmont Report, p. 2.

17   De Grazia, 'Moving forward in bioethical theory', p. 515.

18   Beauchamp and Childress, *Principles of biomedical ethics*, 4th edn, p. 45.

19   Sullivan, *Immanuel Kant's moral theory*, pp. 46, 104, 105, 203, 207, 208, 234.

20   Mill, 'On liberty', pp. 94, 96.

21   Lustig, 'The method of "principlism"', p. 498.

22   Pellegrino, 'The metamorphosis of medical ethics'.

23   Cox, 'Stories as case knowledge'.

24   Barker, 'What is a profession?', pp. 73–99.

25   Gert, 'Morality, moral theory', p. 19.

26   Freckelton, 'Enforcement of ethics', p. 134.

27   Solomon, 'Rules and principles', p. 410.

28   For a discussion of utilitarianism and deontology, see Beauchamp and Childress, p. 45.

29   Sullivan, *Immanuel Kant's moral theory*, p. 214.

30   Solomon, 'Rules and principles', p. 407.

31   Tomaszewski, 'Ethical issues from an international perspective', p. 31.

32   Knultgen, *Ethics and professionalism*, pp. 212, 213, 215.

33   Jonas, *The imperative of responsibility*, pp. 5–6.

34   Sullivan, *Immanuel Kant's moral theory*, p. 29.

35   Tomaszewski, 'Ethical issues from an international perspective', pp. 131–5.

36   McDowell, 'The excuses that make professional ethics irrelevant', p. 157.

37   Berlant, *Profession and monopoly*, pp. 29, 48, 55, 64.

38   Grace and Cohen, *Business ethics*, 3rd edn, p. 179.

39   See the discussion of the work of Joseph Butler in Collinson, *Fifty major philosophers*, p. 79.

40   Seal, 'Patient advocacy and advance care planning'.

41   Antiel et al., 'The impact of medical school oaths and other professional codes of ethics'.

42   Malley, 'Professionalism and professional ethics', pp. 407–8.

43   Rawls, *A theory of justice*, pp. 20, 48, 120, 579.

44   Nakajima, 'Health, ethics and human rights', p. 3.

45   Alexandra and Woodruff, 'A code of ethics for the nursing profession', p. 242.

46   Moreno, *Deciding together*.

47   Harman, 'Moral relativism defended', p. 3.

48   Yarborough et al., 'Interprofessional education in ethics', p. 794.

3

CARING AS SERVICE PROVISION

- Accepting a job to provide service
- Rights and interests
- Models of justice
- Applying the three models of justice
- The business of provision
- Further tools for considering fair distribution

OBJECTIVES

This chapter is on professional caring in terms of service availability and the principle of justice. You will develop an understanding of the practical models of justice: justice as fairness, comparative justice, and distributive justice. Examples of different models in action are applied to the structure and delivery of health care services, in terms of both availability and access.

By the end of this chapter you will have encountered the following terms and concepts: claim, interest, **liberty**, right, health, need, entitlement, and utility. The ethics theory of libertarianism is explained and you will rehearse some concepts of utilitarianism, a theory that you will now feel familiar with from earlier chapters. The analysis tools of cost–benefit analysis and cost-effectiveness analysis are introduced. Remember that these terms are gradually added to the glossary.

Liberty
Freedom of will, as expressed in choice of thought or action.

ACCEPTING A JOB TO PROVIDE SERVICE

When you are applying for a job, you should consider the values and objectives of the institution and the aims it pursues; in other words, the way the institutional services are delivered. Even though health care institutions all aim to provide goods and deliver health care, how they define goods and how they deliver health care can vary subtly. Sometimes this is because of the underlying ethic or morality system of the institution, such as in Catholic and Seventh Day Adventist hospitals. You may be able to discover from statistical summary documents that the hospital offers day surgery and specialises in skin treatments, or in fertility treatments. What is offered is only part of the information that you need. Values may be expressed in mission statements and visions as they relate to the institution's strategic objectives.[1]

Make a note of the goals or mission statement of a hospital near you, and of your own prospective or current place of employment. Once you discover these values, you need to decide whether these objectives and how they are achieved are compatible with your ethics and belief system.

Employees are part of the team that goes about distributing health resources. At some point it would be useful to reflect on the model of distribution that is applied where you work. Taking time to think about how the organisation is set up will inform your reflection on any difficulties you face in securing resources, or in making your idea of a health service a reality for your clients.

The way resources are distributed is a justice concern. You will remember that this was touched on in Chapter 2, in the discussion on definitions of the principles of beneficence, non-maleficence, autonomy (or respect for persons), and justice. The idea of justice has many underlying assumptions. Generally speaking, it is about the fair distribution of burden and benefit. How you think about justice depends on your values and what you think health care should achieve.

EXERCISE 3.1 THE SHARING OF RESOURCES

Take a moment to answer the following questions:
What is the good that you think health care should aim for?
How do you think that good should be shared around?

Your answer to the first question will depend on a value judgment of what is a good. Your answer to the second question will depend on whether you think people have a right to receive that good. Bear in mind that the word 'good' is used as a noun here—it is generally speaking a thing or concept when we talk about justice—not an adjective.

Many people would write something like 'health' or 'life' or 'quality of life' or 'health care' or 'treatment' in answer to the first question. Value judgments such as 'when needed' or 'when available' or 'when reasonable' or 'shared equally' are frequent responses to the second. Thinking about how the way services are delivered shows us what sort of distribution is in action. If your health care institution has a queue system, or waiting times before a booking can be made, some ordering of patients is happening behind the scenes, before you, as a health practitioner, even see them.

If you wrote 'when affordable' or 'when reasonable' in answer to the second question you are assuming that there are competing **claims** on health resources. Competing claims on the system is the reality of modern health care. Before we can decide what is reasonable, we may need to know how large the pool of resources is, including the source of funding that fuels the system, and what and who else requires resources from the pool. The question of who decides on how to prioritise resources is also a crucial justice question. Should it be a clinician or someone who doesn't deal directly with clients?

Your own idea of when you are available to work makes a difference to the type of work that you will do as well. Is 2 a.m. within your idea of proper availability of services? If it is, do you work that shift because your view is that that service should be available? Examining your own individual commitment to the type and availability of services that will be provided becomes part of the system. A system is, after all, made up of many people like you who have chosen to become health care professionals. Ethics can help with these difficult questions by examining the good that is aimed for and the models of justice that guide the distribution of that good.

Doing good is the basic premise of being beneficent, of caring. To 'do good' requires understanding what 'good' is, and then acting to the extent of your responsibility to that good. It is an active obligation. Each profession has its own definition of 'a good' (the word 'good' here is being used in the general sense of 'aiming for good' and avoiding harm; it is not restricted to 'good' used as a noun—for example, delivering a 'good', where 'good' means health care services). To an obstetrician or midwife it may be the preservation of life; to a palliative care specialist it may be an 'easy death'; while to a rehabilitation team it may be 'quality of life'. Getting consensus on what a good is (within a profession, or group of professions in the one system) is the first step in deciding reasonable beneficence responsibilities. Since that good must then be distributed, this consensus is also important in deciding responsibilities concerning justice. The definition arrived at is an ideal, so while the good might not be achieved all the time, the ethical position is to continue to aim for it, thereby maximising the possibility of doing good and minimising the possibility of doing harm.

You may take the view that the profession should not define what a good is at all, and that nobody can really define the good to aim for except the client. If you take that view, you would be an extreme **libertarian**. As J. S. Mill, the most quoted libertarian, writes, each person can and should decide for themselves what is in their best **interest**; having decided what is in their best interest, that person has a right to

Claim
Implicit or explicit demand to receive a good, as one's due.

Libertarianism
An ethics theory that aims for the greatest good for the greatest number, with good defined by each person pursuing their own defined wishes and liberties.

Interest
That which is to one's advantage or benefit.

it, unless it conflicts with similar rights of others or threatens the fabric of society.[2] This position places autonomy first, unless it can be argued, under fairly limited circumstances, that autonomy cannot be granted. The extreme libertarian position would place client choice first, rather than the current or available professional view of what is the best treatment. Whether or not autonomy and the client's wish, or choice, should override the professional's view of beneficence (what they think is reasonable care, or the best care to provide) is discussed in Chapter 4.

However, most health care systems, by definition, do not respond only to what each individual wants. They try to decide what is a good, thereby anticipating what people will want and need, and make resource allocation decisions on the basis of providing that defined good. Most systems are, therefore, not strictly libertarian. However, the limits that Mill identifies as reasonable limits to autonomy are useful in that they may well help to define rights that we are prepared to acknowledge within an existing health care system.

RIGHTS AND INTERESTS

Thinking about an everyday ethics issue of what is owing or due to you can help you to distinguish between rights and interests.

EVERYDAY ETHICS

Imagine that Sally is out shopping with her two primary school-aged children. They return to their car in the shopping centre car park, to put their shopping in the car and head home. They are surprised to see, lying on the ground, neatly behind their car boot, two absolutely brand spanking new twenty dollar notes. No one else is in sight in the car park. They are really in a rush, hoping to be home within a few minutes to get ready for an activity that afternoon.

Well, two children, two notes, you think, and that $20 is a lot of money in the eyes of the two children. So what should Sally do? It clearly is an opportunity to think about whether the children should claim the money as their own. What would you allow them to do, or would you even keep it as your own, being the adult?

Sally asked the children how they thought the person who had lost it would be feeling. They then thought about the options: keep it, look around for the person who might just have dropped it then keep it if they can't find them, or go and hand it in to the centre's lost property to see if the owner contacted the office. They agreed on the latter, with parental encouragement, but not enforcement, from Sally. She tried to impart the values of honesty as well in the process, and the idea that doing what restores the money to the other person is really reward enough.

The money was handed in to an impressed manager, who praised the children for their action. There was also an offer by the manager that, in keeping with the centre policy, if it was not claimed by the rightful owner within a week, she would contact the children as the new owners. In fact, it was picked up that afternoon by an elderly shopper who had rung in, quite distressed about the loss. The children were called by the manager to pass on the grateful thanks of the owner of the money, who had then been able to do her shopping with that money. She had expressed a renewed faith in the honesty of the young people of today as well.

Try to identify the values that were evident in the process. Try also to identify why an interest in keeping the money was not necessarily a right of 'finders-keepers'.

Now, try to analyse another everyday situation.

EVERYDAY ETHICS

After having a quick lunch at a café, you line up to pay your bill. It is very busy, and the crowd around the till is restless, with many people in a hurry to get back to work. The cashier seems flustered. When your turn to pay comes up, you give your table number. The cashier reaches for the details of what you ordered, as written on the waiter's order notebook, and asks you for $10.50. This is substantially less than what you have just eaten, having had an extra order of dessert and then coffee, which on your quick calculation hasn't been added to the bill. What should you do? Should you pay just what is asked, or disagree with what is asked, and suggest paying more?

Try to examine the issues of rights, interests, and duties, from the perspectives of you as patron, the waiter, the cashier, and the café owners, before you make your decision.

As you work your way through the chapter, return to this exercise to see if your reading helps you to further unravel the complex interplay of roles and duties.

You may decide that acting beneficently is only required when someone has a **right** to whatever good you would be promoting. You would be correct because there is a difference between rights and interests. That can be illustrated fairly easily with an exercise that works best in a group. First, ask 'Who owns a car?' Many hands will probably go up. The rest of the group may have an interest in those cars, but they don't necessarily have a right to them ... or do they? The people with the goods (the cars) might be caring for others by giving their cars to people without them, but is that an obligation? Ask the people with the cars: 'Who would give their car to someone who doesn't have one?' Wait, and watch the hands disappear. So what interests are reasonable? Perhaps if I told you that I want your car so that I can get to work more easily, or so I can get to university to study, you might feel swayed. Can I have it? I have shown you a good reason why I want it. I have asked, and made my autonomous decision clear. Do you have a duty to give the car to me?

Under our current societal structure, the answer to this question is 'probably not', and the same applies to whatever else I ask for, unless there is model of justice operating that obliges you to fulfil that wish or want. You will see more on wishes and

Right
Claim that is recognised as imposing obligations on others to fulfil it.

autonomy in Chapter 4. If I were to take your car, I might be depriving you of your similar interest in getting to work or to university. There is also the consideration that you have probably earned the car by buying it. All is not lost though. Society does acknowledge my interest in coming to work, or university, and makes public transport available at a reasonable cost. There are some human-rights agreements—for example, the United Nations Convention on the Rights of the Child—that regard education as a basic right, but only to the level of a decent minimum of primary school level, with encouragement for states to develop different forms of secondary education.[3] Studying or working is seen as a good, so my interest in pursuing that is reasonable, but getting there quickly or more conveniently may not be pursued to the exclusion of others' interests. There is a similar limit to obligations relating to beneficence in health care. Like access to education, it is thought that we only have a right to certain levels of care; beyond those levels our right becomes an interest only.

The two-tiered nature of the Australian health care system reflects this division of health care into 'rights' and 'interests'. There is a publicly funded, government-provided sector and a privately funded, privately provided sector. While these are designed to operate in parallel, there is constant debate about what should be publicly available, and how much public provision should be available to those who can afford private care.[4] In some countries, such as Australia and England, publicly funded care is available to all, regardless of income, automatic cover for many aspects of basic, or decent, minimum health care but not for 'extras' like private rooms in hospital or patient choice of doctor. Patients who are not privately covered must pay for extras somehow. Thus we could say that the minimum publicly covered care is considered a right within the community, but this does not extend to the 'extras'.

To complicate this further, some people in a community may not seem 'entitled' to access care at all, so have no **entitlement**. Usually, before people become your patients, they have been deemed to be 'eligible' to be treated in some way. So in a clinic they might be eligible to receive publicly funded care. In a private practice they may be covered by insurance or public funding or both. Or they may be in a position to pay the full cost. Try to imagine a situation in which a person is not entitled to access subsidised health care (in a given community) and does not have the resources to pay the fee upfront before receiving care. This is the situation for people in the USA, who are caught between government-subsidised health coverage for the very poor and employer-subsidised coverage for middle to upper income earners. Their interest is in being treated, but is it their right? Political refugees can also be in the invidious position of not having joined a community officially and not having access to that community's health care. Despite universal basic health coverage provided in many countries, the public system is for citizens and residents, and not necessarily for those on temporary visas. So the right to access health care is not granted to all. It depends on membership of the community that holds the resources for distribution. Illegal immigrants are in a dubious position in every country that provides care on the basis of right of recognised citizens to access care.

Entitlement
Recognised need to create community obligation to fulfil interest or claim.

Short supply and immediate priorities

Contributor: *Jenneke Foottit*

You are the registered nurse on the afternoon shift in an acute hospital. There have been problems with the supply of dressing packs and you do not have enough dressing packs to complete the dressing changes needed. You do have all other standard sterile and unsterile requirements. There are three dressings that urgently need to be changed, but only two dressing packs left, and you cannot borrow another one from elsewhere, so you need to compromise and modify what you do.

Mrs Smith had a cholecystectomy two days ago and has a wound drain. The dressing consists of gauze packed around a draining tube. The wound dressings are wet and need replacing. She has no signs of infection or complications.

Mrs Chiu has leg ulcers that are being treated with compression bandages and bed rest. The bandages are changed weekly and are due for changing today. Her ulcers are healing well and have reduced in size considerably.

Mr Jones has had an amputation of the forefoot for complications of diabetes. His wound is healing well but very slowly. His blood glucose levels for the past three days have been high. He has daily dressings.

How will you solve this dilemma? Describe your thoughts and your decision-making process using the principles of ethical care you have learnt about.

Distinctions between rights and interests can be illustrated by considering prevention and treatment issues. Advice on diet to prevent heart disease is a good that is so fundamental to health that it is currently seen as a right in Western countries; publicly funded dietary advice begins in early childhood clinics and at primary school. In contrast, transplant of a diseased heart is not seen as a right; we know this because this treatment option is not made available to all. Looking into the future, a life-saving heart transplant may one day be seen as a 'right' (if sufficient hearts are available), but repeated heart transplants may not. Medical treatment after life-threatening injury is, under our current system, a near absolute right because life itself is threatened, and our concept of an interest to health holds our right to life to be fundamental. However, we may not have such an absolute right to receive counselling after injury, because although it could be argued to be essential to recovering a decent minimum of health, it may not be available in places that are convenient to the client, or at hours that suit them perfectly. It may even be left to state or regional bodies to decide how much of a right or interest counselling is.

As a rule of thumb, when there is strong agreement that service obligations are mandated, that service will be a right. When there appears to be considerable discretion about whether or not to provide the service, the service is meeting a strong interest (or claim), not a right.

Raanon Gillon has noted the difference between institutional and moral rights: institutional rights are simply claims that have been justified. The institution can decide, collectively, to grant such things as free medical care, but equally it may take those things away. Moral rights, on the other hand, cannot be taken away. Gillon also notes that only some rights impose obligations on others to act in a particular way.[5] This distinction between rights that impose obligations and those that don't is not new to the field of law, which tries to clarify which of our obligations are contractual, and therefore enforceable, and which are merely goodwill. Jurist and theorist W. N. Hohfeld outlined the difference between wishes, or liberties, and 'claim-rights'. The latter imply an obligation on others to satisfy those claims; the former do not.[6] Daniel Callahan, an eminent ethicist from the USA, also notes that there are limits to our ability to satisfy health interests. He argues that before we talk in terms of health rights, we must re-examine the fundamental goals of medicine (paying particular attention to how realistic and affordable those goals are) and countries must meet agreed goals.[7]

Applying the concept of good, whether it is an absolute or decent minimum, is an illustration of the breadth of responsibilities to do good that health care professionals undertake. Many codes of ethics mention acting in the patient's or client's best interests, and thereby furthering the health of the community. A professional's responsibility is not only to treat each client, but also to ensure that others have the opportunity to be similarly treated. In other words, the individual treatment that a professional gives to their client should not compromise the availability of such treatment to others. In simple terms, questions of individual client care, and doing good for them, come under the concept or principle of beneficence. The community obligation that is part of beneficence is also related to the principle of justice, in that it is about questions of the distribution of, and access to, health care.

By now you will have realised that accepting a job as a health care worker, and providing care, has a professional, community, institutional, and societal context. If you are to remain responsible by world standards, you may need to check, every now and then, that your approach to the business of providing care is consistent with the expectations that are expressed in international documents on human rights. Those expectations can appear to be quite stringent.

Health
State of physical, mental, and social well-being.

The World Health Organization has defined **health** as 'a state of complete physical, mental, and social wellbeing and not merely the absence of disease or infirmity'. WHO's health goal for your clients and potential clients, which is essentially the good we should all be striving for, is expressed in the preamble to the constitution of WHO: 'The enjoyment of the highest attainable standard of health is one of the fundamental rights of every human being without distinction of race, religion, political belief, economic or social condition.' These objectives were viewed as ambitious at the start of the new century but are used as a guiding mandate to tackle such issues as the preventable transmission of human immunodeficiency virus (HIV), malaria, and tuberculosis, and more recently the containment and tracking of potentially pandemic influenza, and attainable improvements in basic living conditions and health care access for all people.[8]

All health care workers struggle to provide 'a good', however they define it, in a context of competing claims on resources and seemingly diminishing pools of those resources.

There are a number of philosophical choices to be made, under the principle of justice, in deciding just how to distribute what is available. Spending is reported by the Organization for Economic Co-operation and Development (OECD) as a proportion of gross domestic product (GDP). The USA spends an estimated 17.4 per cent of GDP on health care, which is very high compared to the UK, at 9.8 per cent of GDP, and Australia, at 8.7 per cent of GDP. The European countries of Netherlands and France spend 12 per cent and 11.8 per cent of GDP respectively.[9] Economists note that recession may reduce spending growth in the short term, but spending will continue to rise with the increased routine use of medical technologies in health care.[10] There is some evidence to suggest that survival rates from serious illnesses, such as cancer, are better in higher-spending countries.[11] That puts the USA, theoretically at least, in the lead. Even so, some would argue that there is great inequity in that system, despite the higher proportion of GDP available, and there is a constant review of how to distribute care better. The proportion of funds available for health care in any given country is unlikely to change quickly. So the question is, given the current pool of resources, how can we distribute what we have in an ethical manner?

MODELS OF JUSTICE

The three justice models discussed most often are justice as fairness, comparative justice, and distributive justice. They derive from the philosophical writings of three well-known philosophers, and as the discussion progresses you will notice that each model has different ethical theories or frameworks supporting it. All these theories and frameworks are about what a society might regard as a fair distribution of limited resources that are in demand by the members of the society.

The philosopher John Rawls writes about the concept of **justice as fairness**. It is a concept of absolute equality and fairness. The model has been applied by others to health, and is the justice model that is closest to the WHO definition of health.[12] Disparate treatment based on the financial circumstances, race, or any number of other distinguishing features of those to whom services are being provided is unacceptable under the justice-as-fairness model. The justice-as-fairness model cuts across lines created by nations or regions: nationality or place of residence do not determine rights to health care. Under this model of justice, differential treatment is

Justice as fairness
Justice model of equality, in which goods are distributed with the aim that community members are restored to equivalent levels.

justified only to compensate for disadvantages suffered by some people. The aim is that all people should end up roughly equal.

Think about what limits your clients in achieving health. Should the removal of barriers to health be part of the health care agenda?

Indigenous education models are now incorporating culture and community into a holistic approach to health. This is only one example of services that aim to alleviate historically accrued disadvantages and barriers as well as putting in place physical health measures in the pursuit of health.

Comparative justice, as its name suggests, involves assessing the relative importance of people's interests in receiving the health resource. This is a compromise between justice as fairness, in which the ideal is providing treatment based on nothing else but **need**, and acknowledging the limited pool of resources from which to provide that treatment. The triage system of health care delivery is an example of the comparative justice model in action: need assessment is carried out and treatment is given accordingly. Minor complaints wait longer, and more serious cases are rushed to the top of the queue.

A type of triage system exists in our emergency/casualty departments. It also exists in our waiting lists for public hospital care. The following extract from policy guidelines on prioritising patients on elective waiting lists is an example of the assessment of need that is the key to the triage system. Emergency admissions are excluded from this, as they are assumed to take place immediately.

Comparative justice
Justice model of need in which goods are distributed on the basis of demonstrated most need, compared with the demonstrated needs of other community members.

Need
Demonstrated interest in receiving a good.

PAUSE & REFLECT

What do you think about the following categories in the policy for elective admissions? A referring doctor completes the recommendation for admission form, obtains the patient's consent, and assigns a clinical priority category. Categories 1,2, and 3 are deemed 'ready for care'.

Category 1—'Admission desirable within 30 days for a condition that has the potential to deteriorate quickly to the point that it may become an emergency.'

Category 2—'Admission within 90 days desirable for a condition which is not likely to deteriorate quickly or become an emergency.'

Category 3—'Admission within 365 days acceptable for a condition which is unlikely to deteriorate quickly and which has little potential to become an emergency.'

A fourth category is used for patients who are either clinically not yet ready for admission (staged) and those who have deferred admission for personal reasons (deferred).[13]

The modern application of **distributive justice** often takes comparative justice one step further. It allocates resources not just on need, but on what our society regards as an appropriate distribution of benefits and burdens. Distributive justice is really just the broad societal consensus on how to allocate rights, duties, and burdens among community members.[14] The important point is that the burden is distributed according to the ability of sections of society to cope with it, and the benefit is given to sections of society that need or deserve it. This means that need is not the only deciding factor. There is also some sort of social assessment of worth and deservedness going on here. If Rawls's model is applied in this assessment, then 'distribution' is interpreted as 'justice as fairness' or 'equality'. In distributive justice, any social difference can be the discriminating feature that decides whether or not a service will be provided, or at what level it will be supplied. For example, resources could go to the wealthy, if we judge they deserve it, and less to minority groups. Or the wealthy could be asked to bear more cost burden for the same care. The distinctions made between different social groups highlight the contemporary political and social divisions of the society that applies this justice model. You may like to revisit some of the ethics theories in Chapter 1 to help you decide how best to make a societal judgment on who deserves what treatment.

Distributive justice
Justice model of need and entitlement, in which goods are distributed based on demonstrated and comparative interest and entitlement to receive community benefits and the expectation or capacity to bear burdens.

APPLYING THE THREE MODELS OF JUSTICE

Once a system is in place, and is mandated by the institution in which you work, the real question for you, as a professional health care worker, is what discretion you have in applying that model. When professionals disagree violently with the model that seems to be operating, they may decide to protest. Our health care history is replete with examples of professionals protesting about the resources provided for them to get their job done, or about the way in which some types of treatment seem to be undertaken (or some clients treated) but not others. Patient groups too can voice dissatisfaction with how resources are shared, how some treatments are developed and others not, and how long it seems to take for their health care needs to be met. The concerns can demonstrate a clash between individual autonomy and a community concept of fair distribution, under justice, as you will read further in the section 'The business of provision', and also in Chapter 8.

EVERYDAY ETHICS

In an everyday setting, we live with queues. We queue at the bus, we queue at a café, we queue at various offices, and so on. So, what if we jump the queue? Are we 'entitled' to, or not? Think about how you feel if people jump queues. Also, if you have ever jumped a queue, think about why you felt entitled to do that. Was it your need? Or was it some other deservedness? You will probably find that the social agreement of waiting in line for a resource that everyone is waiting for is an accepted one, but that there are certain exceptions that people may feel justifies allowing others to go the head of the queue.

Justice has at its heart our everyday sense of ethics of what we should do, and how we should behave towards one another, in taking our share of community resources or ensuring others are able to benefit from their share. As you read the next section, consider the issue from the patient's perspective by raising reflective questions for them. Remember that the answers could be quite different in a context that is different from the one that you are used to, such as in a country in the developing world, or a situation of crisis.

FROM THEORY TO PRACTICE

Staffing and care decisions

Contributor: *Jenneke Foottit*

You are the registered nurse on the morning shift in a residential aged care facility. A number of staff are away on sick leave and have not been replaced. You are short of carers to shower residents. The following residents still need showering. Which residents get showered, and which ones get a wash and a shower the following day?

Mrs Jones has dementia and is incontinent but wears continence pants. She is mobile but does not like a shower and it takes a long time to shower her.

Mr Peters is bedfast after a stroke, incontinent and unable to speak. He needs two people to provide his care.

Miss Smith, who is cognitively not impaired but frail, is continent with regular toileting but due to staff shortages she was not taken to the toilet and she has soiled herself. She is able to shower with supervision but needs the staff member to stay in the shower with her. She is chatty and loves pampering, which can make it difficult to shower her quickly.

Mrs Chang is of Chinese origin and speaks no English. She is frail, and gets very impatient with staff when they don't understand what she wants. She has not had a shower for two days.

Mr Wong is from Taiwan and speaks excellent English, but he has Parkinson's disease which is affecting his vocal cords and he is difficult to understand. He has significant stiffness which is relieved considerably by a long hot shower in the morning, improving his mobility for the day.

You can provide showers for three residents. Using your understanding of ethical principles, choose the three residents who will be showered and give a reason for your choice.

PAUSE & REFLECT

Consider these reflective questions as you read further:

What community am I in?

Can my community help me with health care?

What sort of health care is available to me?

What do I owe my community in return as part of my duties of belonging?

THE BUSINESS OF PROVISION

Being in the business of providing health care involves charging money and buying human and other resources. Australia has Medicare, a Commonwealth system that covers basic medical consultations, basic pathology services, and public provision of health care in public hospitals. Medicare pays health service providers with money collected from Commonwealth income taxes. Providers are paid predetermined amounts for each service they provide. Medicare is set up so that medical care is available when needed (and to a reasonable level) without financial considerations impeding that care. Some health care practitioners choose to charge only the Medicare rebate, which is 75 to 85 per cent of the scheduled fee for any particular service (depending on the provider and where the service is received). These providers are termed 'bulk-billers': their service is largely paid for by Commonwealth Medicare funds. Providers can enter bulk-billing agreements with the government, ensuring that no money changes hands between the patient and provider. The number of providers prepared to bulk-bill has fallen dramatically over the last few years, but there are some federal government schemes for GPs who bulk bill patients in vulnerable groups, and safety net provisions for individuals who have high costs for prescription medicines and medical care.[15] Medicare is not meant to be used in instances when compensation may be claimed, and when medical bills will effectively be the responsibility of the person who caused the injury to the other person. Exceptions are provided for emergency treatment, even if the injury stems from motor vehicle or work accidents in which compensation or insurance claims may be routinely sought. Ambulance officers arriving on the scene of an accident need not worry about who will pay for the service. The bill is worked out later, making it possible to institute essential care and transport patients to hospital immediately.[16] Emergency departments receive casualties with the same expectations.

The routine services for which patients' costs are covered are tightly defined under Medicare and the Medicare Benefits Schedule. What is included changes from time to time as new treatment options become available, of course, but also due to budgetary consideration. Entitlements can be further restricted if a larger than expected outlay is encountered for a particular service item number. For instance, in relation to a rebate for a particular psychiatric condition, the following proviso was added: 'it is not sufficient for the patient's illness to fall within the diagnostic criteria. It must be evident that a significant level of impairment exists which interferes with the patient's quality of life.' Also implemented at the same time was a restriction on the availability of benefits for the removal of broadly classified skin lesions. This change was due to a '30% increase in Medicare outlays above that anticipated'.[17] The rebates that are publicly funded are effectively altered from time to time so that areas of need are balanced with areas of demand to ensure equitable distribution of the limited available public funds.

While Medicare is federally budgeted, state governments have their own budgets to run hospitals, including inpatient and emergency services, and provide numerous other community and public health services. Both state and federal government budgets are routinely available. When tabled in Parliament, they provide an insight into what the current government's key objectives are in delivering health care, and how money is spent to achieve those objectives. Debating a budget for a service makes little sense unless the good that is trying to be achieved is also discussed.

The following exercise illustrates the breadth of one state government's health department budget. This exercise demonstrates the difficult budget decisions that must be made when resources become even more limited than usual, or when primary objectives change. Inevitably, some services lose money as that money is shifted to other services or is cut from the budget entirely. This is a macro exercise: it steps away from individual treatment decisions and asks you to think about what resources the system, or large service units, have at their disposal. Once budget cuts or rearrangements are instituted, those running the services have to examine the objectives of the service, agree on how best to distribute what they have, and, more fundamentally, decide whether they can still provide the 'good' that they believe they are there to provide.

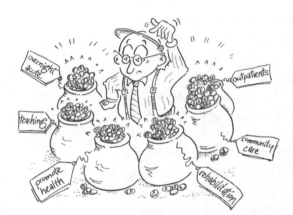

EXERCISE 3.2 BUDGETS AND PRIORITY DECISIONS

This exercise uses a budget for the provision of health infrastructure, programs, and services in public hospitals, and the stated objectives of the budget. Examine the budget and consider the ministerial directive that priorities should change slightly. Think about how to achieve these changes in priority without allocating additional money. You may move money, but not add more. Before you start, put a 'hat' on, and adopt the role of stakeholder. Stakeholder roles can include health professionals (for example, doctors, nurses, and others), consumers of health services/clients (for example, patient advocates, particular client groups), planners (for example, chief executive officers, government representatives), and the general community (for example, local councils, mothers' groups). You may be able to think of other stakeholders as well. This stakeholder exercise is fun in a tutorial or lecture format, with the groups not only implementing the ministerial directive, but also bringing their own agendas to the budget rearrangement.

The hypothetical ministerial directive for this exercise is that aged care and Aboriginal disease prevention programs should be a focus in the coming year, and that operations that can be achieved in day surgery should be carried out in that setting rather than with pre- and post-operation overnight stays.

A budget rearrangement can be combined with the additional scenario of a forthcoming pay increase for nurses, and a pay decrease for visiting medical officers (a similar exercise is found in an early ethics text[18]). This exercise prompts you to find out the objectives of each program, as the good each is aiming for, and to consider them before budgets are rearranged. The detailed objectives can be found in the parliamentary papers.[19]

Some health care workers are very uncomfortable about justice decisions being made as part of treatment decisions about individual clients, but others are less so. It could be argued that the duty to care for the individual client is paramount, and therefore should not be subject to broad budgetary discussions. On the other hand, with a limited resource, health professionals' obligations are also to other potential clients whom they have not yet met, but who might walk through the door and need treatment in the near future. That is why professional codes of ethics emphasise duty to society as well as duty to the individual client, as we saw in Chapter 1. The modern business of health care forces you to consider others as well as those whose health needs are right in front of you.

BUDGET EXERCISE

NSW Department of Health, Total Expenses, Budget 2011–12	$000
Primary and community-based services	1 186 912
Linkage to results: 'improved access to early intervention, assessment, therapy and treatment services in a home or community setting' and 'reduced rate of potentially preventable hospitalisation'.	
Service description: 'provision of health services to persons attending community health centres or in the home, including health promotion activities, community based women's health, dental, drug and alcohol and HIV/AIDS services. It also covers the provision of grants to Non-Government Organisations for community health purposes'.	
Aboriginal health services	97 297
Linkage to results: 'building regional partnerships to provide health services to raise the health status of Aboriginal people' and 'promoting a healthy lifestyle'.	
Service description: 'provision of supplementary health services to Aboriginal people, particularly in the areas of health promotion, health education and disease prevention. (Please note that this program excludes most services for Aboriginal people provided directly by area health services and other general health services which are used by all members of the community)'.	

(*Continued*)

Outpatient services	1 665 318

Linkage to results: 'improving, maintaining or restoring health of ambulant patients in a hospital setting through diagnosis, therapy, education and treatment services'.

Service description: 'provision of services provided in outpatient clinics including low level emergency care, diagnostic and pharmacy services and radiotherapy treatment'.

Emergency services	1 767 349

Linkage to results: 'reducing the risk of premature death or disability by providing timely emergency diagnostic, treatment and transport services'.

Service description: 'provision of emergency road and air ambulance services and treatment of patients in designated emergency departments of public hospitals'.

Inpatient hospital services	7 728 235

Linkage to results: 'timely treatment of booked surgical patients, resulting in improved clinical outcomes, quality of life and patient satisfaction' and 'reduced rate of unplanned hospital readmission'.

Service description: 'provision of health care to patients admitted to hospital, including elective surgery and maternity services'.

Mental health services	1 340 004

Linkage to results: 'improving the health, wellbeing and social functioning of people with disabling mental disorders' and 'reducing the incidence of suicide, mental health problems and mental disorders in the community'.

Service description: 'provision of an integrated and comprehensive network of services by Local Health Districts and community based organisations for people seriously affected by mental illnesses and mental health problems', and 'the development of preventive programs which meet the needs of specific client groups'.

Rehabilitation and extended care services	1 265 395

Linkage to results: 'improving or maintaining the wellbeing and independent functioning of people with disabilities or chronic conditions, the frail and the terminally ill'.

Service description: 'provision of health care services for persons with long-term physical and psycho-physical disabilities and for the frail-aged' and 'coordination of the Department's services for the aged and disabled with those provided by other agencies and individuals'.

Population health services	554 647

Linkage to results: 'reduced incidence of preventable disease and disability' and 'improved access to opportunities and prerequisites for good health'.

Service description: 'provision of health services targeted at broad population groups including environmental health protection, food and poisons regulation and monitoring of communicable diseases'.

Teaching and research	805 608

Linkage to results: 'developing the skills and knowledge of the health workforce to support patient care and population health and extending knowledge through scientific enquiry and applied research aimed at improving the health and well-being of the people of New South Wales'.

Service description: 'provision of professional training for the needs of the New South Wales health system' and 'strategic investment in research and development to improve the health and well-being of the people of New South Wales'.

In the UK, basic universal health care is available. Limited resources, rationing, and managed care, and therefore limitations on the funds available to specific regions, have been a reality for over 15 years. While there are many forms of managed care, in essence it involves reducing health care costs by directing funds for specific services, or for particular patient communities, towards certain health care providers who are able to provide those services at below a designated cost. Patients 'join' a practice as a patient, and they do not have the flexibility of attending multiple practices for their primary care. There is a trend to make general practitioners the 'commissioners' of services for their local populations.[20] Of course, not all GPs want this funding responsibility, as the time and financial responsibility involved is considerable. Throughout the system refinements, there has been an early and ongoing concern that the UK system harboured inequality.[21]

Waiting times for patients for elective services are routinely scrutinised when reforms are introduced.[22] Waiting list systems for treatment in budgeted categories of care can cause exasperation at local levels. Children, for instance, may have changed significantly by the time their appointment for assessment of particular problems arrives. A qualitative interview study of access to cardiac rehabilitation services in an area of socio-economic deprivation in the UK demonstrated that waiting times were lengthy, and many people slipped through the care net due to limited service capacity and difficulties in accessing hospital-based services from small towns. The patients and their families experienced frustration at still being on rehabilitation waiting lists, sometimes for months, after cardiac episodes. Some people avoided the public system queue for services in the National Health Service (NHS) by seeking specific advice or using private rehabilitation services.[23] The government is tackling the waiting list delays in a number of ways. For hospitals, the ratings received for care and waiting times partly determine funding for those hospitals. Patients have a significant input into the ratings, with large-scale patient surveys of care received in acute care and outpatient settings being conducted regularly and the results incorporated into the ratings. In one survey program, 59 000 patients in NHS acute trusts and 123 000 patients in primary care trusts were involved in rating services.[24] This rating system is itself debated, but seems to be here to stay.

Limited dental services are included in the NHS public rebate system, with a set fee available to dentists for certain provision of services. There is some evidence that treatment plans for difficult or complex treatments can be altered by dentists to minimise the cost burdens to the practice.[25] There was also earlier evidence of dentists electing not to accept new NHS patients on their practice lists. So care was on a private basis, if no public treatment place was available, with the patient paying the full dental care bill to the dentist. The 'opening' of a list to public patients could prompt local media coverage.[26] Perhaps the question should be asked whether the burden placed on dentists and their businesses is simply too high, and amounts to a transfer of public responsibilities for funding care to the private practitioners.

How a system is funded and structured can challenge the way individual health care workers relate to clients, as has been debated in New Zealand, where district health boards organise the public funding and provision of health, public health, and disability services. When district budget holding was trialled, there was a concern that the health professional needed to have good, coordinated information available to protect the clients and their interests in an increasingly competitive environment.[27] The Association of Salaried Medical Professionals in New Zealand has stressed the importance of the 'internal morality' of professionals, who strive to provide the best health care they can under different budget constraints and externally imposed limits, and through times of changing structures and systems.[28] Ongoing attention is given to poor life expectancy and outcome figures for New Zealanders from a Maori background, compared with those from an Anglo-European background. As the health services need to be culturally sensitive so that they are viewed as '**culturally safe**' and people do not then delay seeking treatment, there is considerable effort in New Zealand to be aware of culturally specific issues in the organisation and delivery of health services.[29] Culture and community are addressed further in Chapter 10.

In the USA, a managed care system is quite common, as many patients are insured with managed care providers. Defining entitlement is clearly a requirement before any care is received. Managed funds share money from the funding pot of the insurance provider, and very low income earners are granted access to public monies if they become entitled by satisfying certain residential and income requirements.

Cultural safety
Acknowledging and abiding by the social expectations and norms of a specific community.

Different models of managed care can place the rationing decision with one primary provider, usually medical or nursing staff, who then coordinates their own service provision with the services of other professionals. A number of models that help determine who should exercise that rationing decision have been proposed. In all these models, the value of the personal provider–client relationship remains extremely important.[30] That relationship clearly faces new challenges, including threats posed to the trust that clients place in their carer, as the professional strives for the best possible care for all clients under their ambit and care.

PAUSE & REFLECT

To add to your reflective questions that were posed earlier in this chapter, those people will be wondering:

Am I in the community which is provided for by that specific funding?

Can I expect that my request for the funding of my care will be seen as an equitable and affordable use of the funds?

A gatekeeper in such managed fund arrangements is effectively positioned between the provider and the patient, and these questions will be answered before care commences.

Can you say which justice model is applied in this process?

Hospitals can be nominated as care providers by insurers, and they negotiate contracts for reimbursement for care provided. These contract negotiations can be heated and difficult, as hospitals seek to ensure they have sufficient funds to cover anticipated care costs properly. The large US government-funded plan for very low income earners (Medicare—not to be confused with the Australian universal scheme of the same name) once provided a buffer for hospitals as contracted care providers, but a context of falling Medicare rates, tighter margins with insurance contracts, and a continuing backlash against managed care developed.[31] Practices can be nominated as providers of 'capitation contracts' to provide care for certain insured people. The physician needs to balance care and care costs—both those generated in a setting and those outsourced through referral. When asked about their practice in a managed care setting for a study in the USA, many physicians expressed concerns about

- the request for referral or use of outside care
- when to authorise treatments that would help, perhaps more 'socially' than medically
- patients' requests for specific treatments that may be expensive and that may require specific criteria to justify the expense under a managed care plan
- feeling a pressure to provide services outside their own level of expertise
- wanting to give additional service, advice, or supply of goods for free, but feeling obliged to limit expenses for the sake of the practice.[32]

Many of these concerns are about trying to contain costs and services in one setting. This is a common theme in different countries' settings. The limited referral process, or more strictly controlled and budgeted referral process, means waiting lists and longer waiting times for patients to access those secondary services.

Working in managed care brings decisions like drug prescriptions, hospital admission, referrals, and affiliated resource use into sharp focus. The 'budgets' that have to be balanced can be at area level, or, in the US system, at insurance coverage level. The different style of practice implicit in this organisation of care delivery is now taught in resident training in the USA. The case discussions during rounds involve clinical issues, but also issues of referral that could lead to problems in resource use. Use of expensive procedures and specialty referrals are scrutinised.[33] This is clearly a different style of practice from that focused solely on maximal care of individuals using any or all available technology and resources.

The care received in hospitals is constantly assessed. Legislation in mid-2003 set required patient–nurse ratios for Californian hospitals. While care units can vary between three and ten patients per nurse, the aim is for an average of six patients per nurse. This follows research that shows that a higher nurse ratio, and subsequently better surveillance of a patient's condition, leads to lower mortality figures and better job satisfaction for the nurses.[34] Human resources are as much in the debate about expenditure as procedural or treatment resources, as your earlier work on the budget exercise showed.

Asch and Ubel have also described the way that, under the managed care system operating in the USA, doctors are forced to take responsibility for choosing the cheapest treatment that accords with the 'standard of care' set by the managed care policy. They describe how the government 'caps' (puts a limit on) the costs of particular services; this forces the physician to think beyond the individual client, appeal to the standard of care (which in most cases is the most commonly used treatment rather than the best), and, finally, make do with less than the best, unless other options have failed. Their vignette was written to demonstrate how the most reliable option is often the last considered because it is the most expensive. This vignette could be used for discussion in class. Any routine treatment could be substituted to make the vignette appropriate for particular professions.

PAUSE & REFLECT

Ms Cooper sees her general internist, Dr Kelley, about her seasonal allergies. Dr Kelley explains that although he believes a non-sedating antihistamine is likely to be better tolerated, he thinks it is reasonable to try a less expensive conventional antihistamine first and to use the more expensive kind only if Ms Cooper is troubled by sedation.[35]

Note your list of the goods achieved for the client, and for the other potential clients in this scenario.

EXERCISE 3.3 PRIMARY CARE DECISIONS

Now try the following exercise:

GPs in a budget-holding context in the UK are encouraged to prescribe generic drugs rather than brand-name drugs whenever possible. Those prescribing brand names consistently are 'visited' by representatives of the budget team for their area to try to encourage more cost-effective patterns of prescribing.

What should the GPs be asked to do, and what should the GPs' response be? Try to set out your reasons, and explain them to a fellow colleague or friend.

In Thailand, where there is a similar funding problem, patients pay a set affordable contribution for each treatment, and the local hospital covers all further treatment costs. There has been controversy over the 30-baht health care scheme, when referral to a tertiary care specialist or intensive treatment facilities for complex or chronic conditions is likely to be costly, and there is a reported reluctance by some local hospitals to refer their patients for that further treatment.[36]

In Australia, various initiatives have been trialled that encourage coordination and care planning that goes beyond episodic service provision. The early trials focused on care management and budget coordination for high-service clients, such as elderly persons with dementia, who are unable to manage their own care in the current system. The focus was on complex and chronic conditions, which by their nature consume enormous amounts of the health budget, and particularly chronic asthma, diabetes, and heart conditions, as well as for people with chronic disease in Aboriginal communities.[37] The GP has been viewed as an ideal care coordinator for people with complex care needs or chronic conditions, and the significant time needed for planning, coordination of care between multidisciplinary professionals, and review is partly acknowledged by a public funding item number. Planned and coordinated care for high-need patients has emerged in dentistry, with a quantum of money available from the public purse for particular chronic and complex care needs of patients who are referred by their GP.[38] A similar model is used for the funding of a process of psychological assessment and treatment by a psychologist, on referral from a GP. So Australia is effectively building a quasi-managed care system, with the GP commonly a gatekeeper of public care by a range of health professionals.

In the UK, US, and Australian systems, with their different approaches to budgeted health care, it will take some time for health carers to come to terms with the notion of managing resources as well as providing episodic care.[39] The managed care system, however it is formulated in each country, relies on trust that pursuing the best possible care for each patient is the shared aim of the carer, the health service, and the funder. Managed care members interviewed by researchers have spoken about how important it is to have trust in the doctor, and also trust in the hospital and, now, trust in the insurer, that the best possible care will be made available.[40]

FURTHER TOOLS FOR CONSIDERING FAIR DISTRIBUTION

There are tools that can be used to decide if a service is worth offering, and if society can afford to make it available. These tools focus on the likely benefit of the service, and then compare the benefit with the likely demand for the service and the drain on available resources that offering the resource or service would cause.

Cost-effectiveness analysis
A comparative assessment of costs in achieving an agreed objective or beneficial outcome.

Cost–benefit analysis
A calculation of the cost of delivering a service with demonstrated and calculated financial benefits.

Utility
Quality of usefulness for a desired purpose or outcome.

Two of these tools are **cost-effectiveness analysis** and **cost–benefit analysis**. Cost-benefit analysis compares the cost of a program with the expected benefits in dollars. The way that this analysis quantifies outcomes as hard currency makes it controversial in health. It is hard to quantify how much an improvement in health or lifestyle, or life years, means in real dollars. Cost-effectiveness analysis compares alternative ways of achieving a specific set of objectives or outcomes. Cost-effectiveness analysis is being increasingly used to decide program rationing in large health systems, such as in the US system. Its ethics are also being examined.

You will note that the definition of good that is chosen for the assessment in Exercise 3.4 is a broad concept of 'good': of detecting cancer in the greatest number of people in a certain population, or sub-section of a population. This is the common approach of utilitarian analysis. A 'good' is defined, and the process of achieving that 'good' for the greatest number of a defined group is then designed with the primary objective being the desired purpose or outcome. The issue is what testing process is most useful, or delivers maximum **utility**, for the express purpose of detecting cancer. So utility is a concept of usefulness, applied in a previously defined notion of benefit or good. Under utilitarianism, defining the good and utility aimed at is essential. It is then maximised according to the overall aim of delivery to the greatest number of the recognised community or portion of the community that is agreed to be in potential need of such delivery. The effect on those who miss out is acknowledged, but that is deemed to be an acceptable part of the process of working towards the greater utilitarian outcome.

EXERCISE 3.4 PREVENTIVE TESTING BUDGETS

A paper by Ubel, DeKay, Baron, and Asch reported on a study that posed the following scenario to experts in medical ethics and medical decision making.[41] Consider their scenario. What do you think should happen?

The federal government has set up a program to test for colon cancer in people enrolled in Medicaid, a government program that offers health insurance to low-income people and their families. The test allows doctors to find colon cancer at an early stage. So far the federal government has offered the test to people at high risk for colon cancer, and this has prevented many of them from dying of colon cancer. Now the government wants to offer the test to the rest of the people receiving Medicaid, all of whom are at equally low risk for colon cancer.

A group of doctors was formed to help the government decide which of two tests to offer the low-risk people. Test 1 is inexpensive but does not always detect cancers in their early stages. Test 2 is more expensive but is better at detecting early cancers. The decision is complicated by budget limitations: the government only has a certain amount of money available to pay for the screening tests. After evaluating the costs and benefits of each test, the doctors have reached the following conclusions. The budget is just large enough to offer test 1 to all the low-risk people. With this approach, everyone can receive the test, and 1000 deaths from colon cancer will be prevented. The budget is just large enough to offer test 2 to half the low-risk people. With this approach, half the people can receive the test and half cannot, and 1100 deaths from colon cancer will be prevented.

The ethicists and decision makers who thought about this problem were told that the persons selected for screening, if the second scenario were to be followed (test 2 is offered to half the low-risk people), would be randomly selected on the basis of their social security numbers. The ethicists who responded to the survey were uneasy about the assumption underpinning cost-effectiveness analysis: that 'it is best to maximize the total benefit per dollar spent, even if this is achieved by offering a health care intervention to only a portion of a population that might benefit from it'. They rejected the more effective test, in favour of making a test equally available to all potential recipients. In doing so they implicitly challenged the utilitarian basis of cost-effectiveness analysis (that is, achieving the greatest good for the greatest number).

One critic of this hypothetical has pointed out that it does not consider the possibility of moving money across from other budgets to be able to deliver a better test to all the low-income Medicaid recipients.[42] This alternative is really the process that was outlined for you earlier in this section, of rearranging budgets and budget priorities on a large scale.

The controversy associated with tools such as cost–benefit analysis and cost-effectiveness analysis is the way it requires decision makers to make value judgments about who, or what groups of people, should receive treatments. Its controversial nature also stems from the fact that the decision of worth is made before the actual consumer or patient enters the treatment context. The decision is made at a different time (for example, when setting up the service) or is made hypothetically (for example, for the type of situation that any given patient might one day be in).

An early experiment in limiting the costs of public programs was conducted in the state of Oregon in the USA. Before decisions were made about how many of certain types of services should be offered to public patients, the community was asked to rate how successful these services were in adding quality life-years. The Oregon experiment in consultative rationing has been discussed at length in the literature. The controversial aspects—such as making health outcome or quality life-years the focus, considering the worth of the expected lifespan, and making assumptions about the worth of health care programs—have also been debated. Kitzhaber and Kemmy, who were key figures in the Oregon experiment, describe their personal experience of the budget dilemma they were faced with:

> In the interim spring of 1986, a variety of factors combined to produce a budget shortfall of $35 million, and the E-Board took steps to bring the budget back into balance—among them, a decision to drop over 4300 Oregonians from state medical coverage.
>
> ... Not many months later, however, some of those human consequences began showing up in my emergency room—people who had delayed seeking timely treatment because they now had no way to pay for it.[43]

There is now a readiness to learn from the Oregon decisions. Despite the controversy surrounding it, it was one of the first social programs to acknowledge the limitations that health budgets pose to the goal of achieving health for all.

The above discussion focuses on the decisions involved in making a service available. The development of the service is also crucial. This aspect of resource development is discussed further in Chapter 8.

Whether people are 'entitled' to have the goods that their society offers is often hotly debated. This is, in essence, a debate over whether people are entitled to consume the goods or services that are available. It is squarely a matter of justice. The use of publicly provided health care resources can also involve personal decisions, which are open to ethics scrutiny and reflection.

Try the following exercise, as a revision of the consideration of personal need and entitlement in the context of the specific community that a person belongs to.

EXERCISE 3.5 PUBLIC PURSE AND DWINDLING PERSONAL ASSETS

Imagine that your uncle is quite ill and may need long-term nursing care. He lives in a small town in the USA. Most of his money is tied up in his house, which he shares with his wife. His children have grown up and left home. They worry about how the nursing care is to be paid for. One of your cousins secretly worries also that there will be little left to care for their stepmother in her old age, much less any inheritance for the children or grandchildren. All of your uncle's joint cash savings have been used up already in his convalescence from a fall injury and a worsening heart condition. He is still quite weak and unable to care for himself. His wife is also elderly and has health problems, so is unable to care for him at home by herself. He wants to return home, and worries about the nursing home fees, which will slowly and surely whittle away the nest-egg of stocks he had hoped to pass on to his children. He worries that even the house may have to be sold if he is in nursing homes for much longer, as the bills keep coming in. The difficulty is that the US national insurance Medicare can cover hospital costs for seniors, but not long-term care costs, and the state government cover for the poor and permanently disabled can only apply once assets and income are both reduced.

What would you suggest be done ethically?

We have grown used to looking back on earlier health care as characterised by paternalistic beneficence. We may look back on the 1980s as the decade of autonomy. In the 1990s, our enthusiasm for patient and client autonomy was tempered, and the financial realities of modern times have brought the limited availability of resources for public funding into sharper focus. The new kind of beneficence imposed by the system, and then practised by health care professionals, is increasingly limiting the available client choices as the health care professions and the surrounding regulatory system impose limits on client wishes according to which wishes they are comfortable with and are able to grant. In the modern health care context of stretched resources and fluctuating financial situations, justice concerns were predicted to dominate health care ethics in this century.[44] In the context of global financial uncertainty, that trend of budgeted and managed care is set to continue. The restrictions are posed either by the public purse holder or the private fund manager, with a similar effect of limitation on complete patient autonomy. Care is delivered and received in a context that recognises health resources as a valuable asset to be conserved and used wisely.

SUMMARY OF KEY ISSUES

- Institutional goals and values
- Defining a good to aim for
- Development of goods
- Sharing limited resources
- Interests and rights
- Justice models: justice as fairness, comparative justice, distributive justice
- Balancing risks and benefits for clients and others.

SHORT NOTES

1   As a start, search your government health department website, and follow the links to specific hospitals.
2   Mill, 'On liberty'.
3   United Nations, 'Convention on the Rights of the Child'.
4   Peabody et al., 'The Australian health care system'.
5   Gillon, *Philosophical medical ethics*, pp. 54–8.
6   Devereux, *Medical law*, pp. 450–2.
7   Callahan, 'Achievable goals'.
8   World Health Organization, 'Preamble to the constitution of World Health Organization', p. 1; and Lee, Speech to the Fifty-sixth World Health Assembly.
9   GDP figures presented here are from a number of different sources: OECD, *OECD health data 2009*; Levit et al., 'Trends in U.S. health care spending, 2001'.
10 Smith et al., 'Income, insurance, and technology'.

11   Evans and Pritchard, 'Cancer survival rates'.

12   Beauchamp and Childress, *Principles of biomedical ethics*, 4th edn, p. 340.

13   New South Wales Department of Health, 'Waiting time and Elective Patient Management Policy', (PD2009_018/9), <www.health.nsw.gov.au/policies>.

14   Dickens, 'Legal approaches to health care ethics and the four principles', p. 315.

15   For current schemes, see the Department of Health and Ageing website, <www.health.gov.au>.

16   Motor Accidents Authority, *New South Wales Health bulk billing handbook*.

17   Commonwealth Department of Health and Family Services, *Supplement to Medicare Benefits Schedule Book*, pp. 7 and 3.

18   Mitchell and Lovat, *Bioethics for medical and health professionals*, p. 136.

19   Parliament of New South Wales, 'Budget Paper No. 3', pp. 6-14–6-22.

20   Mannion, 'General practitioner-led commissioning in the NHS'.

21   'Health inequality: The UK's biggest issue', editorial, *Lancet*.

22   Lewis and Appleby, 'Can the English NHS meet the 18-week waiting list target?'

23   Todd et al., '"I'm still waiting…"'.

24   Commission for Health Improvement, 'National patients survey programme: 2003 results'.

25   Davies and Macfarlane, 'Clinical decision making by dentists working in the NHS General Dental Services'.

26   Morris, 'County dental care is in crisis'; Morris, 'Queuing for NHS dentists'.

27   *New Zealand Medical Association Newsletter*, 108, 1994, p. 3.

28   Powell, 'Providing quality healthcare under funding constraints'.

29   McPherson et al., 'Ethnicity, equity, and quality'.

30   Urbina et al., 'The managed health care scenario'.

31   Benko and Bellandi, 'The rough and tumble of it'.

32   Pearson et al., 'Caring for patients within a budget'.

33   Gomez et al., 'Preparing residents for managed care practice'.

34   Aiken et al., 'Hospital nurse staffing and patient mortality'.

35   Asch and Ubel, 'Rationing by any other name', p. 1670.

36   Lyall, '30-baht health care a fatal prescription'.

37   Acute and Co-ordinated Care Branch, Commonwealth Department of Health and Ageing, 'Primary care initiatives'.

38   For these and other initiatives, see the Department of Health and Ageing website, <www.health.gov.au>.

39   Magney and Berglund, 'Co-ordinated care: Ethics debate as part of the trial process'.

40   Dorr-Goold and Klipp, 'Managed care members talk about trust'.

41   Ubel et al., 'Cost-effectiveness analysis in a setting of budget constraints', p. 1176.

42   McCombs, letter, *New England Journal of Medicine*.

43   Kitzhaber and Kemmy, 'On the Oregon trail'.

44   Berglund, 'Bioethics'.

ENTER THE PATIENT

- Meeting the patient/client
- The beginnings of treatment responsibility
- A dynamic relationship
- Negotiating treatment
- Seeking consent

OBJECTIVES

This chapter focuses on the ethics involved in the immediate client–carer relationship from the time the client enters the treatment context and becomes the carer's patient. In this chapter the reader will grapple with the dynamic nature of the client–carer relationship. The individual client's input into their treatment is explored, and different approaches to negotiating treatment are discussed. Models ranging from paternalism to liberalism are examined, as are philosophical choices involved in information disclosure. Informed decision making by the patient, and informed consent, are key focuses.

The conceptual terms that are added to your glossary include respect, dignity, wishes, privacy, risk, benefit, personal morality, social morality, doctrine, duty of care, consent, informed consent, and informed decision making. The ethics theories of casuistry and communitarianism are encountered, and an example of a doctrine, the doctrine of double effect, is explained.

MEETING THE PATIENT/CLIENT

When you meet a client for the first time, you meet a new person. A first rule of thumb is to try to respect people for who they are, not who you would like them to be.

We should try to respect everyone we meet, no matter who they are. If you were to make a list of how you could respect a person (and you could do this either alone or in a group), your list would probably include ideas on how you can respect or uphold that person's dignity, wishes, and integrity.

EXERCISE 4.1 PEOPLE YOU MEET

Take a moment to think about the last client, or person, whom you met. What did you notice about them? What did they tell you about themselves? What makes this person different from other people? What makes them them?

Make a note of what you noticed about the last client you met.

Respect
Hold in high regard and esteem, and to refrain from interference with a respected person.

Wishes
Desired states, thoughts, or actions that would bring happiness if attained or realised.

Dignity
Quality of worthiness.

The principle of '**respect** for persons', otherwise known as the principle of autonomy, is about respecting the **wishes** and **dignity** of each person. When asked to respond to the question 'How do you respect people?', many people would write down matters such as 'acknowledge them as people', 'listen to them', 'treat them with dignity', 'ask for and listen to their opinion', and 'give them privacy'. In practice, the principle of 'respect for persons' often revolves around individuals' freedom to plan and choose what will happen to them—that is, their right to be autonomous. Autonomy, derived from the Greek *autos* and *nomos*, means self-rule. In the context of health care this refers, of course, to the client having a degree of power over treatment decisions. A frequent misunderstanding among students is that it is about professionals deciding what should be done in any given treatment situation. While there is such a thing as professional autonomy, generally, when the terms 'autonomy' or 'respect for persons' are used, they refer to client autonomy.

To be able to uphold people's autonomy, to uphold respect for persons, you need to know a little about them. But first you need to put them at ease. Clients entering your health care service are likely to feel sick or anxious or scared, or all three. As a good professional you should strive to put people at ease. Once you have done this, you can begin to hear the client's story and understand them as a person. You need to know what has happened, what their symptoms feel like, what the client values, and what they would prefer. First things first: What is the problem? What brings them to a health care context?

The initial decision to tell others about private information, to allow someone to touch us to see what is wrong, and to tell others something that is personal is at the heart of health care. We all have different thresholds of privacy, as the following exercise demonstrates.

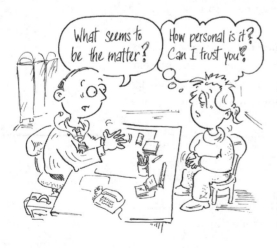

EXERCISE 4.2 PREFERENCES FOR PRIVACY

In a group, turn to the person next to you and tell them a secret about yourself. Tell them something that you don't necessarily want everyone to know. Before you tell them, alert them to the sensitivity of the information by asking them not to tell anyone else. If you think of something but decide you really don't want to tell anyone, let them know you'd rather not say anything. Then count how many people had a secret that they decided to tell, and that they therefore entrusted to their neighbour.

In your health care relationships, your patients make decisions all the time about what secrets to tell, what to let you see, and how much to trust you, the health care worker, to use that information constructively and to respect it as private and confidential.

The relationship between a counsellor and client could be a useful way for you to think about meeting and getting to know your own clients or patients. A good counsellor–client relationship involves establishing trust and ground rules, before tackling the difficult issues that have prompted the client to seek counselling. The initial stages of a counselling relationship have been identified as follows: meeting the client, during which time both the counsellor and client are on their 'best behaviour'; discussion of surface issues, in which the client feels able to discuss everyday issues; and then revelation of deeper issues, which occurs in the context of a developed relationship in which the client feels confident and trusts the counsellor. The counsellor's skill is in setting the client at ease through the initial stage, and gradually encouraging self-revelation.[1] It is a subtle art, and one that counsellors must master, as it is required for an ethical relationship with clients to develop. So much depends on understanding both your client and the problem at hand. You may, like counsellors, have the luxury of more than one meeting to achieve this. If you don't, your bedside manner is all the more important.

A similar appreciation of **privacy** is expected in relation to exposure of the physical body. A practitioner becomes used to draping patients so as to expose only as much of their bodies as necessary, and to letting patients dress and undress in as much privacy as possible.

As clients disclose information and give you access to their personal thoughts and feelings, you begin to get to know them, and try to understand what has happened to them and how serious it is. You tend to make running notes in your head about what you could do to help. You start a medical record, or add to one that has already been started. The initial records that you make about someone are a crucial piece in any treatment relationship. They should be accurate and complete; they can be initiated or added to by any health care worker; and they become the basis of noting and assessing progress as the client is engaged in treatment.

Privacy
State of secrecy or concealment.

Health departments generally recognise the importance of health records, and issue guidelines like the following.

A health record is a documented account of a patient's health, illness and treatment during each visit or stay at a hospital, nursing home, community health centre or other health care facility. For example:

> A health record shall be started and maintained for every person receiving health care services in a hospital, nursing home, community health centre or other health care facility.
>
> Health records must be kept confidential, current, accurate, complete and readily available for patient care. Every attendance or service provided must be recorded in the health care record.[2]

Making medical records is not just the responsibility of medical practitioners. Records are produced by different client care providers in different clinical settings. Yet the basic requirements apply to all: entries must be legible and non-erasable, identified as relating to a particular person, organised chronologically, and made available to authorised persons. The accuracy and completeness of the records you make is relied upon by others, and is an essential supplement, but not replacement, for a full verbal handover between staff.[3]

Taking notes and making records is one of the key skills of health professionals. It is vital in terms of effective teamwork. Other health carers dealing with that client need to know what has happened and be able to refer to detailed information about the client without asking for the information all over again. (The delicate personal balance between disclosure and trust is explored further in the next chapter.) Concerns about privacy, and understanding when it is ethically acceptable to breach privacy, tend to focus on the notes taken by health care professionals. It is the information in these notes that will be made available to others.

There is a model of ethical decision making that centres on understanding the nature and extent of a medical condition. The model was proposed by Jonsen, Siegler, and Winslade and has the following main elements: medical indications, preferences of clients, quality of life, and contextual features.[4]

You have treatment options available to you as a health care worker. Some of those options are predetermined for you, as discussed in Chapter 3. Some options are decided by the type or level of training and skill that you have achieved, as discussed in Chapter 2. Some are decided by you, using your considered professional judgment, in consultation with the client. The difference that social context makes to this consultation process, and the accompanying partnership between health care workers and clients, receives considerable attention from ethicists.[5] It is a delicate and complex partnership that requires an atmosphere of mutual respect and attention if it is to develop in a healthy way.

You read earlier that getting to know clients, at the same time as you begin to understand what has happened to them, is crucial. Unless you know a little about them, it may be difficult to respect and promote their autonomy. You might need to know whether when faced with difficult decisions, for instance, they would simply prefer to be left alone to think things through, or whether they would like to talk things over straight away. You might need to ask directly to find such things out, and you might need to undertake gentle questioning, or negotiating, to come to an understanding of what treatment or management plan the person would like or prefer (given a reasonable choice), and how they would like to receive it. Some standards of disclosure of treatment information rely on this mix of questioning and negotiating, as is discussed later in the section 'Negotiating treatment'.

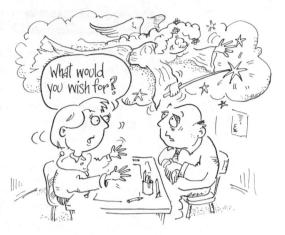

EXERCISE 4.3 MAKE A WISH

We all have different thresholds in relation to being able to think about what we want, being able to express it, and being able to ask for something. We also have different thresholds as to how inclined we are to further other people's wishes. This is at the heart of who we are, and consequently it is crucial to how what we want might be achieved. This brief exercise illustrates how very different we are from each other.

In a group setting, ask the following question of the person sitting next to you: If you could wish for anything, what would you wish for? (Make it clear that you want them to tell you only one wish!) Make sure both of you get to tell each other your wish.

Whenever I have supervised this exercise, I have noticed that a hush falls over the group, as people sigh, try to think of a wish, and then try to work out how to tell it. Some people have trouble thinking of a wish. Should you, if you believe in autonomy, help them to think about what they want? Or is it their right not to think of anything? If they have thought of something, but feel shy, should you help them to tell you? Or should you leave them be? (More discussion on privacy is included in Chapter 5.)

To return to the group exercise above, once the wish is expressed, group members should think about whether it is in their power to grant the wish they heard fully, or whether they could help the person part-way towards their wish. In other words, do they agree it is a good wish, and do they feel able or obliged to help? Ultimately, do they feel obliged to help the person in their pursuit of that wish? Their answers will indicate something about how much they value autonomy in its own right. To further autonomy as an absolute right is to further the client's wishes regardless of whether it would be the professional's preferred wish.

You routinely make promises in everyday life. For instance, you promise to do the washing up. You promise to meet your friends at a certain time and place. Do you keep your promises? Think of an occasion when you did not keep a promise that you had made to a friend or family member. How did the other person react and feel as a consequence? How did you feel?

Promises that are made without your intention to keep them place other's trust in you at risk. How much is in your power to promise is also crucial. Do you give others the impression that you can do more than you can, and so not keep promises? When someone asks you for a favour, to help them achieve a wish of theirs, should you promise to help regardless of whether you agree with their wish? Or is it less hurtful in the long run to state your disagreement, and unwillingness to actively help? If you do agree, but doubt how much you can do, a useful technique is to say 'I will try my best' rather than promise absolutely, making it clear that while you would hope to fulfil their wish, you may not be able to. You will have plenty of practice at this as a health care professional. Wishes are not acted on without professional consideration of objectives and logistics.

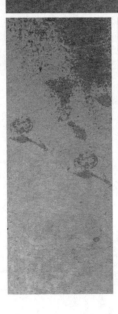

FROM THEORY TO PRACTICE

Trust and promises

Contributor: *Leanne Boase*

Does trust solely rely on what promises we make? Will a client be more likely to engage openly in the client–carer relationship if promises are made?

List the reasons why promises in the health care setting can have both positive and negative effects on the relationship.

Are there 'good' promises and 'bad' promises? What are some examples of each?

You could focus on making promises realistic and achievable, as opposed to making promises in order to meet the emotional needs of the patient. Is the intention of your promise relevant if you fail to keep it, and what effects could this have on the relationship?

What could influence the patient to seek a promise from a carer? Think of yourself as the 'expert', and how that may convey power, and affect the client.

Benefit
Positive effect or outcome.

Some clients are risk takers, others are not. There is a difference between how much risk people are prepared to take for a perceived likely **benefit**. For instance, cautious people might not want to go parachuting on their days off, but risk takers might, because for them the thrill of the activity and the sensation of being airborne is worth the possibility of physical injury. How people approach their everyday health, health risks, and treatment, when they become clients, varies in just the same way. The likely positive and negative effects or outcomes of different treatment or management plans is weighed up by individuals. This is a weighing of risks and benefits.

John Stuart Mill, the famous early libertarian, thought that individual liberty should be allowed, within certain limits. This applied to the different liberties of consciousness, thought and feeling, expressing and publishing opinions, tastes and pursuits, and the liberty to unite with others for any purpose. The limits to liberty allowed by Mill were, broadly, serious and imminent harm to others, threatening other's similar liberties, and threats to the fabric of society. These limits take into account the respect that we should afford others (as well as expect ourselves) and the need for all to live in a society that has established structures and boundaries. Interestingly, Mill did not think that liberty should be limited on the sole grounds that the person's choice would harm themselves. He thought that competent adults should be free to **risk** their own health and well-being without interference.[6]

We are used to limiting autonomy in an institutional context. If you think of our society, we have rules that tacitly limit autonomy on a number of grounds. For instance, a person who likes to drive will be allowed to do so, but only on the road. If the person likes to drive fast, we might say that that type of driving should be done on freeways and not in suburban streets. Why? One explanation is that we have judged it too dangerous to others if these limits to driving are not imposed. So that person's wish or preference for fast driving should not be to the detriment of others. Another example is the person who likes to drive but also likes to drink. We say yes to each of that person's wishes, but stipulate that these things should not be done together, as we judge drink-driving to be too dangerous to both the driver and others. Institutional bounds to autonomy and liberty are explored further in Chapter 10. Try answering the following questions. They will prompt you to reflect on the way you value autonomy, and how autonomy is limited or promoted.

Risk
Chance of negative effect or outcome.

PAUSE & REFLECT

Think of a situation in which it has been difficult for you to accept the autonomy of an individual patient or client. What did you do? Were you satisfied that you acted properly?

Now think of a situation in which the client's autonomy was limited, not by you but by the institution or resources. Were you satisfied that the principle of 'respect for persons' was upheld?

Now think of a situation in which you have promoted someone's autonomy. How did you do that? Were you satisfied that you acted properly?

Personal morality
Significant lessons prompting reflection to identify a virtuous, right, or acceptable course of conduct of an individual, largely affecting that individual.

Social morality
Significant lessons prompting reflection to identify a virtuous, right, or acceptable course of conduct of individuals, with significant implications for the choices then available to others in society.

The choices of an individual are made within a social context. Such decisions are therefore subject to social limits. Such limits are termed 'social morality limits'. Mill's essay 'On Liberty' suggests a difference between **personal morality** and **social morality**. That is, if something affects no other person, it should be in the realm of their own choice. However, if it affects others, by threatening the fabric of society or by threatening other people, then it is a social issue, and the liberty can be legitimately constrained by social decision.[7] As a further exercise, you could make a list of what you think constitutes personal morality decisions and what constitutes social morality decisions, in a health and medical context. You may like to consider the limits placed on the choices that an individual can make in relation to a public-health issue such as smoking.

In our health care system, treatment choices made by clients are usually interpreted as questions of personal morality. In practice, we allow autonomy that is consistent with Mill's position. People can choose what type of treatment they would prefer, given a choice, and they can even choose not to be treated at all. Provided they are not harming other people too greatly, by for instance spreading an infectious disease, their choice about treatment is their own, and their reasons for making that decision must be respected.

One of the practical limitations of client choice is that such choices are often made within an institution. The institution may offer only a limited range of treatment options. In setting up institutions, we show our concern for the health of all people in society, and most limitations imposed by institutions are intended to protect the integrity and health of all people rather than any one individual. These limitations may be interpreted as social limitations protecting the social structure of the health care institution. For instance, under our health system, a public patient in hospital may not be able to choose their own doctor, while a private patient can. If individual public patients wanted to choose their own doctors, but could not pay for the doctors' services, we may feel justified in denying them that choice on the grounds that the system, as our society has set it up, can stretch to allowing them treatment options, but not their choice of doctor.

We may accept that it is more important to protect the social system than to promote autonomy. In Mill's terms, this means that we are prepared to limit personal choices in relation to the allocation of resources because the question is one of social morality. In a less strict sense, we have decided that people cannot have unlimited choice of health care and, consequently, unlimited spending on this health care because this would affect other people in society to an unacceptable degree. You will remember that distribution of resources was discussed in terms of justice in Chapter 3.

The key to this is that autonomy and client preferences, or wishes, are not absolute. They must be weighed against competing liberties and interests. Professionals have their own threshold for allowing individual autonomy before they begin drawing boundaries to this autonomy. Philosophical stances can guide us as to when to place those bounds. Libertarianism is at one extreme, and even it acknowledges some limits on liberty. Paternalism is at the other extreme. And there are choices in between. These choices are set out in the 'Negotiating treatment' section later in this chapter.

So far we have established that what the person is like, what has happened to them, and what they would wish for or prefer is ethically important. Their autonomy is important but it is not absolute, and there may be circumstances in which you are not obliged to promote it, and even some circumstances when it should be curtailed. In any situation in which you are deciding to promote, allow, or limit autonomy, you need to consider the accepted standards relating to the extent of client choice. Sometimes there are clear standards to refer to, sometimes not. Legal and administrative limits can help, but as professional ethics is about reflection, these standards must always be assessed from an ethics stance as well. If you disagree with the standards on ethical grounds, you should challenge them.

Non-judgmental harm minimisation approaches are quite well accepted in health care when a patient poses a risk to themselves, such as in illicit drug use. Gaining trust and understanding what substances are being taken is important, then different strategies can be used towards the goal of reducing use, while also monitoring health. One physician's advice is that in treating sports people who use performance-enhancing drugs, the first step is encouraging disclosure of dangerous practices and understanding why people choose to engage in them. If the sports people are elite and using drugs as a tool towards performance goals, they may only be engaged in reducing their usage over time. Recent gym users can be amenable to information about effective diet and training that can achieve the results hoped for more safely. For recreational users, other illicit drug use can be common, so different strategies may be needed. One physician acknowledges the illicit or dangerous drug use and works towards keeping each patient as safe as possible.[8] Can you work out which philosophical stance this harm minimisation practice is compatible with?

Different clients want different types of care. So do different sub-groups in our society. You need to ask yourself continually whether you are equipped to provide the care they desire. The Western model of care, which attempts to maximise choice, views each adult as an individual agent, and which has the prolonging of life as one of its aims, may not be culturally appropriate for some health care recipients. For instance, Qiu argues that Chinese culture reinforces group responsibility over individual choice: self-interest should not be pursued to the exclusion of the interest of one's family or community, and one's duties assume greater importance than one's rights. He notes that this communitarian approach does not occur so much in the West, where generally an individualist approach prevails.[9] Under **communitarianism**, a very limited definition of personal morality issues would apply, with issues of social moral import emphasised.

These days, health professionals are trained to work in different contexts and to serve different cultures. You have the benefit of a more comprehensive knowledge of other cultures by your ability to travel, live, and work in different countries, and by the fact that you live near a rich diversity of ethnic communities in your own home towns. So you are partly prepared for the fact that people are different from you.

Yet we should still be aware that our culture shapes our expectations and understanding of illness, health, and care. Clients' expectations and understandings

Communitarianism
An ethics theory in which the relationship of a person to a specific community is identified, and the interests and needs of that community as a whole take priority over individual interests and needs.

may be different from yours. Professionals' expectations should include getting to know the clients a little, understanding them for themselves, and beginning a health care relationship with them that is based on respect for their difference. Only then are you ready to take on some responsibility for caring for them.

THE BEGINNINGS OF TREATMENT RESPONSIBILITY

The decision to take on the responsibility of caring for someone underpins health care. The responsibility to take on their care can be expressed as an obligation of doing good, also termed beneficence, as you will remember from Chapter 2. 'Beneficence' is a tricky word, but its meaning is quite simple. It is pronounced a little like beneficial. Many students and professionals have trouble pronouncing it. Try saying beneficial a few times out loud, then change the 'ficial' bit to 'fecents', and put less emphasis on the middle of the word at 'f', and more on the 'n'. It is useful to remember that if something is beneficial for someone, it has often been brought about by an action that is beneficent.

You will also remember, from Chapter 3, that doing good can be defined in different ways by different professions, and that we may only be obliged to deliver that good if someone has a right to it under the model of justice that operates in our society or institution. Bear in mind, though, that ethics is an ideal and optimal standard of behaviour, so even if there are constraints it is plausible to aim to maximise what is regarded as good. The principle of beneficence implies an ideal level of care. It goes beyond what is accessible or affordable, or a just claim.

> **EXERCISE 4.4 IDEALS OF CARE**
>
> You could reflect on what sort of care you would like to provide, given an ideal environment for providing that care. Try completing the following statement.
>
> In an ideal world, the sort of care I would provide is . . .

Consider this case from the UK, in the context of reorganisation of aged care and home standards, public assistance for fees for residents, and allocation of subsidised care placements in designated homes. At the start of this reorganisation, an elderly woman was required to move from the aged care home she had been in for some years. Her doctor opposed her move, believing the 90-year-old's best interests were to remain in what she knew to be her home. Five days after the move, she died, and the GP reportedly entered the cause of death as 'acute stress reaction to the move', refusing to list natural causes of old age on the death certificate. He championed her care, and continued to champion her interests in opposing the authorities' decision, despite the public interest in imposing financial constraints on public monies for each individual's care provision. An inquiry ensued. The media coverage of the case extended over many months, and became a public petition for further government attention to the needs of old age pensioners and, specifically, individuals in aged care.[10] The commitment by the local doctor illustrates the nature of the strong responsibility the health professional feels to the individual patient. It is above the constraints of justice and resource allocation debates.

The heart of beneficence, of taking on a responsibility to care, is:

- the micro level of what is beneficial for the client
- the delivery of that benefit
- working towards that benefit in the context of the partnership between the health care worker and the client.

Health professionals routinely take on new patients or clients, or refer them on to others if they feel they either cannot provide the care sought to the standard required, or cannot provide as effective or timely care as another professional. The ethical issue is how hard you should try in providing care, and what care you should offer.

You also have a choice about whether or not to take on care—for example, whether or not to disclose your health care skills in everyday situations in which they may be called upon, and whether or not to disclose the extent of your capabilities in the course of caring for a client. On a group holiday, would you disclose that you are clinically trained? Would you be prepared to adopt your professional role if it could be helpful in the course of the trip (for example, for a broken arm or a serious allergic reaction)? Think about what you would be prepared and able to do in such situations. Of course, answering this depends on what resources you have around you, how serious the situation is, and who else is available to care. (Taking on treatment responsibility in emergency situations is also dealt with in Chapter 8.)

Once you settle on the scope of what you define as beneficent, you may be obliged to assist in that way. On a broad level, once you train as a health care professional, you may be obliged to use your training where your skills are needed. Clearly, the definition of beneficence has some force because it creates a responsibility. That responsibility can be interpreted as an obligation to assist and rescue whenever anyone is in need. The Australian philosopher Peter Singer believes that beneficence means that you must always act to prevent what is bad, unless something of comparable moral importance must be given up by performing the action—such as leaving yourself worse off than your potential clients. In Singer's framework, other people's interests are equal to our own.[11] This is not quite a positive duty (an obligation to actively seek out ways of doing good), but it is a duty to intervene to prevent harm occurring. For example, if harm is about to be experienced by someone because of lack of food, shelter, or medical care, then preventing the consequent harm may require positive action, such as giving them some of your food, which could be said to imply some degree of self-sacrifice. Another example of this prioritisation of duty to others is the way in which religious orders and volunteers working in some countries place themselves in living conditions similar to their clients, and suffer great physical ordeals so that they can improve the lives of others. It often takes particular skill and special commitment to work in dangerous or exacting conditions. For instance, the rescue training for the ambulance paramedic service has been described as particularly 'physically and mentally demanding, very intense and demanding'.[12]

It is up to you to decide whether you think the level of service promoted by Singer is an obligation or a sacrifice. If you see it as a sacrifice, then you would view those who make this sacrifice as good Samaritans. More importantly, not to do it would not reflect badly on you at all.

Duty of care
An obligation to take reasonable care in dealings with a person, once there is an undertaking to provide care or advice, or contribute to such specific benefit for a specific person.

The limits of a **duty of care** are more palatable to the professional if Singer's position is seen as a sacrifice, and this seems to be the professional consensus. For instance, few health care workers would envisage their responsibilities to extend to 24-hour vigilance, or treatment for all people in all parts of the country or world. Being a counsellor doesn't necessarily mean that you are obliged to work in crisis situations that you find too stressful. You can fulfil your obligations to beneficence by finding your own niche, and satisfying yourself that the work in crisis situations is being done by someone else.

Yet this commitment is sometimes tested in your routine job, in unusual times of crisis.

EXERCISE 4.5 DUTY AND LIMITS OF CARE

As a group, work on the following scenario. The facts have been changed slightly from a real example from early 2003, when the SARS (severe acute respiratory syndrome) epidemic was reaching its peak. At the time, it was unclear whether the epidemic of the flu-like illness was peaking, but what was clear was that it was racing through many populations in Hong Kong and other areas of China; people had died in Singapore and Canada and there were isolated cases in the USA and Europe. The sudden acute illness was affecting front-line health workers significantly, and schools were being closed and sections of the community quarantined. Daily updates on numbers of people who had contracted suspected symptoms, as well as numbers of people who had died from suspected or confirmed SARS, were issued by the World Health Organization and local health authorities.

A local practice receptionist and health nurse, living and working in Hong Kong, with two young children, became worried that her work was becoming increasingly busy and demanding. She had seen her hours increase dramatically, as people flocked to the local doctor to have any symptoms checked and ask about the symptoms of SARS. One of the practice doctors, an expatriate Australian, decided to take his family home, thus leaving fewer doctors and an increased workload for the practice. Those remaining were under stress, and were increasingly worried about their families if they should contract an illness from one of the patients coming to be checked. As the receptionist, she was the first to see any patients. She felt she had to make a decision whether or not to keep working, for her family's sake. What should she do? How could you advise her to go about making her decision? If she is a receptionist, does she have the same higher duties as a health professional? How far do those duties extend if she is practising as a nurse? And what do you say about the doctor who returned home?

Clearly, the extent of duties needs to be assessed by each person, given their own context, family responsibilities, and professional roles that they have undertaken.

It is not sufficient just to define beneficence and try to do good. Being a health care worker also carries with it an obligation not to cause harm. This is termed an obligation of non-maleficence. To be maleficent is to intend to harm, like the word 'malevolent'. Health care workers must try not to cause harm. There is philosophical debate about whether actively causing harm, or allowing harm to occur by not intervening, is equally morally reprehensible.

EXERCISE 4.6 RESPONSIBILITY FOR HARMS

Thinking about a scene from a murder mystery novel by P. D. James may help you to decide if you think there is a moral distinction between acting and not acting, when harm seems to be the outcome of not acting.

In the scene, two children of about 11 and 9 years old, Alex and Alice, are playing in the garden while their father clears out a part of the shrubbery. He is using a sharp-bladed hook, called a billhook, to cut and pull the overgrowth away. Suddenly the children hear him yell in pain and call for help. They both look from a distance and see him bleeding heavily, with a large gash on his thigh. The older child, a boy, drags his sister after him, but instead of pulling her towards their father, he pulls her out of sight and away into the orchard. She asks him to let her go so they can get help, but he holds her still against a tree. They wait there for a few minutes, until the brother releases her, and says that they can go now. When they reach their father he has died. The boy simply says that she has nothing to fear from now on.[13]

Try to list why you think each person, in this case each child, is morally responsible for the harm or not, and why.

There are times when you, as a health care worker, have a choice about whether or not to act. You could, as an exercise, do a role-play of a health care situation in which there is a choice of acting or not acting, and demonstrate why you think each person in your role-play is or is not morally responsible.

'Smith and Jones' is a shorthand way of referring to a well-known scenario illustrating a particular type of philosophical conundrum: the moral import of acting or not acting; of killing or letting die. In one version of this scenario, a cousin

(Smith) actively drowns his younger cousin (Jones); in the other, Jones watches and does nothing while Smith drowns. Inheritance is a key part of the scenario: in both versions, one person stands to gain from the other's misfortune. Rachels argues that the bare difference between killing and not killing is not, in itself, morally relevant.[14]

Doctrine
Tenet or lesson held out or taught as a true guiding rule.

There are a number of philosophical **doctrines** to help us decide if harm is morally our responsibility, and to what extent that harm is our particular responsibility. One is the doctrine of 'double effect', which involves a distinction between what one foresees and what one intends. Harm may be morally forgivable if it is foreseen, but not if it is also intended.[15] For example, a psychologist who encourages a client to face their phobias, intending to, in the long term, lessen their fears, may in fact cause the client to experience short-term anxiety. The psychologist can be forgiven if they have not intended to cause that anxiety, even if it was foreseen as part of the healing process. However, if the psychologist intended to cause anxiety for its own sake, they may be regarded as unethical because there was intention to cause harm.

Doctrine of double effect
Ethics doctrine in which the intention of likely positive effects is considered to excuse morally certain foreseen negative effects.

The **doctrine of double effect** may also be used in more extreme cases—for example, a pregnant woman with a cancerous uterus may be told that, in the absence of intervention, there is a high likelihood that both she and her unborn child will die. The woman may decide to have a hysterectomy, and it would be an unintended, though foreseen, consequence that the unborn child would be aborted. Under the doctrine of double effect, it would be unethical if the bad effect (the abortion) were the means to the good effect (the curing of the cancer). It could not, however, be said of this situation that the abortion would be the means of curing the cancer. Rather, it would be the hysterectomy (in conjunction with further therapy) that promises to achieve that good effect. The doctrine of double effect attempts to achieve a balance between, on the one hand, the good pursued, and on the other, the harm that may accompany an attempt to do good. The action taken (in this case, the hysterectomy) must be good in itself, just as treating the woman for her cancer is good.

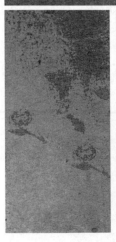

FROM THEORY TO PRACTICE

The doctrine of double effect

Contributor: *Leanne Boase*

A well-known double effect in the health care environment is that of giving pain relief medication or analgesics to dying patients. A commonly used analgesic is morphine. Often dying patients suffer severe pain, but there is concern around causing earlier death through the administration of the high doses of morphine sometimes required to relieve the client's pain effectively. Morphine has the effect of relieving pain, but it can also cause sedation, and can depress or slow the breathing rate—the double effect. Very high doses can cause respiratory arrest and death.

Doctors or nurse practitioners write legal orders for morphine. A doctor, nurse practitioner, or registered nurse may administer the drug to the client. This can occur in the hospital or institutional setting, or in the client's home. Sometimes family members, as carers, may also be responsible for administering analgesics within the legal orders.

The aim of administering morphine to dying patients in pain is to relieve their pain and suffering. While this may always be controversial, it is the *intent* that is important, and whether the action was *reasonable* in the circumstances. A higher dose of morphine given to a client who has required a gradually increasing dose over time to relieve their pain effectively is reasonable. The intent is to relieve their pain in the safest way, and the action or decision must be informed by all of the circumstances and facts. Administering a high dose to a client under different circumstances may not be reasonable, for example, a patient with mild pain, or pain that may have been relieved by a lower dose.

Some modern philosophers, such as Philippa Foot, think that the crucial point is whether something is deliberately allowed, and this concept of deliberately allowing something encompasses both intended and foreseen consequences.[16] They would encourage us to acknowledge that harm from actions is often unavoidable, and they advocate weighing up the rights of the parties before deciding whether one is entitled to bring about some benefit for one person when that person or another may be harmed.

Deciding what you can do as a health care worker depends on what can be achieved by what you can offer. The crucial test is whether it can bring about good; whether it really is beneficent. This decision as to whether or not it is good involves taking into account the other options available to the client. What you have to offer may not be appropriate. Jennett has provided a test (essentially rules of thumb) for deciding when a specific treatment is inappropriate. He proposes that if the treatment satisfies any of the following five criteria, then it should not be used:

1. It is unnecessary because the patient is not seriously enough affected to need it or the desired objective can be achieved by simpler means.
2. It would be unsuccessful because the patient has a condition too advanced to respond to or benefit from treatment.
3. It would be unsafe because the risks outweigh the probable benefits.
4. It would be unkind because the quality of life following the treatment is not likely to be good enough or long enough to justify such treatment.
5. It would be unwise because it would divert resources from activities that would benefit others to a greater extent.[17]

This test has been used not only in individual treatment decisions, but also in debates on resources because it takes into account the good that may be achieved for one person, as well as the good that may be achieved through the same or other means for others.

Health carers assume that there is a right to receive treatment and that a comparison of rights and interests should be part of the decision. Because rights carry with them obligations on us to act, comparing rights is, in essence, a weighing up of our duties. Some rights are positive and some are negative. Those that are positive oblige us to act in a certain way, and those that are negative oblige us to refrain from acting. The concept of rights and duties is also referred to in Chapter 3.

Beneficence is tied up with autonomy in that a client is free to choose a definition of good, determine what an acceptable risk of harm is, and make a choice between types of health professionals accordingly. For instance, someone who does not perceive mental health as part of their health would probably never go to a psychologist, and people who think that only active medical treatment can provide adequate physical care would not elect to go to a palliative care unit if they were diagnosed with a terminal illness (they would probably pursue active treatment as long as possible). So the client makes choices both within health care relationships and before even visiting a health professional. As the treatment responsibility is accepted and care begins, negotiation about the type of care begins, as does the real test of both the professional's responsibility to be beneficent and their commitment to autonomy.

A DYNAMIC RELATIONSHIP

There is a debate in ethics about which principle—autonomy or beneficence—should take priority. There is really a need to consider this only when these two principles come into conflict: when the professional definition of caring and the client definition of what care they would like to receive diverge. Most beneficence models either give way to autonomy when the client's idea of good is very different from the professional's, or include autonomy as an integral part of the principle of beneficence.

If you were a paternalist, you would believe that your idea of good, and therefore your interpretation of the principle of beneficence, applied to everyone. There would be no need to change your view on good or your interpretation of beneficence, no matter how different your client's views were from yours. That means beneficence could always override autonomy. In extreme paternalistic stances, there may be little need to ask clients for their **consent** before doing something that you believe is good for them, nor would there be a need to tell them all the options before asking them to agree to something that you think is good for them. Many people associate this with the old style of health care, particularly the old way of conducting medical practice.

Consent
Agreement.

The paternalism associated with medicine, as practised in the past, cannot be entirely attributed to professionals: patients also abrogated responsibility and autonomy. This attitude is captured in the phrase 'Doctor knows best'. The move away from this position has involved a developing sense of shared responsibility and the development of the model of a dynamic relationship between health care worker and patient. The modern rejection of paternalism amounts to a belief that the patient has a responsibility to double-check that the good being aimed at by the professional is compatible with their definition of a good.

The model of beneficence that builds in autonomy still has something of that paternalistic attitude because it lets the professional define what the good is that they will offer. Ultimately, it is up to the client to make decisions within the limits set by the professionals, but the basic good that the professional is willing to help their client towards does not change. Pellegrino and Thomasma argue for 'autonomy within beneficence' as a model that is distinct from paternalism.[18] This model acknowledges the complexity of the illness of the client, as well as the professional input in determining what could be beneficent.

Many modern philosophers, such as Beauchamp and Childress, maintain that beneficence and autonomy are separate principles that can outweigh each other, but in different circumstances.[19] When they do depends to some extent on the type of decision being made and the broader philosophical framework you choose to work under. A dramatic example might be a person who is terminally ill, and who wants to be removed from life support. Autonomy may be upheld if that is done, but if you think that beneficence includes the concept of sanctity of life (regardless of quality of life), you may not be satisfied that turning off the life support is beneficent. If you are a deontologist, you will be less likely to switch off the life support because, under deontology, fundamental rules such as observing sanctity of life must be obeyed irrespective of the circumstances. If you were a utilitarian, on the other hand, you might decide that the present and future happiness of the person, their family, and even other members of society is best served by switching it off. So you solve the dilemma by placing autonomy above the importance of preserving life, and justify this prioritisation of values by arguing that, overall, everyone would be better off if the life support were to be turned off.

An alternative balance between autonomy and beneficence is found in the 'enhanced autonomy' model, which encourages both health worker and client to exchange views, information, and their respective understandings of that information. This raises the question of the interpretation and value judgment of medical facts. If this is instituted solely by professionals, it is paternalistic; the enhanced autonomy model has the client participating actively in the interpretation and judgment of medical facts.[20]

In some ways, adopting a framework that gives autonomy primacy challenges the role of the health professions in defining good at all. If there was perfect liberty, a client could decide what outcome they wanted and what process they wanted to achieve it by, and could then seek out a health professional to deliver it.

EXERCISE 4.7 TREATMENT PROCESS AND DECISIONS

In clinical situations, ethics issues centre on a real patient. Choose a case in which a decision of some sort needs to be made, and in which there are different views on what should be decided. If you or your fellow students have access to a clinical setting, try this exercise with the decision faced by a real patient, being careful not to identify the patient. You could also use a hypothetical patient by constructing a case as a group. The discussion process has been suggested for a training program for nurses who train in a clinical setting.[21]

Gather as much information on the issue as you can from the perspective of the patient and the family. Analyse and interpret this to help in defining the dilemma. Then list possible alternatives for actions, checking these with colleagues, supervisors, and a doctor on the team. Identify the most likely solution to the dilemma, and the advantages and disadvantages of each option. Try to keep your own views separate from the analysis of what the parties think. In a clinical setting, the next step would be to consult each party to see if a consensual decision can be reached, or if there is one course of action with the most agreement.

Each treatment decision you make is tinged with this debate over defining care, doing good, and the extent to which the views of health care workers and clients should be taken into account in coming to decisions about treatment. The process of making treatment decisions is therefore dynamic. The same balance is not necessarily achieved in all decisions.

Our cultural context is crucial in striking an acceptable (Western) balance between promoting client choice and choosing the best care on offer; in principlist terms, this is a balance between beneficence and autonomy. However, we should at least be aware that in some cultures striking this balance is not considered so important: doctors and health professionals simply do the best they can for the client, and the client makes very few real decisions about their own care. In some cultures, informed consent is not seriously pursued. It is not that health care workers are intentionally trying to limit autonomy or cause harm to clients, but simply that they do not think full information and choice will be most beneficial for the client. At a time of great vulnerability for patients, health professionals want most of all to care for the client; they want to take the burden of decision making so that the client can feel secure and gather their own resources for recovery. In some cultures, when a patient is terminally ill, professionals routinely would not disclose the prognosis, or even diagnosis, to the patient. This has been noted to be a feature of health care in some Asian countries such as Japan.[22] Health care professionals may instead inform the family so that the family can ensure that they can make the patient comfortable.[23] Patients in these cultures may appear to be less self-determining and may be reluctant to decide any serious matters without consulting their family.[24]

That we, in Western health care, find a lack of information and lack of choice for the patient unsatisfactory is a product of our preference for liberty. However, we would do well to remember that it was not all that long ago that our own patients were not told of their diagnosis of cancer at all, and even now the process of preparing the client before disclosing the diagnosis can be fairly long-winded. It is not that professionals in other cultures are less committed to care, but rather that we Westerners place a higher emphasis on autonomy, and have a different way of expressing caring.[25]

Our own emphasis on autonomy challenges our commitment to beneficence and non-maleficence. You must continually decide whether, as health professionals, you can collude in the facilitation of harm if clients want something that you regard as harmful. We must decide whether allowing and promoting autonomy is a good in itself, along the lines of libertarianism, or whether the good we value is something more derived, like health.[26]

NEGOTIATING TREATMENT

Joint input is needed for treatment decisions to be made. The health care worker and the client exchange and discuss information. Each continually takes stock of the situation facing them. This is where good notes can be invaluable. These medical records serve as a record of what happened, what has been explored, and thoughts on what might be useful to pursue.

Information is so central to the assessment of conditions and options that it assumes key ethical significance as well. Information disclosure on both sides becomes a key dynamic in negotiating treatment. Health care workers often hold significant pieces of health information as a result of their knowledge of health sciences, their ability to interpret test results, and their conversations with other health professionals.

Information disclosure from a health professional to a client is probably best understood in the context of a consultation. A role situation such as described by Beauchamp and Childress entitled 'Non disclosure of prostate cancer' is useful as a starting point.[27] In this situation a retired man has just had tests done as part of a routine physical work-up. His doctor knows that these indicate 'inoperable, incurable carcinoma'. The man has recently lost his wife, and is planning a trip overseas. The man, as yet unaware of the test results, visits the doctor, who says nothing of the indications. After he has left the doctor's office the man returns to ask, 'I don't have cancer, do I?' The doctor answers, 'You are as good as you were ten years ago'.

This type of scenario is essentially weak paternalism in action. The doctor's response to the man's question is not the only possible response. It was the response chosen by the professional, for the moment, perhaps to put off telling the patient at a later date, perhaps because the professional wished to avoid imparting bad news. Telling bad news is part of health care, and it is dealt with in more detail in Chapter 5, in the section 'Veracity on both sides'. The essential part of the dilemma is that the doctor had access to information that could have affected a patient's decision about treatment or management plans and also life plans. Should the practitioner have told the man about his condition when the man asked, 'I don't have cancer, do I?'

EXERCISE 4.8 STANDARDS OF INFORMATION DISCLOSURE

Three information disclosure standards have emerged in recent debates about disclosure in the health professions:

- *The professional practice standard:* information given to patients by professionals that is that normally disclosed to other patients, and as disclosed to other patients by peers undertaking similar procedures.
- *The reasonable person standard:* information given to patients that a reasonable hypothetical person (in legal terms this person is referred to colloquially as 'the person on the Bondi tram', or in a British setting, 'the person on the Clapham omnibus') would want to know before consenting to the procedure.
- *The subjective person standard:* information given to patients that is normally disclosed by the health professional, or reasonably desired by the client, but tailored by the professional to suit the individual client's situation or specific concerns.

Returning to the Beauchamp and Childress scenario, in a tutorial situation divide into groups, with each group taking one of the three standards. Try to think of the response that the doctor would have given under each standard. Here are some ideas that other groups have come up with in the past. The 'professional practice' group often has the doctor talking to colleagues to hear their view on what to do. The central notion here is that peer practice in similar situations determines acceptable disclosure. The 'reasonable person' group often speaks in terms of what people usually want to know to make x, y, or z decision. A fairly common approach in disclosing information is then taken. The 'subjective person' group most often advocates entering into a conversation with the patient to find out whether he really wants to know (or if he is asking not to be told). If he does, the doctor then needs to find out how much he would want to know before disclosing further information. This group requires an atmosphere of negotiation between patient and doctor.

The information disclosure part of the consent process can be contentious, with the type and amount of information on material risks (material to the patient) at issue. This is an example of the testing of appropriate and feasible autonomy. Standard information is of course more efficient to deliver than tailored information. A balance between the two approaches is sought. How much information to provide on routine matters can also pose professional dilemmas. Consider the next exercise, and what you would do.

EXERCISE 4.9 ADMINISTRATIVE INFORMATION AND DECISIONS

At some times of the year, wards have fewer beds available. Staff holidays are planned for, and fewer elective procedures are done over that time. There can be administrative decisions, however, in units such as intensive care, that close beds for periods of time. This means that those beds are not available for critically ill people. Most critical care incidents are difficult to plan with any certainty, so the bed closures cause considerable concern. The availability of back-up beds in intensive care units is relied on by clinicians when they undertake even routine operative procedures. This information on bed closures has an ethical dimension, and forms part of the background of material risks—the information that may need to be made available to patients considering elective procedures.

Consider an administrative decision to close one-third of the 12 intensive care beds available in a tertiary care hospital over an upcoming holiday break. As a small group, discuss the ethical elements of that decision. Then decide what information should be given to health care personnel working in the hospital, what information should be passed on to acutely ill patients, and what information should be given to patients planning elective procedures.

In an ethics study on this topic, perceptions of clinicians and managers on the consequences of bed closure decisions were analysed. Concerns were raised over fairness, accountability of the decision, and poor prior publicity of the decisions to key staff.[28]

How much information clients should have before they make decisions depends on the philosophical framework that clients, carers, and our society is prepared to support. For instance, under a libertarian framework, in which each person decides what is best for them and pursues their own best interests and happiness, the maximum information, and therefore the maximum corresponding choice, would be available to them. Max Charlesworth writes that under a liberal society, restrictions on autonomy would be limited. Governments could still discourage excessive individualism, and could promote 'altruistic concern for others' and 'a recognition of community values', but the basic autonomous agent must have the opportunity to make real choices.[29] Under a paternalistic framework, on the other hand, lesser information and choice could be supported if such restriction was for the client's good. Strong paternalism, in which a client's expressed wish is overridden, is less common than weak paternalism, as Pellegrino and Thomasma write. Weak paternalism occurs when someone cannot give full informed consent or is not given the full range of options, and the physician decides in advance what might be in their best interests. Limited or sole options that correspond with this are then presented.[30]

It is the reason for the lack of full information disclosure that is ethically critical here. The time available in consultation, knowledge of medical jargon, and so on could be presented as reasons for the presentation of limited information by a physician. Should any of these reasons be enough to impinge on the client's interest in full and informed consent? You could reflect on why you presented fuller information for one client, or one procedure, and not for another.

While issues in health ethics are often 'considered in abstraction from the social and political context in which they arise', informed consent and the issue of information disclosure has succeeded in reuniting theory with practical context.[31] Informed consent and information disclosure is most usefully considered as a process that occurs in a social context; it is undertaken in the context of knowledge of acceptable political norms. Therefore the best way to learn about it is not in textbooks but in everyday societal interaction and transaction. The exercise on informed consent in the next section highlights this everyday context.

SEEKING CONSENT

Informed consent
Agreement given contingent on information and understanding of the proposed process, significance of decision, and potential benefits or risks entailed.

Informed consent is really a process, not a discrete event. It is a process of information exchange and autonomous decision making. The patient or client needs to understand the key issues in a proposed or sought treatment, and then, before that treatment is given, the client must have made an informed, voluntary, competent decision to go ahead with it. Patients often sign a consent form, but this signing is not, in itself, informed consent. It is merely one way of documenting a whole process. Particular issues involved in understanding information and competency are followed up in Chapter 7.

The responsibility for information disclosure falls largely to the health care worker. As the 'expert', the health care worker knows how to describe the process, and knows its risks and benefits (and their likelihood), as they are known to the profession. These risks should be communicated to the client so that a decision can be made about whether to go ahead with the treatment or management plan.

Some of the issues relating to information disclosure were addressed in the previous section, 'Negotiating treatment'. The present section concentrates on the process of informed consent for procedures. (Note that in the health care context, the word 'procedure' has a particular meaning: it refers to intervention processes performed on patients by health care professionals.) However, not all the responsibility for information disclosure falls to the health care worker. Some information about the client's values, preferences, or wishes needs to be voiced also, as this may make a difference to the type or range of treatment offered. Ideally, this information should be voiced by the client.

Informed consent to medical treatment lies at the heart of concerns in ethics for client autonomy. Informed consent is about clients giving permission for examinations or procedures, with the optimal amount of information available to them. It is the quality of health care that is being given increasing attention in health care contexts and in the training of health practitioners. Health students, medical students, and health practitioners can find the theory behind differing information disclosure standards difficult to grasp. The following exercise has been written with that in mind.

What do you consent to in your everyday context? You will find that the key feature of whatever situation you think of is that you seek something, or agree to something, and another person provides something to you. Write down everything you know about that process (and have experienced in it). Then turn the tables: imagine that you are the one who is about to provide the service or process to others, and write a consent form explaining that process. The reality of health care is that health care workers provide something that others seek. They understand the process involved in the thing that is sought. Before they can provide it to others, most of whom will probably have never experienced it before, they have to explain it in sufficient detail so that the potential patients or clients can decide whether or not to go ahead.

EXERCISE 4.10 CONSENT FORMS FOR THE EVERYDAY

Try writing a consent form for these everyday processes: having a haircut, getting your legs waxed, having your ears or other body part pierced, having a sandwich made, taking a bus ride, and going on a plane. You might like to think of others too. Before documenting the process and transforming it into a consent form that might be used for other people contemplating seeking these services for the first time, it is important to think about what you have experienced in these situations, and describe it in detail. Those contemplating engaging in these activities will want to know the risks and benefits, the likelihood of these occurring, and perhaps the cost and future effects. The law terms this information 'reasonable knowledge of risks', and in ethics it is said that to know such things is to 'maximise autonomy'. Providing such information is, in effect, enabling a full and informed choice.

When used in a class or group setting, the consent forms make for a lively tutorial-style discussion and some entertaining presentations when each form is read out. You will find that your colleagues are quite efficient at providing a range of information levels in relation to what the process or procedure would be like for the client, the expected risks and benefits, and avenues for further information.

A consent form documents the patient's condition, the proposed or required treatment, the general nature and effect of the treatment, the significant risks or side effects of the treatment, reasonable alternatives and their risks, the views of the patient, how much the patient understands about the treatment, and whether they are able to consent.[32] There may be only a small space for writing these things down on the form. It is a shorthand document that points to a larger process.

Re-examination is a consistent theme in health ethics. Guidelines on informed consent and information exchange are issued to articulate current standards and guide practitioners. Advice includes allowing patients to ask questions uninterrupted and express their concerns so the practitioner becomes aware of issues that are important to the patients; and then, how to deliver information to maximise comprehension of all risks, and how to allow further time for questions at the end of the consultation.[33] This is in keeping with prior advice that informed decisions rely on the availability of complete information about their condition, treatment options, and the risks and benefits of the different courses of action.[34] The process is perhaps more properly termed **informed decision making** than informed consent. An alternative and more modern term for informed consent, informed decision making also encompasses the active participation of both parties in determining options to be potentially agreed to, and in identifying significant material risks and benefits to be explored. The end of that process should be an informed consent, as routinely documented on a consent form. It is worth remembering that the consent form is just one form of documenting that an informed decision-making process is likely to have taken place.

As well as capturing ethicists' attention, given the obvious autonomy implications of exchanging relevant information, there has been considerable discussion of the appropriate standard of information disclosure in the law. Risks are part of all treatment processes. The courts have sought to balance the extent of the practitioner's duty to warn their patient about undesirable outcomes as part of their general duty of care. The discussion and court decisions reflect a societal expression of fairness, so can subtly change over time, but the decisions are guided by past decisions on appropriate fulfilment of duty of care. **Casuistry** is a pragmatic theory in which previous value-laden decisions are examined with reference to their factual and cultural context, with an objective of aiding future decisions. This is essentially the approach of legal reasoning, in which the facts of the previous cases help decide the principles to be applied to future decisions. The approach is to consider past decisions and reflect on whether a similar decision or conduct is acceptable in the new situation. When treatment risks that were foreseeable befall a patient, and the deficient information process may have altered a patient's decision to undertake the treatment, the courts generally regard the lack of disclosure of information to be negligent, but the material risks are interpreted more narrowly than they were in a landmark case.[35] Nevertheless, each professional in each clinical situation must ask themselves, 'What further information is this client asking for beyond the standard information?' Deciding this may be difficult, particularly as clients do not use the same language as trained professionals. They may not use the language of ethicists to say they want to maximise their autonomy. They may not use the language of health care workers to express their particular health concerns. Yet even a hint of concern, or questioning in an indirect way, is now an indication that professionals should at least think about offering more information for clients to use in their decision making. This legal redefinition of

Informed decision making
Alternative term for informed consent, also encompassing the active participation of both parties in determining options to be potentially agreed to, and in identifying significant material risks and benefits to be explored.

Casuistry
Ethics theory in which previous decisions are analysed in terms of values, and factual and cultural contexts, and used to guide future decisions.

acceptable standards illustrates how standards can change. It is perhaps not surprising that this judgment was handed down more than ten years after patients began to be called 'consumers' and began to be encouraged to become progressively more active in their own health care and health care decisions, with ethicists championing autonomy. The decision process of each patient must come under further scrutiny for a case to be proven. Also note that state legislation can limit recourse to negligence claims. Legal texts can explain the current legislation and approach of the courts further.[36]

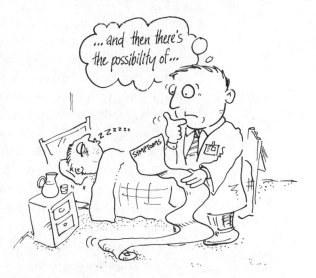

After you have considered the standards for information disclosure expected in your context, you may wish to check whether the consent form you wrote as part of the earlier exercise includes:

- information on the processes involved in the everyday action you chose as the subject of the consent form
- information on the risks and benefits involved in taking that action
- options for further information.

Of course, a balance needs to be struck between informing a client and overwhelming them. If there is too much information, they may not understand, or attend to, any more details on the proposed procedure or treatment processes. The challenge is to be able to communicate essential information, have opportunities for requests for further information, and ensure that each client understands and remembers crucial pieces of information so that their decisions are informed. If a minor risk or effects of small likelihood do not concern them in the slightest, then listening to all of the effects may be more of a burden than a help in their informed decision. On the other hand, if the ethical significance of a process is important to them, such as the use of blood products in one part of a treatment (the religious significance of this is referred to in Chapter 10), then much more information may be needed. The ethical consequences, the social and personal significance, and the relevance of information are increasingly part of routine information disclosure in health care work.

The key point is that you should try to look through the everyday nature of what you are doing when you provide a service. To people who are receiving it for the first time, it is not 'everyday'. You need to take the time to consider what it is that you do, in an everyday sense, and then try to explain it to others and discuss what it means for them. After all, it is in the everyday that health professionals work. For you as health care workers, a 'simple' operation is as straightforward as buying a sandwich or having a haircut. The challenge you face is to unpack the process and the things you take for granted about it; the process, risks, and benefits must be documented in minute detail so that they can be communicated and discussed with the client.

There is a subtle re-emergence of weak paternalism in acknowledging the special knowledge and experience that health carers have, and consequently their great importance in helping to direct patients to sensible treatment options. Decision making entails a shared role, to work towards reasonable and achievable goals. This has probably always been the case, but it is now explicitly argued that the balance of decision making should shift back to the health care professional in different circumstances, depending on the urgency and gravity of the decisions at hand. The complexity of technological options for care may have also influenced this shift. The ethical justification for such paternalism is discussed in the professional literature. In caring for children with cancer, for instance, a health care team have written about how the balance in sharing of decisions between parents, clinicians, and (mature) children can vary depending on the likelihood of cure for the ill child and the range of reasonable options the clinician considers to be available. The clinician could feel justified in strongly directing the family to one realistic course of action, based on the clinician's knowledge and experience. The child's preferences may be more practically important when two or more reasonable choices are available for their care. The child assumes greater decisional authority with maturity, and is expected to have greater capacity for understanding complex issues.[37] More on the child as decision maker is included in Chapter 7.

SUMMARY OF KEY ISSUES

- Respect
- Developing a relationship
- Being trusted
- Taking on responsibility
- Acting and not acting
- Taking notes
- Choice and autonomy
- Paternalism to liberalism
- Informed consent.

SHORT NOTES

1   Burnard, *Counselling skills for health professionals*, 2nd edn, pp. 96–7.
2   NSW Department of Health, 'Health records and information'.
3   O'Brien, 'Making a note and handover'.

4   Jonsen et al., *Clinical ethics*, 4th edn.

5   Momber and Rueda, 'Bioethics and medical practice'.

6   Mill, 'On liberty'.

7   Ibid.

8   Dawson, 'Drugs in sport'.

9   Qiu, 'Bioethics in an Asian context'.

10   McVeigh, 'Violet Townsend Inquiry reaction'; 'We're improving our care services'.

11   Singer, *Practical ethics*, pp. 13–19.

12   Smith & Nephew Surgical, *Hospital and health services year book 1995/96*, 20th edn, p. 34.

13   James, *Devices and desires*, pp. 92–3.

14   Rachels, 'Active and passive euthanasia'.

15   Honderich (ed.), *The Oxford companion to philosophy*, pp. 204–5.

16   See, for example, Foot, 'Killing and letting die'.

17   Jennett, 'Quality of care and cost containment in the U.S. and the U.K.'.

18   Pellegrino and Thomasma, *For the patient's good*.

19   Beauchamp and Childress, *Principles of biomedical ethics*, 4th edn.

20   Quill and Brody, 'Physician recommendations and patient autonomy'.

21   Zeleznik et al., 'Teaching ethics to students in the University College of Nursing Studies in Maribor'.

22   Hoshino, 'Information and self-determination'.

23   Brahams, 'Right to know in Japan'.

24   Hoshino, 'Information and self-determination'.

25   Berglund, 'Bioethics'.

26   Max Charlesworth puts forward the libertarian position in *Bioethics in a liberal society*.

27   Beauchamp and Childress, *Principles of biomedical ethics*, 5th edn, pp. 418–19.

28   Rocker et al., 'Seasonal bed closures in an intensive care unit'.

29   Charlesworth, *Bioethics in a liberal society*, pp. 3, 5, 6.

30   Pellegrino and Thomasma, *For the patient's good*, p. 7.

31   The quoted text is from Charlesworth, *Bioethics in a liberal society*, p. 1.

32   For an explanation of practitioner responsibilities in gaining patient consent, and a sample consent form, see NSW Department of Health, 'Health records and information', p. 9.246.

33   National Health and Medical Research Council, 'General guidelines for medical practitioners'.

34   Skene, 'What should doctors tell patients?'

35   *Rogers v. Whitaker* (1992) 175 CLR 479.

36   Clarke et al., *Torts*, 2nd edn, pp. 364–9.

37   Whitney et al., 'Decision-making in pediatric oncology'.

THE CLIENT AND CARER RELATIONSHIP

- Expectations and responsibilities
- Privacy and confidentiality
- Risks facing community
- Veracity on both sides
- Trust in the hands of the professional
- Risk to client or carer
- Risk to others
- Terminating a relationship

OBJECTIVES

As the relationship of caring progresses, the expectations and obligations associated with it become increasingly defined. This chapter explores the boundaries of risk and the negotiated limits of care. Challenges to the relationship and different approaches to resolution are canvassed. The carer's broader responsibilities to others are discussed, particularly in relation to the risk posed to others by clients or the treatment process. The expectation that carers will respond to this risk is also discussed. Public health issues of risk, risk assessment, and containment are explored further.

The following terms are added to your glossary: virtue, trust, confidentiality, public interest, private interest, public health, veracity, mandatory, and compulsory.

EXPECTATIONS AND RESPONSIBILITIES

Clients expect to receive help when they are sick, and they expect to receive help so that they do not become sick. Our society is set up to provide this within reasonable limits, as discussed in Chapter 3, and some of you have chosen to become health care workers to provide this societal benefit of health care, as discussed in Chapter 2. When you become health care workers, others expect certain things of you, and you take on the responsibility of meeting those reasonable expectations.

In broad terms, we are all part of a reciprocity of interactions, expectations, and benefits. This reciprocity was explored by the philosopher David Hume. Hume made a distinction between natural **virtue** and artificial virtue. However, Hume's use of the word 'artificial' did not imply that he thought artificial virtues were not truly virtuous. He used the term to indicate actions that furthered the system of reciprocity that underpins society and aims to ensure the well-being of every individual.[1]

Virtue
Worth or quality of particular moral excellence.

All members of society expect to receive the benefits that living in our society promises. As a health professional, you also play a role in delivering those benefits to others. To be successful, you will need to communicate clearly to clients what it is reasonable for them to expect, and what responsibility can be shouldered by the health professional.

Sometimes clients seem to have wildly inconsistent notions of which treatments work and which do not. What do you make of the following quote from a novel? 'His first heart attack had followed soon after, and Henry, half inclined to envisage his doctor as a personification of his illness, had declared himself much improved since the doctor had ceased to pay regular daily visits.'[2]

Some humour is being made of the patient's feeling that he gets sicker when the doctor comes. This is quite different from the doctor's own probable perception that the client gets well under his care (and then does not need further regular home visits). Checking perceptions and expectations every now and then might be useful.

You need to find a way to work together so that the expectations of clients and carers are similar and you understand each other's responsibilities. Professional responsibilities have been expressed, and are continually developing, in professional codes, as is discussed in Chapter 2. Patient responsibilities and expectations are now visible in patient codes, statements of patient rights, accreditation manuals, and patient handbooks.[3] There is increasing emphasis on the active obligation of clients to be a part of the management plan, to take responsibility for attention to their treatment, and to take responsibility for their recovery and future health. The availability of information about professions and institutions may be crucial in forming appropriate client expectations.

Trust
Confidence in another person, or persons within an organisation, to act in an expected manner.

Clients and health professionals engage in client–carer relationships with certain expectations of each other. One expectation held by carers, and addressed in Chapter 4, is that clients will **trust** you and will reveal their problem in detail, so that their care can progress. This disclosure on the part of the client requires them to trust the carer (this trust is discussed later in this chapter).

Within health care teams, different professions have different responsibilities. Each team member expects the others to work within their skill, with due care, and to shoulder their fair share of the responsibility in caring for the client. If something goes wrong, there is a team, as well as an individual, responsibility to minimise the impact on the client. You need to check that each member is properly responsible and skilled.

EXERCISE 5.1 ACCURACY AND RECORDS

Think about the following example, which is from a Masters course in clinical ethics:

A nurse makes a mistake with the amount of medicine he dispenses to a patient. He realises the mistake, as does a fellow nurse. The patient's records show that the correct amount has been given. Neither corrects the records, or reports the mistake to the charge nurse or the attending doctor.[4]

What do you think could be the effect of the mistake?

What responsibility is being degraded by not rectifying the records?

It is part of health care workers' responsibility to be vigilant about and aware of the expectations placed on them and the responsibilities they bear in their professional role.

There are many opportunities for clarifying these responsibilities and for encouraging a team to live up to them. Generally, internal mechanisms have the potential to be educative, as discussed in Chapter 11.

PRIVACY AND CONFIDENTIALITY

You know you are in a private domain as health care workers because you hear personal details and see personal things that are not routinely disclosed or seen. You are in this privileged position so that you can help. The initial disclosure of such information by clients is discussed in Chapter 4. Think back to Exercise 4.2 that asked you to disclose a secret to your classmate. Those people who chose not to tell their neighbours anything exercised their right to privacy, and we might think of those people as being inherently private. Those people who told a secret now have to trust that their neighbour will not tell anyone else, and that the confidentiality of that secret will be upheld.

EVERYDAY ETHICS

Imagine a friend tells you a secret, which you know is quite personal and has been difficult for your friend to discuss. Soon after, you and your friend have a falling out. When chatting with some mutual friends a few weeks later, you use your old friend's situation as a humorous example of the problems people can get themselves into. Everyone has a laugh, but you feel terrible afterwards, convinced that what you did wasn't 'right'. So what is the problem with that type of gossiping and breach of earlier confidence? Perhaps you can express it in terms of potential harms, or in previously agreed obligations.

We can and do choose to keep some secrets in our social interactions. Yet we also know that some information needs to be disclosed in the course of everyday life. We seem to accept that this is so in relation to dealings with many institutions, such as when we disclose details to our bank, the taxation department, our employers, and so on. Some health information needs to be disclosed for treatment to be selected and provided. Some of this information is private, but that does not mean that clients need to tell everybody everything, or that health care workers should expect to know everything about their clients. You need to know as much as is necessary to provide proper care, and no more. Your respect for your client's individual integrity is demonstrated by allowing the client to make a decision about what is too private (or unnecessary or unacceptable) to disclose.

Whenever we have disclosed information that is private and personal—personal even if only because it has our name on it—we do so with an understanding of why it is asked for, and what it will be used for. Personal and private information includes verbal information, information about one's body, and disclosing one's body to view. It is when that personal information potentially becomes available to a wider audience that we become worried about privacy and confidentiality. We are worried because we have lost some control over how and what the information is used for.

Once information is potentially available to a broader audience, we further trust that those who seek access to it are authorised to have this access, and that they will respect it.

EXERCISE 5.2 SECRETS AND DUTIES

Sometimes clients choose to limit how many people know about their medical condition, even when they are quite ill. Consider the following scenario.

An ambulance is called to a house where a woman in her late fifties has had a heart attack. Many of her relatives are over that day for a family gathering, and most of them are highly emotional about the situation and unsure about what to do. The ambulance crew starts basic resuscitation measures, working through a routine protocol, when the local GP, who has also been called, comes rushing around the corner and says 'stop'. The family look totally startled, as do the ambulance crew.

Can you guess why the GP might have said 'stop'? Perhaps the GP knew something that the ambulance officers didn't, and even something that the family didn't know.

What the GP knew was that the woman did not want active treatment in the event of a life-threatening situation. She did not want it because she wanted to die quickly rather than linger, and she was greatly influenced by the fact that she had terminal cancer, which she had not disclosed to her family. She had chosen to keep that a secret so she could enjoy whatever time she had left without them worrying unduly about her. That was her choice, and as it happened, she suffered a heart attack prior to the expected onset of the rapid deterioration in her health. The GP's knowledge of this was the reason he called out to the ambulance crew to stop active resuscitation. Unlike the family, the GP knew the woman's secret, and also knew her wishes. She was unable to inform the ambulance officers of her wishes because, by the time they had arrived, she was almost clinically dead. Whether the GP should have asked the ambulance officers to stop is addressed in Chapter 9, as is the question of when health care workers should stop active care. As will be discussed in Chapter 9, there is a difference between, on the one hand, care and comfort, and on the other, active restorative treatment.

Privacy and confidentiality are integral to maintaining human dignity and so are concerns derived from the principle of 'respect for persons' (otherwise known as autonomy).[5] You may remember reading in Chapter 4 about how respect for persons is essential in ethical dealings with clients and patients. The challenge in modern societies and health care institutions is to balance the commitment to respect, privacy, and confidentiality with the need for information about individuals.

Confidentiality
Limited distribution of another's personal information, due to respect for privacy.

The issue common to both privacy and **confidentiality** is respect for an individual's control over their personal information. Information privacy issues centre on control of access to personal information. Confidentiality issues are derived from privacy; confidentiality relates to control over the use or further disclosure of that information. In practice, privacy relates to what personal information should be collected or stored, while confidentiality is concerned with the storage, security, and use of personal data that has already been stored.[6] It is important to understand the difference between privacy and confidentiality because so many debates and guidelines draw the distinction. You may find the following explanation useful in understanding the difference.

Consider a 'private & confidential' notice on an envelope. The word 'private' implies that there is no public right of access to the information inside: only authorised persons should open the envelope and read its contents. To comply with this instruction is to recognise the interest that individuals have in being able to limit access to information; in other words, their rights to privacy. The word 'confidential' implies that those persons who are granted permission to read the contents have an obligation to guard against further lessening of individual privacy—for instance, by preventing non-authorised persons from reading the contents of the document. It also means that their use of the information should take into account its confidential nature: that its substance should not be revealed to others.[7]

This explanation illustrates the limited direct control that individuals have over their private information, beyond the initial disclosure. Individuals rely on their confidants to maintain desired levels of privacy and to use the information in the expected manner. They also rely on those who are not granted access to the information to respect that situation.

Think about what you might do if you had a letter delivered to you that was not for you. You could return it to the sender, or pass it on to the person who is the rightful recipient (if you knew that person) without opening it. To open the letter would be to pry. That feeling of prying is what you get when you invade someone's privacy. The rule that you should not open or read other people's private correspondence is fairly straightforward. However, you may receive correspondence where the name on the envelope is very similar to both your name and the name of a colleague. What would you do then? One solution would be to open the letter together, and together read one line at a time until you identify whom it really belongs to. That way, neither person would read more private information than is absolutely necessary to identify the proper recipient.

Some simple safeguards with regard to privacy and confidentiality can be undertaken at your work. Keep lockable filing cabinets locked so that only authorised persons can open the cabinet and read files. If you are working with confidential material on your desk, cover it up when you have meetings with other people in your office. Other people do not routinely need to see the contents of all the confidential files in your office. And if you happen to be opposite someone else's desk and a confidential letter is in your line of vision, turn it over and say something like, 'I probably shouldn't see that and it is difficult not to notice it as I talk to you'. If you are discussing clients, you should do it in a private and secure area.

Next time you are in a public area, think about how common it is to hear sensitive information discussed by other people in places such as lifts, walkways, theatres, etc. It is amazing that such sensitive information is discussed loudly in public places; the participants in these conversations seem to be oblivious to the crowds of people around them, many of whom are only too pleased to have something to listen to as they wait for the lift to get to their floor, or for the concert to begin. It is a useful rule of thumb not to discuss work outside the workplace, and especially not to name patients or clients as you discuss their background or particular treatment scenario, unless of course you are discussing the case with health workers who are part of the treatment team and need to know who the person is, and you are in a secure environment.

Within the work context, there are also things that constantly alert us to the presence of private and confidential information. When faxes are delivered, they are essentially opened letters. Only as much of the fax should be read as identifies the recipient; the fax should then be kept securely for that person. Some institutions use a folder, like a large envelope, so that faxes are not left lying on desks or in pigeonholes for others to see. Your institution may have different procedures for guarding privacy and confidentiality. Often faxes have a special message printed on them alerting us to the fact that they are private, in the same way that 'private & confidential' may be written on an envelope. To act on information contained in a fax destined for somebody else is a breach of respect. This, of course, also applies to the situation in which you hear private or confidential information that was not intended for your ears. The same applies to shared email addresses.

Institutions that routinely use fax machines balance the pressure for fast delivery of information against the risk to privacy and confidentiality. Safeguards are used, such as cover sheets, instructions on what to do if the wrong recipient receives the fax, and the practice of telephoning before faxing material (to make sure the recipient is standing by the fax machine ready to receive the fax). Here is one example of a printed message used on faxes to alert unintended recipients that they have duties of confidentiality.

> This facsimile contains confidential information that is intended only for use by the addressee. If you have received this facsimile in error, you are advised that copying, distributing, disclosing, or otherwise acting in reliance upon this facsimile is strictly prohibited. If you are not the intended recipient, could you please notify us immediately.

Once information is disclosed and written down or distributed, we need to guard against the lessening of privacy and confidentiality.

Some information needs to be written down during the provision of health care. Notes based on the information gathered about the client are called medical records, or health records. Those records are stored for further reference. As is discussed in this chapter, those notes should be accurate and complete so that they provide a good basis for following a client's progress and making future treatment decisions. There is little ethical debate about that. It is when those notes are not safely stored, or when they are made available for a wider purpose than treatment of the individual, that ethical concerns arise. Professional associations for medical records personnel are acutely aware of this responsibility. In large institutions, organising files and computerised records for easy access and protecting unauthorised access to them are the primary roles of medical records personnel or health information management professionals. Their codes of ethics acknowledge this responsibility of safeguarding confidentiality. The responsibility is usually expressed in terms of a duty to respect and secure the information, within legal and regulatory limits, such as: 'Preserve, protect, and secure personal information in any form or medium and hold in the highest regard the contents of the records and other information of a confidential nature, taking into account the applicable statutes and regulations.' The American Health Information Management Association Code of Ethics has also stated: 'Both handwritten and computerized medical records contain many sacred stories—stories that must be protected on behalf of the individual and the aggregate community of persons served in the healthcare system.'[8] This wording explains the sensitive personal nature of the information that you are responsible for.

EXERCISE 5.3 MOVEMENT OF INFORMATION

Identify a piece of personal health information in your professional work and track its progress. Take a blank page and draw a box labelled 'information'. Draw a circle for each place that this information moved to, using arrows to denote the movement of the information. On your diagram, note who collected the information, who knows about it, who accessed it, and how it was used for the client's treatment. Then look back through your trail and note the potential points at which information could be leaked or used for an unapproved purpose. Those leakage points may be at handover, at moments of minimal security, and so on.

You may also like to discuss if the following situation, or a similar one, would be likely to occur at your health care workplace. This vignette was developed in a general-practice ethics project, in which general practitioners and consumers nominated their concerns and then met to discuss vignettes such as this one.[9]

A GP walked into the staff coffee room of his group-practice surgery and found the staff discussing (with a great deal of amusement) the diagnosis and circumstances of a patient of his who happened to be a well-known television personality. They were passing around a fax that had just been received with a report on the patient from a specialist consultant. The doctor remonstrated with his staff about confidentiality.

The real danger of each potential leakage point in the information trail you constructed for the last exercise is that while each person may genuinely need access to the information for the primary reason of client care, they may not understand the importance of privacy and confidentiality; in other words, they may not understand how important such ethical obligations are in a large institution or in society.

FROM THEORY TO PRACTICE

Tearoom chat

Contributor: *Jenneke Foottit*

You are in the staff tearoom and you overhear one of your colleagues talking about the complicated care of a patient in your unit. The person uses the patient's name. You know this breaches confidentiality and you know you should interrupt the conversation, but you choose not to. Later you approach your colleague alone and try to speak to her about the issue. She gets very angry with you and shouts at you that you have no right to tell her what to do. This is not the first time she has breached confidentiality rules.

What are your responsibilities as an ethical nurse? How would you address this issue, and who can you approach?

What may be some of the consequences of your actions? How would you deal with them from an ethical perspective?

The lack of individual control over personal information, and the demand for this information by others, is of particular concern when information is collected in institutional settings, and when it is centralised and stored in computerised data banks. The danger is that if stored personal information can be used for another purpose, privacy interests will be overridden without adequate consideration of the importance of that further use, or in spite of professional concerns that confidentiality should be maintained.[10] A Swedish project linking 1500 individuals' medical, educational, and financial records, and an Icelandic study holding detailed genetic information in a database were frequently cited as ethically debatable.[11] We rely on others, usually professionals or administrators, to use their discretion in deciding whether or not our information privacy interests should be overridden. In health care, clients rely on health care workers and records administrators to protect their privacy interests and treat their personal information with respect.

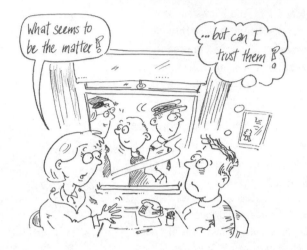

EXERCISE 5.4 REGULATED INFORMATION

Different privacy protection applies in different contexts, but there is a trend in most jurisdictions to protect the privacy of an individual's information, and to improve security to ensure this. The information should not be transmitted further unless the individual consents to specific further use of the information, or there is explicit outweighing of public interests in this privacy to justify the transmission and use. In the USA, the professionals would need to keep in mind the federal regulations, and particularly the latest Department of Health and Human Services Privacy Rules, which came into effect in April 2003. They support patient privacy in the context of a sufficient flow of information for quality medical care. This regulation has had implications for the way organisations store their information, further refined due to the Security Rules for standards for confidentiality, integrity, and availability of electronic health information, in force as of April 2005. The Privacy and Security Rules are enforced and administered by the Office for Civil Rights. Their implementation has prompted the generation of standard consent forms for potential further use of the information, which practitioners can give the patient to sign if further use is anticipated. It can be very difficult to recontact all patients at a later date to seek their permission, so it is sought upfront.

As an exercise in keeping up to date on regulations, try this internet exercise. You can generally get access to the internet at public libraries, if you do not have access at home, work, or a university. Look up the summary Privacy Rules and Security Rule under the Department of Health and Human Services at <www.hhs.gov>. Search for the web address under the department name, or go through the US government link. Then look up one profession's response to the regulations. Journals are a vital discussion forum, as practitioners share their views on how to comply with the regulations in professional practice, and what difficulties they face as practitioners dealing with confidential information.[12]

It is important to realise that individuals could suffer harm if a promise of confidentiality of personal information is not upheld. For example, if police were able to access research data that identified persons involved in criminal activities, those persons might be jailed. In the 1970s in the USA, a number of commissions into research participation collected instances of embarrassing situations that were caused by clinical information being disclosed in other contexts. The following extract is from the report of one of these commissions. As one witness told the Commission:

> a researcher was doing a follow-up study of people who had been enrolled in a methadone maintenance program . . . The contractor had the name and address of one particular individual who had been enrolled in the program several years previously, and the contractor went to the individual's residence. It was a Saturday night and the person was having a party and the contractor said, 'Hi, I am so-and-so from such-and-such an organization, and we are doing a follow-up study of patients who had been enrolled in the methadone maintenance program.'

Another such incident which came to the Commission's attention involved the recontact of patients who had received treatment at an abortion clinic. On both instances the recontacts were unwelcome, resented, and extremely embarrassing to the persons contacted.[13] Remembering the sensitivity of personal information has been a feature of guidelines for modern research practice.

It is a separate philosophical decision whether any disclosure and any harm or embarrassment is justified, as will be discussed soon. The key point to note here is that there is potential harm in any breach of confidentiality.

On a broader level, the disclosure of personal information could also threaten the public's trust in the confidentiality of certain relationships such as banking, employment, and health care relationships. Health care relationships in particular are based on trust in the confidentiality of the information provided. A threat to an individual harms not only that person, but also others because it erodes their trust in similar relationships.[14] The essence of privacy and confidentiality is that information is disclosed under certain conditions, which consist of particular promises of confidentiality and particular expectations as to how the information will be used. Truthful information is given in exchange for that trust. The professional's obligation to maintain the confidentiality of the information continues until the informants give consent to the further distribution of the information.[15]

The conflict is, however, that interests in privacy and confidentiality, just like interests in autonomy, are not absolute. The problem for all health care workers is in deciding when obligations to maintain privacy and confidentiality can be overridden by other obligations. These obligations can in turn be overridden by competing interests.[16] The following are some examples of public interests:

- Society has an interest in the release of information that will assist in preventing other members of society from suffering harm. Societies need some personal information to assess the welfare of their members and to protect others from harm caused by infectious diseases.[17]

- Health care systems need access to personal information in order to assess their own effectiveness and efficiency, and to improve so that others may be better served.[18] Access to information is justified if research is directed towards preventing harm to others in the future (this would be the kind of argument put forth by research organisations to support their access to information).

You can probably think of some more examples from other professional spheres.

There are some general rules for health care workers to consider in relation to the confidentiality of their health records or medical records:

- Confidentiality should be maintained, and consent sought for further use or disclosure of information, unless there is an overriding public interest. (This interest is generally mandated by another body, not just by the health care worker.) Thus when public interest overrides the duty of confidentiality, it is legitimate to breach confidentiality. These interests include the reporting of infectious diseases and the provision of evidence in criminal trials in response to a subpoena (and at the discretion of the court).

Private interest
Issues of importance and significance to an individual, defined on an individual basis to be in that person's best interest.

- Confidentiality should be maintained because otherwise there is the potential for harm to be done to the client, which would contravene the health care worker's duty of care to the client.

It is difficult to specify the precise circumstances that would justify an infringement of privacy and confidentiality, apart from the sorts of extreme public interest provisions mentioned above. The primary question in relation to the release of information in the ordinary course of health care is: 'Does the information disclosure serve the purpose of the treatment that the patient originally agreed to?'

Public interest
Issues of importance and significance to the structure of a community, and to the general benefit of a significant group of a community's members.

Whenever there is a request for the disclosure of information, professionals need to identify the full extent of their obligations both to keep information confidential and to disclose it. Consideration of the distinction between public and private interests may be a useful part of this process of identifying the extent of these obligations.

The distinction between public and **private interests** in privacy is similar to Mill's distinction between social and personal morality, which was discussed in Chapter 4. Generally, **public interests** affect groups of people as a whole, whereas individual interests affect individuals in particular circumstances. Individual interests in privacy are generally upheld, except where there is a substantially greater public interest that cannot be achieved if that private interest in privacy is allowed. An example of a public interest in privacy is the need for trust to be maintained in confidential health care relationships so that members of society are not dissuaded from seeking health care for fear that the information they give to health carers will be disclosed to all and sundry. This is a public interest because this safeguard is needed in order to maintain a healthy society. An example of a private interest is the need for information to be guarded carefully because individuals may be harmed socially if their information is disclosed.

J. S. Mill said:

> [A]s soon as any person's conduct affects prejudicially the interests of others, society has jurisdiction over it, and the question whether the general welfare will or will not be promoted by interfering with it, becomes open to discussion. But there is no room for entertaining any such question when a person's conduct affects the interests of no persons besides himself, or need not affect them unless they like (all the persons concerned being of full age, and the ordinary amount of understanding). In all such cases there should be perfect freedom, legal and social, to do the action and stand the consequences.[19]

The codes of ethics of health care professionals generally offer the advice that privacy is not absolute and can be overridden. For example, the Pharmacy Board of Australia's Pharmacy Code of Conduct for registered health practitioners states: 'Patients or clients have a right to expect that practitioners and their staff will hold information about them in confidence, unless information is required to be released by law or public interest considerations'.[20] The codes, however, are unable to provide practical help about which interest should take precedence in specific situations.[21] This means that further professional discussion is essential. From time to time, when professional codes explicitly acknowledge this conflict and admit that the right of privacy is not absolute, there is controversy. The acceptable limits of privacy can be the subject of legislation, and case law and the terminology used often mimics that of J. S. Mill. In one example, guidance for consent requirements for the collection, use, storage, and further disclosure of personal information is legislated, demonstrating a societal commitment to personal integrity and autonomy. The circumstances when the requirement for consent can be waived are limited to the following:

- It will 'prevent or lessen a serious and imminent threat to the life or health of the individual concerned or another person'.
- It is required or authorised under law.
- It is necessary for the enforcement of a criminal law (or the payment of a penalty in the criminal justice system).
- It is to protect the public revenue.
- It is directly related to the initial purpose for which the information was obtained.[22]

A judgment as to the relative merits of different interests is tested in court from time to time. For instance, in 1992 a court was asked to decide if the Red Cross should be granted immunity from disclosing the identities of blood donors to persons subsequently infected by blood donation. The court considered survey results (the survey having been done for the court hearing) which showed that many people would not donate blood without an assurance of confidentiality. The court ruled that the public interest in assuring confidentiality, so that people would continue to donate blood, outweighed the interests that those infected had in the disclosure of the identities of blood donors.[23]

The active consideration of the competing interests to privacy interests is prominent in such deliberations. Some public interests rely on the flow of information, such as in human rights protection, for social interests and for business interests. Individual liberty and, in this case, privacy are supported, but social limitations are placed on both due to public concerns over the welfare of other members of society, and over the strength of the fabric of society.

Finding this balance is potentially complex when personal health data is sought for use in health research. National funding bodies and professional associations generate their own guidelines and discussion papers about the balance between the public interest in access for research practice purposes and the public interest in privacy, bearing in mind the requirements under law. Generally, there is guidance on the circumstance in which the use of personal data for research may constitute a specific exception to the general requirement for a consent process, such as when there is minimal risk gaining consent would be impracticable, and further, the benefit is likely to justify the harm associated with not seeking consent.[24] The exception is not granted lightly. Ethics committees are required to decide this, and in doing so to consider if the public interest in the promotion of the research 'outweighs to a substantial degree the public interest in adhering to that Information Privacy Principle'.[25] Usually, people other than the health care worker make the judgment as to whether one public interest outweighs another. The health care worker still needs to consider any request for confidential information and should refer it to the appropriate authorities if the request is clearly not consistent with the purpose of treatment.

RISKS FACING COMMUNITY

When health issues pose a risk to others, the information can become 'notifiable', which means that it is mandatory to release to a relevant public authority. The severe acute respiratory syndrome (SARS), which began in November 2002 and reached the most serious epidemic proportions in China by mid-2003, was legislated as a notifiable condition in many countries. Quarantine provisions—that is, limiting the movement of people affected, or people in contact with those affected—were also made on the grounds of public interest. The World Health Organization requested international cooperation and central reporting of SARS cases and infection patterns. Health outcomes were made available routinely on a public website, as soon as they became available to the WHO.[26] The WHO also became involved in issuing descriptions of symptoms to be vigilant for, travel warnings, and containment advice, as it tracked the epidemic in countries worldwide. In ethics terms, the measures were justified on grounds of serious and imminent risk if the information was to remain private.

EXERCISE 5.5 ORGANISATIONAL REGULATION

As a tutorial exercise, find out what one organisation's policy was on SARS. You could use your university, workplace, or local school as examples. See if there were travel restrictions, limitations on attendance after travel, exclusion based on symptoms, and so on. Find out how the policy was argued in terms of ethics, and take particular note of any wording on risk and interests.

If you had an opportunity to rewrite this policy, what would you suggest? Take into account the symptoms and health consequences (including the mortality and spread of SARS). You will find crucial facts to consider on the WHO website (www.who.int), or in local health authority warning or alert documents.

Can you think of any other identifiable and potentially catastrophic transmissible diseases? How about bird flu and, in particular, one form of avian influenza named H5N1?

Bird flu (H5N1 strain) raised similar issues to SARS in terms of the importance of identification and containment of risks and the need for rapid response. An epidemic in birds, affecting large wild bird populations worldwide and many domesticated flocks, poses a potential risk not just to further birds, but also to humans. Bird handlers have predominantly been at risk of infection, with serious life-threatening infections reported in some people. These have largely been in the developing world so far. Avian flu is potentially a large-scale threat to the human population if it mutates into a virus that is easily transmissible between humans. Mass culling of birds has been undertaken in areas where the bird flu has been identified. Quarantine provisions apply to affected areas in terms of trading in birds. Infected people are ideally treated in quarantine conditions.

Some flu drugs (e.g. oseltamivir) are likely to be used for the rapid onset of symptoms, once bird flu is identified, but the worldwide stocks are limited and governments have tried to stockpile certain amounts for front-line health and emergency workers. Prescriptions from individuals without symptoms, who tried to stockpile some in case they might need it quickly, became near impossible to fill. Vaccine trials were under way in 2006 but had not promised high enough effectiveness to be relied on for protection from H5N1 bird flu.[27] There was also a concern that as vaccines became available, they should be equitably available.[28] As a transmissible mutated virus that could initiate a pandemic has not yet occurred, the exact mutated virus that needs to be countered by a vaccine has not yet been developed. The WHO's advice was therefore that a precise vaccine would not be readily available early in a pandemic in any case, and to supply vaccine for the whole world of 6.7 billion people over a six-month period would not be feasible.[29]

Given that background, try the following exercise on risk and assessment of risk from a private (personal) or public perspective.

EXERCISE 5.6 RISK AND ASSESSMENT

Imagine you are a small farmer in a developing country. You rely on the meagre income from your chickens to feed your children. One chicken has recently become sick. List your concerns.

Then, imagine you are a public health official with the WHO, and you hear a rumour about a small farmer with a sick chicken in a remote village. List your concerns.

Compare your lists. Should one list of concerns outweigh or take precedence over the other? Why or why not? Try to justify your position, and make use of the ethics theory you have learnt in this and previous chapters.

Public health
Field of health care concerned with assessing and improving health and preventing illness or disease on a population basis.

Note that **public health** practice is compatible with assessing individual and community risk, and setting and imposing limits in the public interest. This broad notion of care, and taking responsibility for deciding what is in individuals' best interests, is a form of paternalism. The notion of paternalism in fact underlies much of public health practice in instances of serious risk. Factors are identified and acted upon for the good of a community, independent of individual preferences. As risks decrease in magnitude and probability, more individual choice is offered.

It is likely that we will always have to live and work with the reality of both the duty of confidentiality and the demand for access to health care information. This will continue to pose challenges, with rapidly developing technology, communication over great distances, and ever-growing networks of health care workers involved in the care of individual clients.

VERACITY ON BOTH SIDES

In a treatment relationship there will be points of progress and points of decline. There will be good news to tell in relation to progress, and bad news to tell if the prognosis, or diagnosis, is grim or is not what was hoped for. Some health care workers are better at being frank with their clients than others, and some clients are better at hearing the truth than others. The willingness to relay bad news—for instance, to discuss imminent death with a patient, and the emotional preparation for it—is increasingly regarded as part of professional skill. If you choose to have an open and frank relationship with your client or patient (and this is a culturally influenced decision, as is discussed in Chapter 4), you are upholding **veracity**. Upholding veracity does not necessarily mean telling a client all the bad news in one sitting. When unfavourable results become available, it is common to have a number of meetings with the patient so that the information and its implications can be discussed, and future management can be planned, as the patient gradually comes to terms with the bad news.

Veracity
Truthfulness, accuracy, and completeness in information relied on by others.

Breaking bad news was the subject of a vignette in Chapter 4. Any bad news told to a client needs to be relevant to the client and must be information that is used in the further treatment or management of the client's condition. How risk or information is conveyed can dramatically alter the dynamics of the client's recovery process. It is important not to destroy a client's hope, as hope is essential for recovery and for achieving the best quality of life possible.[30]

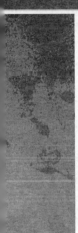

FROM THEORY TO PRACTICE

Direct questions

Contributor: Jenneke Foottit

You are showering Mrs Jones, a patient being treated with chemotherapy for metastatic breast cancer. You know her prognosis is poor. Her family has been avoiding talking to her about it and keeps up an artificially cheerful front. The medical team pays only short visits. She says very suddenly: 'I am dying, aren't I? Nobody wants to talk about it, but I know I am.'

How do you respond to her, and what ethical principles do you keep in mind while you think about what you would say to her?

There is some concern that professionals are not trained to uphold veracity, or be truthful, with sufficient vigour. This has been noted particularly in competitive training settings, such as medical school. While senior researchers have, with some surprise, discovered instances of cheating and lying by students, students themselves do not register the same level of surprise at these findings. Students report doing what they can to get through. In her prize-winning essay on ethics, medical student Tara Young reflects on the way in which some of her fellow students lied and presented a false picture of their ambitions when trying to secure training placements in particular fields of medical practice.[31] She observes the discrepancy between this behaviour and the centrality, to medicine, of honesty in dealings with colleagues and patients, quoting the American Medical Association's code of ethics: 'a physician shall deal honestly with patients and colleagues, and strive to expose those physicians deficient in character or competence, or who engage in fraud or deception.' Veracity with colleagues and clients is part of the trust-forming relationship between society and professionals, and between individual practitioners and their clients.

People are increasingly asking how, if veracity is routinely degraded in personal lives, can it be upheld with clients. Attention is now being given to reinforcing veracity in all dealings between those involved in health care—students, professional peers, educators, clients, and the general public—as a first step towards veracity in health care relationships. In the context of health care education, we should encourage students to say if they don't know something, rather than having them pretend that they know (and try to bluff). There is a danger, as there is for all professionals, that in pretending to know something, you may overstep the bounds of your own skill and make a mistake: a client may be given the wrong information or a procedure may be conducted incorrectly. It is ethically responsible to acknowledge that you don't know something. Such an acknowledgment is an active reflection on the limits of your skill, similar to the skill-limit exercise you did in Chapter 2. When this happens, it is your professional responsibility to ask for help, but then also to remedy the deficit in your knowledge, to apply your new-found knowledge to the problem at hand, and to implement proper treatment once you know what to do. In short, it is acceptable not to know and to admit it; but having done so, it would be ethically irresponsible if you then failed to remedy the gap in your knowledge or skill.

The previous chapter focuses on consent and the disclosure of important information by the professional to the client. Some of the information disclosed could be test results, the client's physical status, and what treatment options were available and their concomitant risks and benefits. Recently, ethics and law have also focused on whether clients are entitled to see their own medical records for themselves and whether they have a right to access those records. It is generally acknowledged that the client does not 'own' the record, as it was made in the course of treatment by a professional for the purposes of professional assessment and management. The record includes 'aides-mémoire' (French for memory aids or triggers), as well as personal information about the patient. Yet as it is primarily about the patient, shouldn't the patient be able to see it? Shouldn't there be frankness and veracity about its contents?

While the National Health Service in the UK is supportive of patient access and control over electronic distribution of their own data, the British Medical Association expressed concern that if patients share their information 'online', they will have lost control over sensitive information, and also that narrative aides-mémoire noted by the doctor may not be easily interpreted or be appropriate for a wider audience.[32]

There is concern that some information could be harmful or distressing to clients, and that the information should only be available if a professional explanation and counselling are also available. This concern amounts to a belief that any disclosure of information in health records should really be done in the context of normal consultative disclosure processes, and is less about veracity than about healthy and full communication between practitioner and client. The main exceptions to a health agency providing access to records when requested by the individual about whom they are written are if it contains private information about someone else, if having access could affect the person's physical or mental health or well-being, or if there is an overwhelming public interest in lack of disclosure. The two interests need to be weighed before such a decision is made. As you read earlier, holding something in confidence has a similar public interest importance and breaching that confidence requires a consideration of interests in doing so.

TRUST IN THE HANDS OF THE PROFESSIONAL

Clients have significant trust in their carers. Whatever process or procedure you are undertaking with your patients or clients, you can probably sense that they trust you are doing the best you can for them. Professional standards bodies and ethics committees are worried if the trust that clients have placed in their carer is abused. The abuse of trust is taken seriously because it goes to the heart of health care. When they need help, people are vulnerable, exposed, and dependent. If their trust in their carer is threatened, they may feel unable to return to the health care situation, even when they need care.

FROM THEORY TO PRACTICE

The client–carer relationship and fidelity

Contributor: *Leanne Boase*

Reflect on your own experiences as a client (or perhaps that of a family member of the client). What is it that has influenced you to trust or distrust the carer or health professional? If you can't be specific about trust or mistrust, perhaps you have decided to 'open up' on a particular occasion.

Specifically list any impressions that affected your decision. Was it appearance, manner, affect, statements, questions, or responses that influenced your decision? Were there other factors that influenced how you responded?

Now put yourself in the same situation, with the same health professional or carer, and consider how you might have responded if you had been in significant pain or distress. Would you have been more or less likely to engage openly with the carer? Would the decision be influenced by different perceptions? What are they?

Finally, put yourself in the position of the carer or health professional. How important is it to establish trust? What could you do to foster a trusting relationship with your client? What indicators would be evidence of a client not engaging well with you as their carer, or not trusting you?

The general public should also be able to trust that decent care will be available to them. Stories of abuse of trust can have a lasting impact on the trust that a community has in a professional, a profession, or an institution. One example of the trust placed by the public in health care workers is trust in maintenance of confidentiality, which is discussed below.

In the late 1990s, a Victorian health care worker was barred from practising medicine because he was found to have breached, on a number of levels, both professional standards and the trust placed in him as a health care professional. The *Daily Telegraph* newspaper reported: 'He has been found guilty of abuse of trust by having sexual intercourse with two current patients, by flagrantly defrauding Medicare, by misusing the doctor–patient relationship to borrow large sums of money from existing patients'.[33] The basis of trust was abused in a number of ways. Even just one of the abuses could have severely damaged the basis of trust. The issue of sex between practitioner and client has received significant attention in the press, and before professional standards bodies, because of its potential for extreme damage to the trust and care involved in the relationship between provider and recipient, as well as its potential to deter other members of the community from seeking help because of fears that the same could happen to them.

On a different level, a hypothetical story of potential abuse of trust in the context of a seemingly routine first procedure conducted by health care students has been published in the *Canadian Medical Association Journal*. (The essay, by Caroline Shooner, came second to the essay by Tara Young, which was noted above.) The patient in the story, John Brown, is to have a chest tube inserted, and the resident invites the third-year (postgraduate) medical student to perform the procedure. When they go into the patient's room, her anxious expression, slight hand tremor, and sweating is observed by the patient, who asks if she has inserted chest tubes before. The resident replies: 'Don't worry, Mr Brown, Jane is familiar with this procedure. I myself have done it many times. We are going to perform it together. Everything will go fine.'

Shooner points out the possibility that the patient has lost trust that capable and experienced medical staff are handling his care, and also that he may not have agreed to the type and manner of the performance of the procedures. In other words, the patient's belief that the doctor has been honest and comprehensive about disclosing the particulars of his treatment has been shaken. In this story, the moment of loss of trust passes, thankfully, as the procedure is performed skilfully, and the student is congratulated on the skill she showed.[34] Nevertheless, the potential for a loss of trust challenges the way students are used in real health care throughout their training. It is usually seen as a matter of truth and veracity that students divulge that they are trainees and disclose their level of skill with a planned procedure. There simply has to be a first time for every procedure.

PAUSE & REFLECT   You may like to think back to the first time you performed a certain process or procedure. Do you think you had the trust of your client? Do you think you deserved that trust?

RISK TO CLIENT OR CARER

Health care is, by its very nature, a risky business. As a health care worker, you will be in contact with people who are ill, or injured, or both. You will be exposed, sometimes, to dangerous situations and you will also expose your clients to some risk. Actively doing good and intervening often entails some risk. Your skill and care can minimise that risk. Institutional factors also influence how risky a procedure may be.

The following exercise explores one type of risk in a health care situation, and asks whether a proposed way of dealing with that risk can be seen as ethical. The risk is HIV transmission in health care situations, either from patients or from professionals. The proposed way of dealing with that risk is mandatory blood testing of patients and professionals. You will have seen this issue aired in the media and no doubt in your professional circles. Exercise 5.7 gives you a chance to try out some of the arguments for and against mandatory HIV testing. It was originally written up more fully as a teaching exercise in the journal *Medical Education*, and if you are undertaking this as part of a class or with colleagues, you may wish to refer to the full paper.[35] This exercise presents a contemporary dilemma that invites discussion of philosophical theory and ethical principles. There is no one answer to the exercise. It is designed to elicit opposing answers so that you learn about ethics as something that emerges from the construction of an argument. If you have a couple of groups working on different arguments this exercise will take about one hour.

EXERCISE 5.7 MANDATORY INFORMATION GATHERING

Undergraduate and postgraduate health students are training in the age of AIDS. They are likely to work with HIV (human immunodeficiency virus) and AIDS (acquired immunodeficiency syndrome), a disease that, now over 30 years after first being identified in the early 1980s, continues to evade researchers and clinicians. It is a long-term disease that poses serious and life-threatening risks to sufferers.[36]

Understandably, in the early years, health carers and health care institutions were very concerned about HIV/AIDS issues and the implications for clinical practice. The treatment of HIV and AIDS patients can be listed by institutions as an ethical concern, along with matters such as 'not for resuscitation' orders.[37] The concern centres on the fact that HIV is a blood-borne virus. Exposure to blood or other bodily fluids that contain the virus could pose a risk to others. Transmission could occur from patients to other patients or professionals, or from professionals to patients. Fear of contagion was a primary concern of health professionals dealing with AIDS, as evidenced by a Canadian survey.[38] Internationally, there has been extensive ethical debate over whether health carers are obliged to care for people with HIV or AIDS, given the potential risk to their own health.[39] Now, it is a routine part of practice, and professionals expect to encounter patients with blood-borne viruses, much more so in some countries and communities.

(Continued)

Patients with HIV/AIDS undergo numerous invasive procedures in the course of the disease, from repeated blood tests to more invasive procedures such as biopsies. It is arguably the more routine bedside procedures that pose the greatest risk of transmission from patient to professional. During the procedure professionals may prick themselves with an instrument that has been used on a patient.[40] Needlestick injuries appear to be very common. One survey found that over a two-year period all surgeons and roughly half of the medical-unit doctors, ward nurses, and emergency staff in a major teaching hospital in Australia had 'stuck' themselves at least once. Students also reported that they had been 'stuck'.[41] Workers not in direct contact with patients, such as laboratory staff or cleaners, are also at risk of occupational exposure.[42]

It is estimated that needlestick injury with HIV-infected 'sharps' carries a 0.4 per cent risk of HIV transmission and the development of HIV antibodies.[43] This is a small but grave risk, given the potential seriousness of the disease.[44] Minor surgery situations have alerted physicians and patients to the risk of transmission from patient to patient.[45]

The HIV status of professionals is also under scrutiny, although no risk of transmission has been calculated. Situations involving dentists and doctors with surgical duties have received greatest prominence.[46] The suggestion is that the likelihood of transmission from a professional is greatest in invasive procedures, when there is considerable exposure to blood and therefore possible transmission to the patient.

Such concerns about possible transmission led to early calls for mandatory HIV testing of patients and professionals.[47] It is worthwhile noting the difference between mandatory and compulsory actions here. A **compulsory** action is that which is required of everyone, and is enforceable. So, for instance, it might be compulsory for all citizens to register the birth of a new baby with a central registry. No exceptions are granted, and the action is enforceable under criminal law. A **mandatory** action is one that is only required contingent on certain choices and corresponding obligations. Dress rules in certain clubs and restaurants are one example. The dress requirements apply to people who wish to dine or socialise there. They do not become 'compulsory' for everyone, nor do they apply in other places apart from those establishments. Yet, if you wish to go in, you can expect to be checked according to the mandatory dress rules, and turned away if you do not comply. In the health care context, the call for mandatory testing is an expression of possible rules to apply to those who choose to make use of the services of health care. The call for mandatory testing was hotly debated on grounds of autonomy and considerations of serious and imminent risk, with many commentators arguing that protecting the rights of persons with HIV/AIDS should take precedence. There is no conclusive evidence that shows that 'knowing' a patient's HIV status reduces the risk of needlestick injury to a professional. The use by professionals of 'Universal Precautions' (the term used for accepted infection-control standards) and routine hygiene, such as handwashing between patients to prevent any cross-infection (even in the absence of knowledge of any viruses), is under scrutiny.

This situation poses an ideal dilemma for ethical discussion, enabling both health care workers and students to learn about ethics as a tool for structured and rigorous debate where complex and emotive issues are concerned.

Compulsory
Required action for all, with enforcement provisions.

Mandatory
Required action, contingent on being under certain command and corresponding enforceable obligations.

From what you have just read, try constructing a few points in the arguments for and against mandatory HIV testing. You could take the writings of J. S. Mill, which are about the philosophical importance of liberty and of not putting others at risk, as a starting point. Mill described different types of liberties, of thought and action, and claimed that all people had a right to exercise these as they wished, and they should only be 'interfered' with if others were at risk: 'The only part of the conduct of any one, for which he is amenable to society, is that which concerns others. In the part which merely concerns himself, his independence is, of right, absolute. Over himself, over his own body and mind, the individual is sovereign.'[48]

The four possible positions in the arguments for and against mandatory HIV testing for professionals and patients are represented by the quadrants in the grid below, which you could make use of in noting your points. The arguments about this really hinge on the definition and perception of harm, and of the risk of that harm. It is quite appropriate that the expected risk of harm is lower for professional-to-patient transmission than it is for patient-to-professional or patient-to-patient transmission. This is because any 'sharp' that has the blood of a professional on it should be immediately discarded and should not be near a patient. This is in contrast to a sharp with the blood of a patient on it, which is routinely discarded by the health professional, before or during which time the professional may 'stick' himself or herself. There are high-risk situations in which professional injuries may occur while the professional is in contact with the blood or fluids of the patient, most commonly in surgery.

Mandatory HIV test: argument grid		
	Mandatory testing	*No testing*
Patients		
Professionals		

The exercise also prompts assessment of the relationship between the particular liberty and the particular harm. For instance, it may be that what is required is an improvement of the universal precautions to prevent cross-infection, rather than knowledge of the HIV status of a patient or professional. This exercise illustrates that in order to construct arguments about ethics, it is necessary to have a good grasp of the facts (in this case, clear information on risk and the benefits of mandatory testing). The factual context can change over time, as clinical practices and standard treatment evolve. Ethical arguments are perhaps best constructed in conjunction with fellow professionals who can provide this crucial factual information.

After you have completed your basic grid arguments, you may feel you want to apply the reasoning to specific vignettes.

On the same theme, you may also like to consider the following hypothetical vignette.

<table>
<tr>
<td>PAUSE & REFLECT</td>
<td>A young man comes to your practice or hospital for treatment. He has injured his leg in a car accident. Conscious and alert, he tells you that he is HIV-positive. He is bleeding profusely, and requires treatment to stem the flow and repair the limb.

You might like to think about how you would have reacted 20 years ago, and how you would react now.</td>
</tr>
</table>

And another hypothetical vignette:

<table>
<tr>
<td>PAUSE & REFLECT</td>
<td>A patient is to undergo minor elective surgery, which you will perform. She notices that you have recently injured your hand, which has been sutured, but also that the injury has not yet completely healed. She asks that you undergo a blood test for HIV, and that she be told the results before the operation.

Consider how you would feel about the request, and what you think you should do, in relation to both your wound and the requested test.</td>
</tr>
</table>

These vignettes raise issues of infection control, and the risks and responsibilities of patient and carer. They also raise the ethically perplexing decision of whether health carers who have ethical objections to a particular form of treatment (or some other aspect of the client–carer relationship) have an obligation to take on the patient concerned and be responsible for their treatment. You can use these vignettes to ponder privacy and secrecy, and to consider whether there is any difference between the risks posed by clients to carers and the risks posed by carers to clients. The issue of privacy is dealt with in more detail in Chapter 4. You could use the same series of exercises with hepatitis C, which is also a serious virus, transmitted by blood contact, such as in reused intravenous equipment. Liver failure can result from hepatitis C infection.

RISK TO OTHERS

Posing risk to others is, in essence, a public health issue. Debate can centre on whether there actually is a risk, and in what circumstances. It is doubtful whether many blood-borne diseases should be described and treated as a significant routine health risk if there is no contagion risk in the course of normal population contact, such as airborne contact. Tuberculosis and influenza, on the other hand, clearly do pose significant public-health risks, as both are airborne. This assessment of risk is crucial. Unless the level of risk is established, the infringement on one person's rights in the interests of the rights of others is very difficult to justify ethically.

In Chapter 4, you read that caring for the client and for others is an important feature of the health care worker's duty to care. Chapter 4 explores confidentiality and trust in a professional caring relationship, as examples of aspects of this duty.

It discusses the fact that while the duty to maintain confidentiality is strong, it is not absolute: it can be breached where risk to others is involved. In some situations of significant and imminent risk of serious danger, there can even be a duty to disclose confidential information. This duty was tested in the famous legal case *Tarasoff v. Regents of University of California*, in which a patient told a psychiatrist that he (the patient) was planning to harm someone. The psychiatrist was found to have a duty to disclose this so that the person the patient was planning to harm could be protected.[49] This duty was said to depend on whether the potential victims are identifiable and whether other protective mechanisms are available.[50]

The client can act to minimise risk to others. For instance, after a person gives blood to a blood bank, their blood is tested for a range of hepatitis conditions. If there are positive results for any of these conditions, the patient is informed and counselled to pursue health care for their own benefit, and they are advised on behaviours that pose risks to others. Their blood is discarded from the donor pool. There is a large degree of trust placed in the individual to minimise their risk to others so that the infection can be contained.

Quarantine wards attempt to balance the aim of treatment with the aim of protecting others in society from diseases. Looking back into the history of quarantine, we can see that there are instances where it has been applied too widely—for instance, the practice of isolating people with developmental or mental disabilities. The balance (between treatment and protection) of risk that society is prepared to accept determines the laws and regulations that health care workers then implement. Private interests have, at heart, an individual's freedom to determine their own interests and therefore their own actions. This balance of public versus private interest is a social issue of ethical importance. Public health is in effect a paternalistic position which seeks to impose 'good' for the community as a whole, within certain limits that are socially determined. The private sphere is intruded upon in the interest of the health and safety of the community.[51] Countries that are comfortable with individual freedoms and risk taking would impose movement restrictions only in circumstances of severe and imminent risks to others. Further discussion on community input into deciding acceptable risks and benefits is included in Chapter 10.

TERMINATING A RELATIONSHIP

The ending of a health care relationship is a natural consequence of the beginning of that relationship. While the process of ending such a relationship is studied by many, such as rehabilitation workers, acute care workers, and counsellors, it is sadly neglected by others.[52]

If the treatment relationship deteriorates for any reason, the patient may need to be referred to another health carer. So a treatment relationship can end even though treatment is not yet complete. A transfer can be effected with the exercise of professionalism and without apportioning blame. The question is determining the best way to proceed with care for the patient, and that takes precedence over individual feelings of disappointment.

Once a task has been completed and the objectives of the relationship have been met, it may be time to move on to a new set of objectives. There can, of course, be reference points for reassessment. You can nevertheless stay in this cycle of defining objectives and monitoring progress repeatedly, as new objectives are set and health is monitored over a long period of time, if your role is to be available long term or if the treatment and management is a long-term process. Your level of satisfaction with the termination stage of a treatment relationship probably depends on the clarity of the goals identified early in the relationship.

To have a client return time and again when there is really no need, other than force of habit, could be viewed as overservicing. The health care worker may be taken to task by their peers—overservicing implies that the service is not being provided to meet a clear and reasonable objective. It may still be financially rewarding for the provider, but may not be giving any real or relevant service to the client. This dilemma highlights the importance of re-examining the good that is intended in any treatment relationship, which was discussed in Chapter 3.

If you, as a health care worker, are asked to do something you cannot or will not do, this may signal that your aims are incompatible with your client's aims, that the end (at least in part) of your treatment relationship is imminent, and that your client should be transferred to another practitioner. It may be useful to ensure that the client understands the full implications of what they seek, and why you feel you cannot be involved as their health care worker. When nothing more can be achieved by active treatment, the focus can properly shift to care and comfort. Health professionals find this particularly difficult when dealing with young patients, but it can be difficult with many other patients as well.[53] Team support in shifting the focus of care supports not only the patient but also the health carers.

SUMMARY OF KEY ISSUES

– Mutual understanding

– Trust in the context of disclosure and care

– Privacy and social limits

– Risk and harm posed by carers or clients.

SHORT NOTES

1   Honderich (ed.), *The Oxford companion to philosophy*, p. 380.

2   Spark, *Memento mori*, p. 140.

3   For a discussion of patient handbooks, see Corsino, 'Bioethics committees and JCAHO patients' rights standards'.

4   Berglund et al., *Exploring clinical ethics*, 2nd edn, pp. 195–6.

5   Flaherty, *Protecting privacy in surveillance societies*, p. 9.

6   Westin, *Privacy and freedom*, pp. 6, 7.

7   Berglund, 'Australian standards for privacy and confidentiality of health records in research'.

8   American Health Information Management Association, 'AHIMA Code of Ethics'.

9   Berglund et al., 'General practice and ethics'.

10 Westin, *Privacy and freedom*, p. 383; Flaherty, *Protecting privacy in surveillance societies*, p. 5.

11 Andersen and Aranson, 'Iceland's database is ethically questionable'.

12 Department of Health and Human Services (US), 'HIPAA administrative simplification statute and rules'; see Flores and Dodier, 'HIPAA', p. 5.

13 National Commission for the Protection of Subjects of Biomedical and Behavioral Research, *Institutional Review Boards*; and see the *Appendix* to this report, p. 309.

14 Beauchamp and Childress, *Principles of biomedical ethics*, 2nd edn, p. 232.

15 Westin, *Privacy and freedom*, p. 374.

16 Australian Law Reform Commission, 'Background report no. 22', *Privacy*, p. 20.

17 Czecowoski, *Privacy and confidentiality of health care information*, pp. 1, 3.

18 Ibid.

19 Mill, 'On liberty', pp. 92–3.

20 Pharmacy Board of Australia, 'Pharmacy Code of Conduct'.

21 Berglund and McNeill, 'Guidelines for research practice in Australia', p. 126.

22 *Privacy Act 1988* (Cwlth), *Privacy Amendment (Private Sector) Act 2000* (Cwlth), Principle 10, section 1(b); and Principle 11, section 1(c).

23 *PD v. Australian Red Cross*, New South Wales Supreme Court, unreported, December 1992.

24 Australian Research Council, Australian Vice-Chancellors' Committee, and National Health and Medical Research Council, *National statement on ethical conduct in human research*, 2007, and as amended 2009, at 2.3.6. p. 24; *Privacy Act 1988* (Cwlth).

25 Section 95, 72(b), *Privacy Act 1988* (Cwlth); Australian Health Ethics Committee and Office of the Federal Privacy Commissioner, *Review of guidelines under Section 95 of the Privacy Act 1988*.

26 World Health Organization, 'Alert, verification and public health management of SARS'.

27 Robotham, 'High-dose bird flu vaccine trial fails'.

28 Gostin, 'Medical countermeasures for pandemic influenza'.

29 World Health Organization, 'WHO News: Pandemic flu; Projected supply of pandemic influenza vaccine sharply increases', 23 October 2007, website press release item at <www.who.int>.

30 Surbone, 'Truth-telling, risk, and hope'.

31 Young, 'Teaching medical students to lie'.

32 British Medical Association, 'Information revolution could mean patients have more access to records'.

33 'HIV doctor struck off', *Daily Telegraph*, article.

34 Shooner, 'The ethics of learning from patients'.

35 Berglund, 'Mandatory HIV testing of patients and professionals'.

36 Centers for Disease Control, 'Revision of the CDC surveillance case definition'; Bacchetti and Moss, 'Incubation period of AIDS in San Francisco'.

37   McNeill et al., 'Ethical issues in Australian hospitals'.

38   Taerk et al., 'Recurrent themes of concern'.

39   Tegtmeier, 'Ethics and AIDS'.

40   Wall et al., 'AIDS risk and risk reduction'.

41   de Vries and Cossart, 'Needlestick injury in medical students'.

42   Centers for Disease Control, 'Public health service statement' on management of occupational exposure to human immunodeficiency virus; Jagger et al., 'Rates of needle-stick injury'.

43   Marcus, 'Surveillance of health care workers exposed to blood from patients infected with human immunodeficiency virus'; Heard, 'Multidisciplinary response of San Francisco General Hospital'.

44   Mallon et al., 'Exposure to blood borne infections'.

45   Chant et al., 'Patient-to-patient transmission of HIV'; Scott, 'Syringe may have held virus'.

46   Dickinson et al., 'Absence of HIV transmission from an infected dentist to his patients'; Larriera, 'Doctors' HIV'.

47   Connell, 'Doctors seek powers to test for HIV'; Di Angelis et al., 'State dental boards'.

48   Mill, 'On liberty', pp. 14–15.

49   Devereux, *Medical law*, 1st edn, pp. 220–1.

50   Coverdale, 'Ethics in forensic psychiatry', p. 67.

51   Beauchamp, 'Community', p. 59.

52   Burnard, *Counselling skills for health professionals*, 2nd edn, p. 103.

53   Sorlier et al., 'Male physicians' narratives'.

AT THE BEGINNING OF LIFE

- Personhood and beginnings
- Genetic issues
- Abortion

OBJECTIVES

This chapter discusses the more dramatic ethics issues at the beginning of life. Classical philosophical choices and contemporary comment are canvassed, and the changing nature of personal, professional, and societal views on issues relating to the beginning of life is explored.

The glossary terms that are added in this chapter reflect the fundamental issues of the philosophical interpretations of the beginning of life that are dealt with: personhood, person, and potentiality. The universal application of rights is reinforced, as in human rights assertions, and caution is expressed about even small exceptions or diminished standards of important principles. Specific terms like stem cell, genetics, and abortion have not been added to the glossary. These are defined within the text of the chapter, and are viewed as subjects of discussion and debate rather than examples of ethics pedagogy.

In this chapter you will see how ethics choices that may be made vary between countries, given the limitations provided by guidelines and laws. Research on specifically produced human embryonic stem cells may be possible in the UK, for instance, but may be prohibited in the USA. That doesn't mean that the ethics debate isn't raging in both countries. It just means that what can and cannot be carried out currently is different in each country, and that a window for full ethics debate is opened when changes to these guidelines or laws are suggested. Some of the ethics debates, and the forums that they are held in, are explained in this chapter.

PERSONHOOD AND BEGINNINGS

At what point do we give life moral and ethical significance? Human beings essentially start as clusters of cells, and, before that, as separate yet potentially significant elements of human life (single cells). The moral and ethical significance of life has been debated since the beginning of early philosophical thought.

The 13th-century philosopher St Thomas Aquinas spent considerable time studying the Greek philosopher Aristotle, who had debated form and matter. Aquinas's position was that the human soul was integral to the **person**. He believed that the soul determined what made an individual a distinct human being, different from all others.[1]

Person
Live human being, or live human being in development, with essential and recognised qualities of intrinsic capacity or function.

Modern philosophers continue the tradition of that debate. There is debate among some over whether life itself is an absolute good (the view that life is itself an absolute good can encompass the notion that even the mere potential for life is significant), or whether there is a particular point in development at which time human life takes on a moral significance.[2] Other philosophers, more controversially, argue that the right to life depends on the desire for life.[3] This may mean that only beings who are conscious, self-conscious, and desiring have a right not to be killed. Such philosophers even suggest that, depending on when this consciousness begins and whether memory is associated with it, all people, at least up to age four, are without a moral right to life, as are those who, by virtue of some degeneration, lose consciousness or their capacity to be desiring beings. Other philosophers have suggested that the indicators of the moral significance of life are brain development and an interest in human life.[4]

Solving this ethical problem is crucial in relation to processes that intervene in natural human reproduction. In vitro fertilisation (IVF) is one such process. It involves the external fertilisation of cells, and then implantation of the cells into the uterus. In order to refine this process, research was needed on human ova and sperm. The risk of damaging cells, and of 'wasting' cells, was ever present. The moral value of cells on their own, and of early embryos, needed to be debated. Mary Warnock, who chaired the British Government's Committee of Inquiry into Human Fertilisation and Embryology, has written a seminal article on this early debate, which occurred in the mid- to late 1980s, at the time when the UK was pioneering IVF.[5]

Personhood
Quality of being a person.

The Warnock committee reached a compromise on the issue of when **personhood**, and therefore moral significance, can be said to come into being, settling on 14 days after fertilisation. You might have a different view of when to begin attaching moral significance to life.

Mary Warnock's book *Making babies* is an excellent essay-style summary of the history of reproductive technology and the choices allowed within that technology. Warnock argues that it is a privilege, rather than a right, to have access to as many opportunities as science now affords us in making babies.[6]

Even apart from the issue of the age of cells and potential reproductive material, heated debates occur about the rapid pace and ultimate worth of modern technological reproduction. Feminist ethics has emerged as a forceful tool of analysis in examining what society is offering women in terms of medically assisted reproduction.[7]

In the early days of IVF, ethics classes discussed issues such as the creation and storage of embryos, and their disposal. Rules to 'flush' unused embryos at the end of five years prompted questions about why so many embryos were being created, and the position of the embryos as potential children if their potential parents changed their minds about their creation—for example, couples who plan to have a child then decide otherwise, or fail to establish successful pregnancy and give up, or who have separated and now have different plans for the embryos. You may like to consider the following dilemma.

EXERCISE 6.1 CHOICES AND LIMBO

In 1992, in the USA, a court case was heard to decide if a divorced woman could use embryos that she and her former husband had created and lodged with a clinic. Her former husband (the potential father) did not want this to happen. One newspaper headline at the time read 'Frozen embryos in legal limbo'. The case prompted debate on the right to procreation, and the right to avoid procreation. The right to life of the embryos was not established, as the embryos (a cluster of cells essentially) were classified as having a legal status somewhere between property and persons. The decision over whether or not they should develop to their full potential was thought to lie with the donors.[8]

Do you agree with this position?

If the donors disagree, should another 'guardian' make a decision on behalf of the cluster of cells?

Similar cases have since appeared in other countries, some regarding circumstances of sperm and/or ovum being stored prior to fertilisation. Does the fertilisation make a difference to your reaction to the significance of the stored cells?

IVF and related technologies have certainly led to myriad ethics dilemmas by virtue of the availability of viable and reproducible human cells. Embryonic stem cell research has captured the world's attention because it involves complex and provocative ethics issues. Stem cells can develop into any type of cell. They are embryonic not only in coming from an embryo, but also in terms of their undifferentiated form. The technology now exists to harvest embryonic stem cells from embryos, then implant them into other tissues to research their development into all manner of human cells. The proposition is that the cell regeneration could aid in the management of diabetes, Alzheimer's and Parkinson's conditions, and possibly even with spinal cord injuries by generating fresh fully functioning cells for affected organs and tissues.

A consequence of harvesting is that the embryo would not survive. So the debate has been about the intentional production of embryonic material, and about the use of those created for another purpose. The concepts of personhood are central to the debate. If you acknowledge the 'personhood' of an early cluster of cells, then person interests and rights would be expected to be respected; the potential for developing into a person can be treated as equivalent to attaining personhood. Even if rudimentary rights are afforded, the intentional creation and destruction of cells would then be objectionable.

Before embryonic tissue can be used for research, there is a consent process that often involves couples who have had IVF therapy. It is these people who have a reason to seek reproductive assistance, and therefore it is their embryos that have been created and stored and are most readily available for such requests. In this context, the embryo or embryonic tissue is regarded as a part of the fertility patient, that is, the potential mother and father, and their consent is needed before the embryonic tissue can be used for other than treatment purposes. You will remember a detailed discussion on consent in Chapter 4, and you will remember that the rigour of consent is open to ethical scrutiny. There is some research on that process of consent to suggest that couples who have agreed to donate surplus IVF embryos for research were generally concerned later about the social status of embryos that hadn't been selected to become a baby. In terms of the research request, they tended to view the donated embryonic tissue as an 'entity' rather than as a person or potential child. Their consent had been given at the start of the IVF treatment cycle, when they were mainly preoccupied with their treatment rather than the research request, and their main focus was on being able to have a baby. They didn't subsequently know if any of their embryos had actually been used in research. A number of interviewees were ambivalent when 'good', 'viable' embryos had become 'spare' and not implanted or frozen for this later use. The prospect of them having been used for research generated strong emotions.[9] Clearly there is more work to be done on this aspect of the embryonic stem cell research process.

We can learn from history, in terms of the debates that have taken place and the decisions that have been made, given the reasoning that was applied in a particular historical context. Much of the debate so far has been on the nature of the cell and the embryo, and their ethical significance. In the USA, there was extensive media coverage of the presidential decision on stem cell research in late 2001, and the ethics and religious advice on the issue. President Bush decided on a compromise: to allow federal funding for research on embryonic stem cell lines already created out of 'spare' embryos no longer planned to be used for IVF, but not to allow further stem cell lines to be intentionally produced for that purpose.[10] It was a compromise that did not satisfy religious objectors to any use of human life for other ends, or the scientists and researchers seeking full research flexibility. The Catholic Church always opposed IVF, as it increased the risk of disrespect for the **potentiality** of each individual life.

Potentiality
Capacity to develop in a certain way, given the opportunity and suitable development conditions.

The President's Council on Bioethics subsequently issued a white paper on alternative ways of sourcing embryonic stem cells (specifically human pluripotent cells), without the intended production, use, and destruction of such cells. The suggested options include deriving cells from dead embryos, biopsy to extract single cells, and other hypothetical manipulation of somatic cells such that their potential development as human embryos is altered. The emphasis was on finding alternatives to creating embryonic cell lines from viable embryos that would then be discarded.[11] On the scientists' front, the National Academy of Sciences in the USA issued guidelines to encourage embryonic stem cell research, with careful surveillance and oversight.[12] The guidelines are amended from time to time as the science rapidly develops and the processes of monitoring evolve. The National Institute of Health actively oversees human stem cell research in the USA. The monitoring systems are particularly scrupulous given that there is caution surrounding this area of science. The debate on allowable research directions was of course far from over and further examples of heated debates are evident, particularly at times of an election of a new president. President Obama removed the restrictions on federal funding of research involving new stem cell lines from leftover embryos from, for instance, IVF.[13]

The Presidential Commission for the Study of Bioethical Issues was formed in 2010 to advise the President on emerging issues in science and on ethically responsible practices in research, health care, and technological innovation, including in its charter the examination of issues relating to the 'creation of stem cells by novel means'.[14] The tone is one of encouragement for exploration of use of synthetic or adult stem cells as an alternative to embryonic stem cells.

PAUSE & REFLECT	We can learn from the debates and discussion of others when forming our preliminary views on a matter. Try the following exercise as a part of your early personal reflection on this topic.

Either individually or as a group, source an article on one aspect of the use of human stem cells. You can look in newspapers, editorial reviews, or professional journals for your article.

Identify the words that have an 'ethics' feel in your article, list them, and find definitions for them.

Try to identify how the words were used in forming an argument or position on the topic.

These words can facilitate your own process of reflection on a topic. You may find yourself in general agreement or disagreement with an argument. Try to identify why you feel that way.

The UK currently allows human embryos to be knowingly created for research purposes, including cloning techniques and stem cell research by licensed researchers. It is permitted up to 14 days after fertilisation, as in IVF research, when the primitive streak appears.[15] Extensions to the originally allowed uses for fertilisation have been added to allow specifically for therapeutic cloning for the development of treatments for 'serious diseases'.[16] These guidelines rely on deeming an early embryo of less than 14 days old to lack 'qualities' and to have 'potentiality' but not actual capacities (for thought, action, communication, and sentience), and so to have limited moral status. There has been criticism that this is objectionable, and that the resulting embryo research is therefore immoral.[17] The UK stem cell bank stores cell lines derived from adult, fetal, and embryonic tissues and makes these available to researchers with international monitoring and oversight by the Medical Research Council.[18]

Other countries have had similar rigorous debates, and alternative cell methods, such as harvesting specified adult stem cells, have been supported. These are differentiated, and specific in function to a specific type of tissue. Then, only ten years ago, it was thought possible, though more difficult, to culture cells from one part of the body and transplant them to other damaged sections, such as from a thigh muscle to a heart.[19] Now, research into this area has burgeoned, with success in rejuvenating various muscles and even with building tissue on a scaffold for a trachea using a person's own cells, which has the advantage of the body recognising and accepting rather than rejecting the reintroduction of the tissue. No anti-rejection therapies are needed, and the ethical debate on harvesting stem cells is sidestepped.[20] In a way, the ethics debates prompted alternative methods of therapy to be explored. There are now multiple options in stem cell research for researchers, with the community actively providing funding and constraint when considering research directions to concentrate on. If the debate had not been so heated on the ethics issues of personhood, potentiality, and sanctity of life, it may have been longer before the adult stem cell field was actively supported.

There is continuing community assessment of the acceptability of the product of the research, as well as its process. For instance, the European Union European Court of Justice was asked by Greenpeace in Germany to consider if it was acceptable to profit from some stem cell research if the commercialisation violated public order or morality. The decision was much anticipated as it would potentially impact on the feasibility of embryonic stem cell research in the UK and Europe. The Court's ruling, in 2011, was reportedly that it was not acceptable to patent research that has involved the destruction of a human embryo.[21] Such decisions may reshape the direction of research endeavours yet again, as it may not be feasible for companies to invest in an area for which they lose commercial credit. As you will now realise, the commercial decision they must make in this case is made in a context of community discussion and debates of ethical significance.

EXERCISE 6.2 CREATION FOR OTHERS

The manipulation of life and of people's lives is at the heart of the personhood debate. The following example provides a useful opportunity for reflection on the creation of and respect for human life. A story reported in the world's media in 1991 captured attention and focused debate on what the limits are for a family trying to help their dying child. A *Time* magazine article recounted how a couple had conceived a child (Marissa) in the hope that she would provide compatible bone marrow for a transplant to save an elder sibling (Anissa) who was suffering from a form of leukaemia.[22] The ethics of conceiving a child for that purpose, and, more generally, of using family members as live donors, were touched on in the media and actively debated by health care workers and ethicists.

The case of Marissa and Anissa is particularly challenging because it forces us to consider the sanctity of life. Marissa would not have been conceived if Anissa's life had not been threatened. Is it acceptable to use, or at least manipulate, life in that way? How important is the obligation to care for both Marissa and Anissa? How far should Anissa's and Marissa's and the family's autonomy extend? As part of your reflection, make a list of the benefits and drawbacks of this bone-marrow transplant. Make separate lists for Marissa, Anissa, their family, and the community.

BENEFITS

- Marissa
- Anissa
- Family
- Community

DRAWBACKS

- Marissa
- Anissa
- Family
- Community

Once you have your lists, try to decide whether the pluses outweigh the minuses. The crucial item on your list that makes you decide in favour of or against the procedure is likely to shed light on what fundamental principles are important to you, and what ethical framework you prefer to use.

As you think further about ethical frameworks, you could try to work out whether you are, for instance, more comfortable with deontological or utilitarian theories (see Chapter 2 for a discussion of these theories). You may remember that the deontologist is an absolutist. The deontologist decides which fundamental obligation is the most important—such as right to life, or right to freedom—and whether a proposed action violates that obligation. A utilitarian, on the other hand, weighs up the outcome of any action or situation and then decides whether it is permissible and/or what action should be taken. A utilitarian takes care to choose the action that is likely to yield the greatest good for the greatest number. The fundamental concern of each utilitarian is reflected in what they use as a measure of 'good'—for example, happiness or health.

It is worth spending time working out which of the philosophical stances you agree with. This will help to determine your reaction to the dilemmas posed by the specific issues that follow in this chapter: genetic issues and abortion.

GENETIC ISSUES

An international genetic project has studied the genetic composition of the human race. Called the Human Genome Project, its aim is to describe, or map, the human genetic structure to determine which genes are responsible for certain physical and behavioural characteristics. All human chromosomes carry DNA (deoxyribonucleic acid), and the Human Genome Project analysed and sequenced this DNA. An international group, the Human Genome Organisation, has coordinated the project's funding and scientific efforts, and the project was declared 'completed' in 2001, after which attention turned to mapping, variation, and identifying applications for personalised medicine.[23] The long-term aim is to improve the health of all individuals, but minority groups began asking whether this project would result in benefits for them. Many others were asking whether it was dangerous to understand exactly what we are made of too well, as that brings with it the possibility that someone or some group will control other people or all humans.

UNESCO cautioned against the misuse of the burgeoning knowledge in the Universal Declaration on the Human Genome and Human Rights, urging respect for dignity and rights regardless of genetic characteristics. As stated in Article 2b of the Declaration, 'That dignity makes it imperative not to reduce individuals to their genetic characteristics and to respect their uniqueness and diversity.'[24]

EXERCISE 6.3 DECLARATION—ENSHRINED CONCERNS

As an exercise, source the Universal Declaration on the Human Genome and Human Rights. This is easily accessed by looking up the UNESCO website (www.unesco.org).

Read through the whole Declaration, and summarise the concerns that are addressed in each of the sections or 'articles'. You will notice that they generally point to the danger of a loss of freedom and dignity, but try to identify what the concerns are specifically and gain an overall sense of the main concerns by reading the whole Declaration.

Compare your list of concerns with someone else who has done the same exercise if possible.

Human rights
Fundamental assertions and expectations of basic rights, thought to be due to all human beings.

Human rights documents are partly aspirational documents, in that they set ideals. Nevertheless they have some legal force because countries that agree to be signatories thereby state that they will endeavour to uphold those principles.

As more is understood about genes, the issue of predictive genetic testing, the availability of genetic information, and the possibility of discrimination or inequitable treatment in a social sense are vigorously debated. Genetic information is generally the subject of privacy protection, and inquiries are held into the implications for employment, insurance (in which risk assessment is vital), law enforcement, and database management.[25]

EVERYDAY ETHICS

Perhaps you know someone who has considered having a genetic test done; either a test on themselves, or perhaps on a child or foetus in utero. It is a complex issue, with personal and social implications. If you do know someone who thought about having genetic testing, what were some of their hopes and fears? How did that person make their decision to proceed or not?

EXERCISE 6.4 GENETIC PREDICTION

A simple genetic test kit became available about ten years ago in health-related lifestyle shops in the UK. For about £100, nine genetically determined metabolism processes could be analysed for your body. The focus was on diet and lifestyle. In the USA, a combined genetic-based test of predisposition to osteoporosis, heart disease, and immune deficiency became available through primary care practices, and worldwide through the internet.

Commercial genetic testing is the subject of guidelines, but these vary in different countries, and consumers decide if they want what the technology claims to offer them.[26] Note that a range of such directly available genetic tests are available to consumers, and professionals would generally prefer that they were only offered in a professional context.[27]

In a small group, consider whether you would be happy to have these tests available at all, and if so, whether they should be available

- in a shop setting
- in a practice setting
- via the internet.

List your reasons for support or objection in order from least to most strongly felt views.

Once an individual decides to undergo genetic testing, the information about the risks they face, or may carry in terms of genetically inheritable conditions, raises perplexing future decisions. Should they tell others or not? Should they change lifestyle or further risk factors? The decision to have a test is generally accompanied by counselling because of the complexity of consequences that may follow for themselves, their family, and their future family members.

David Suzuki has written extensively on the ethics of the genetic manipulation of plant, animal, and human life. His 'genethic' principles are, in summary:

- to understand, in detail, the nature of genes
- to be cautious in claiming to understand the complicated interplay of genes in behaviour and 'defects'
- to accept variation as a natural and desirable phenomenon
- to maintain individual autonomy over genetic decisions that affect us as individuals
- to preserve the distinction between genetic species.[28]

Exercise 6.5, devised as a tutorial exercise, can be worked through in groups or alone. It is a fictitious scenario of genetic manipulation (and genetic testing) that asks you to consider the ethical importance of the genetic process, and to nominate who or what groups might have ethical concerns about the process.

Suzuki's 'genethic' principles can be used as a discussion base for the exercise. You could decide whether they should apply, and if so, what they would mean for the polis proposed in the exercise. Alternatively, other principles, such as those of Beauchamp and Childress (beneficence, non-maleficence, autonomy, and justice), could be used to examine the issues.[29] The ethical dimension of genetic manipulation is partly about control over individuals and species, and partly a scientific debate on what is most beneficial, in the long term, for the reproduction and survival of a species.

EXERCISE 6.5 SOCIAL GENETIC PLANNING

It is the year 2100. A multinational, multifunction polis has been established in space. Its job is to investigate the further use of space in light of the overcrowded and climatically undesirable nature of the Earth. The results of the Human Genome Project have enabled researchers to identify a gene that predisposes people to obesity. Obesity-related complaints would be undesirable in the multifunction polis, from which people will not be able to leave for the next ten years. Too many ill people will drain the resources of the polis to the extent that the project would have to be abandoned. The administrators propose either to limit work permits to those who are cleared of the defective gene, or to rectify the genes of those with the obesity gene before they can gain work permits.

- What do you advise should be done?
- Is it a national or international problem?
- Should the polis go ahead?
- Should Suzuki's 'genethic' principles apply?
- What would be allowed under your country's guidelines for gene therapy?

Using the following justice models—justice as fairness, comparative justice, and distributive justice—advise how a genetic testing service could be distributed. You may wish to come up with different advice for each model, or you may wish to combine the models in producing your advice.

This works well as an exercise in determining what is a good that the society, or international community, agrees with, and then how that good should be distributed. As your good, you can use either the genetic testing for the gene, or the genetic manipulation of defective genes. You may like to look back over Chapter 3, particularly the discussions of resources and justice, before you try this exercise.

Apart from examining, understanding, and 'rectifying' genes, we are also on the threshold of the replication of entire genetic structures. This scientific advance, termed cloning, captured the world's attention.[30] Since 1997, with the creation of Dolly, the sheep cloned from another sheep, the ethics of the creation and re-creation of exact copies of individual humans has been discussed and debated. Dolly was created 'by transferring the nucleus from an udder cell into an egg whose DNA had been removed'.[31] Many countries around the world were prompted to enquire into the process and the reasons for it, and to ask what the ethical limits of such a process were. Should it be allowed at all, and should it be extended to humans? In the USA, President Clinton was very quick to promote public and government debate on the ethics of the process in relation to both animals and humans.

The US Senate Committee formed to consider the subject of cloning expressed a number of concerns about the issues it raised, such as the essence of personhood, the control over life, and the risk and harm resulting from the hundreds of failed attempts that preceded the successful creation of the perfect Dolly. They publicly stated that experimentation on humans would not be allowed.

The progress of Dolly has been closely followed, as has the progress and sudden health failures of other cloned animals. Dolly developed premature arthritis in 2002 and progressive lung disease in 2003, which led to her being put down.[32] Other cloned animals frequently suffer from heart failure and rapidly ageing constitutions. Despite occasional sensational claims that humans have been cloned, the risk of creating many unviable and desperately malformed embryos and babies in the process, not to mention the hidden uncertainties for the resulting live babies, acts as a strong deterrent to human cloning.

There are scandals in all research fields, but when the subject is cloning, coverage is immense. The accuracy of cloned human embryonic stem cell research results, as reported by an eminent Korean researcher, was called into question, leading to considerable media coverage. Researchers in the field then immediately reassessed how many of the earlier reported results they could rely on from that previously leading laboratory.[33]

Genetics institutes are working to minimise the impact that disabling conditions have on the lives of individuals. Further debate is needed on what should be considered a disability, and what is simply a part of the normal distribution and variation of characteristics in humans. The potential to develop a disability is also different from the actual development of disability. Should those with the potential to develop such conditions be thought of differently, and should they even be tested? Should such testing and information only be limited to what is socially and medically agreed to as being serious and disabling?

Early diagnosis of potential genetic disease is itself an ethics issue. It involves assessment of family responsibility for genetic predispositions and family ownership of genetic information, as well as individual autonomy and choice in investigating and controlling one's own health. Family members may well disagree among themselves on whether genetic disease is a collective problem or the responsibility of the individual. The balance between the responsibility of individuals for their own health, and the responsibility of the family (or of society) for the health of larger social units, may vary between cultures. In a position statement on genetic testing, Kare Berg has outlined the importance of family responsibility in serious disease predisposition from a Norwegian perspective.[34] The balance between family and individual responsibility is not the same in all cultures. Nor is the broad societal availability of genetic information uncontroversial.

In China, the policy position that requires couples to follow their doctor's advice to limit the number of children born with genetic aberration worries Western physicians and ethicists. The concern is partly about the use of genetic information and reproductive technologies, and then applying them to concepts of normality and disability, and partly about limiting the parents' autonomy.[35]

The above exercise about obesity testing in a hypothetical work space-station of the future could be changed to include any number of potentially testable characteristics, in any social situation. Genes predispose us to variations in appearance (height, weight, hair colour, complexion, etc.), as well as to internal physical variations, not least in our internal organs (and their effective function), and structural variations in essential organs such as heart vessels and lung capacity.

The debates that occur constantly in relation to the ethics of genetics are a prime example of the often dizzying possibilities that science and health care (either singly or in partnership) present us with. The possibility of changing the very nature of the human race is increasingly real. Every now and then, the community calls for a halt to such developments, and asks for reflection on their ethics and legality. The overall aim is to prevent us from losing control of our future to technology. The community seeks to agree on particular objectives for technology so that it can be harnessed, through agreed means, for those agreed aims. In setting these objectives and means, we can take into account the concerns of both deontologists (in relation to the process of change) and consequentialists (in relation to acceptable outcomes).

ABORTION

The issues of sexual activity, planning children, and pregnancy face most adults, and they test our ethical convictions in our personal lives and our health care work. These issues may raise the dilemmas of preventing or aborting pregnancies for medical, emotional, or social reasons. The following scenario can be used to ponder the ethics choices raised by pregnancy.

EXERCISE 6.6 PERSONAL CHOICES AND INDIVIDUAL DIFFERENCES

A married couple have been trying to have a child for some time. The woman is in her early forties. At last, they conceive a child. The routine ultrasound at 16 weeks reveals a very high chance of both Down's syndrome and various disabilities in the child. The couple pursue further tests, which confirm that the child is severely disabled. They now feel torn between their strong desire to have and raise this child, whatever its disabilities, and the fear that they may inflict a life of pain and burden on the child by allowing it to progress to term and be born.

What would you do in the scenario?

You may wonder whether Down's syndrome should be thought of as a 'disability', and you may wish to know precisely what the other diminished capacities are. Some medically defined disabilities may not be considered disabilities in other contexts, and vice versa.

The cultural context of such decisions may make a significant difference.

Abortion and contraception laws in each country reflect cultural stances and beliefs on the ethics of reproductive choices and the development of personhood. In some cultures, such as in China, abortion is officially seen as part of the range of contraceptive methods available. This is based on the belief that a human being or person comes into being at birth, not before. The Chinese debate over abortion is about the acceptability of late-term abortion rather than the acceptability of abortion itself.[36]

Health care workers who deal with clients in scenarios similar to those above will also feel that their discretion is limited by different laws, depending on where they work. Beyond that, they will make their own ethics decisions about whether or not to be involved. As mentioned in Chapters 3 and 4, if there is a service that an individual health care worker feels unable to provide, they should at least refer to someone who can explore the decision with the client.

FROM THEORY TO PRACTICE

If in doubt, pair out

Contributor: *Beah Revay*

This is a comment on the utility of pairing out your students after first giving them a clear task, a time limit, and often an example to get them started.

Here is a pair-out question which I use regularly in different tutorials:

- Can you think of ten issues which have ethical conflicts at the beginning of life? E.g. abortion.

(Continued)

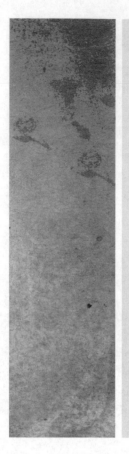

Once a pair says they have the nominated number of responses I get them all to stop. The pairs then have to report back. Every pair is then asked for *one* of their responses. This response is then noted on the whiteboard for working with later, or talked about directly (briefly). How it is responded to is determined by when in the class this occurs (beginning or end) and what I want to do with the points. I usually end up doing two or more circuits.

This pair-out has the effect of getting their heads into gear for whatever exercise I have to follow. It will often bring up one of the triggers I am planning to work on in the body of the tutorial (verbal gold star to that student); it ensures everyone contributes something as some students are really reluctant to speak, it is extremely non-threatening, and it shows the breadth of the topic area. I even make it into a competition—'First to the required number gets a prize'. The prize is the dubious opportunity (but strategic advantage) of calling out the first response. Since I go around the class a couple of times, that is a real benefit as they are not likely to find themselves in the position of having no new response.

I use this pair-out approach for other topics as well. In public health ethics and human rights classes, the initial pair-out questions could be:

- Come up with 12 public health initiatives that you are aware of, for example, healthy eating advice and advertising.
- Before considering further the whole notion of human rights, I want you to list ten things you feel strongly about, which you think have an element of 'human rights' to them, for example, the right to education.

It is interesting to note that the legal stance of each country and each state on difficult issues such as abortion may change from time to time. Also, key players in each side of the debate may alter their views. The *Roe v. Wade* court case in the USA made history in the 1970s as the case in which a right to legal abortion was argued for and was won. The ruling essentially limited the power of the state to intervene or interfere to prevent abortion before the foetus was viable, on the grounds of liberty of personal privacy for the mother. In an article published in 1996, the woman whose right to an abortion was at issue in that case, Norma McCorvey, discusses her changed views on abortion.[37] She became vehemently 'pro-life' (anti-abortion), in contrast to her former 'pro-choice' stance, and since the case she has campaigned outside abortion clinics to stop abortion. One of the things that reportedly made a difference was that she had become a fundamentalist Christian. This is an example of one of the features of ethical reflection. Over time, and given our understanding, convictions, and experiences, we can change our minds.

Government agency decisions and supporting discussion documents can provide an interesting public record of community sentiment and shifting ethics debates on basic bioethics issues. Their rulings provide the benchmark for subsequent administrative implementation of treatment processes. As an example, consider the morning-after pill, an emergency contraception that is routinely available in some countries over the counter. When a New York judge supported its over-the-counter availability to young women over 17 years old in a 2009 judgment, the focus was on the administrative justification for excluding 17-year-olds from access given that the Food and Drug Administration (FDA) had already decided that such women could do so safely, with appropriate consent.[38] So the legal focus of the decision was effectively on safety and autonomy. When the FDA granted general approval for the morning-after pill, the ethics debate on personhood and acceptability was assumed to have taken place elsewhere. A comprehensive critical review of the controversy surrounding the earlier approval process has been carried out.[39]

The same issue was debated extensively in Australian parliaments before being passed to the drug regulation body Therapeutic Goods Administration (TGA) to decide on.[40] The reading of the bill and speeches made by members of Parliament make for interesting reading. The issues raised include philosophical reflections on personhood and the intervention of humans in conception, religious expressions of doctrine and rules of conduct, and practical concerns about the risks that are posed and the benefits to be gained.

The morning-after pill RU486 is available in New Zealand and the USA, but in the latter at least, this availability is likely to be reconsidered by the Senate. The abortion laws are regularly debated again at the level of state legislature in the USA, and each debate generates further professional comment and discussion.[41] So the parliamentary debates in each country can provide an ongoing interesting insight into community sentiment and ethics debates on basic bioethics issues, as well as noting current practices.

Two prominent ethicists, whose work is frequently referred to by commentators in the abortion debate, and who use the paradigms of classical philosophy, are John Finnis and Judith Jarvis Thomson.[42] Thomson asserts a woman's right to choose, arguing that the potential to develop into a human is not equal to a human, just as an acorn is not equal to an oak tree. Further, she claims that a woman should have the right to choose to allow or not to allow an imposition on her body. She makes an analogy between this choice and the choice that a good Samaritan makes in helping another. Thomson uses the now quite famous analogy of a violinist to highlight how one body may be justly or unjustly imposed on another.

You wake up in the morning and find yourself back to back in bed with an unconscious violinist, a famous unconscious violinist. He has been found to have a fatal kidney ailment, and the Society of Music Lovers has canvassed all the available medical records and found that you alone have the right blood type to help. They have therefore kidnapped you, and last night the violinist's circulatory system was plugged into yours, so that your kidneys could be used to extract poisons from his blood as well as your own. The director of the hospital now tells you, 'Look, we're sorry the Society of Music Lovers did this to you—we would never have permitted it if we had known. But still, they did it, and the violinist is now plugged into you. To unplug you would be to kill him. But never mind, it's only for nine months. By then he will have recovered from his ailment, and can safely be unplugged from you.'[43]

Thomson's point is that the woman faces a difficult decision: whether to allow or not to allow another human being the use of her body. She argues that the woman has a moral right to choose what to do on her own terms and in her own way.

Finnis discounts this argument on a number of grounds, not the least being that the concept of rights is a popular concept that is widely used and misapplied. In Hohfeldian terms, a liberty or choice does not equal a claim right, which implies an obligation on another to act. (You may remember that Hohfeldian rights were mentioned in Chapter 3, as was the distinction between liberties, interests, claims, and rights.) Finnis questions Thomson's reliance on a woman's right (to anything), positing that a right does not exist until it has been proven to be a claim right. The notion of when personhood begins seems to be central to the debate between Thomson and Finnis; the earlier the point at which personhood is said to come into existence, the harder it is to discount that being's 'right' or 'claim' to life.

Throughout the parry between Finnis and Thomson, the different ethical frameworks of utilitarianism and deontology are apparent. According to utilitarianism, serving the greater good may justify inflicting harm on others, depending on the circumstances and on the consequences for the mother, the potential child, and society. Under deontology, intending harm is of the utmost ethical gravity, regardless of whether a good outcome may be achieved. Bad actions cannot justify good outcomes.

EXERCISE 6.7 TWO INTERESTS AND ONE IMPOSSIBLE DECISION

As a review of this section, try this further exercise, in a group if possible.

There seem to be increasing reports of conjoined twins. Tragically, in many instances, vital organs are shared and parents face the impossible decision of watching both slowly deteriorate in health, or agreeing to operate to separate them, knowing that at least one may die as a result. The religious background of the parents, the willingness of doctors to intervene, and the capacity of legal systems to make best-interest decisions vary between countries. See if you can think of a recent example of a conjoined twin birth, and research what happened. What were the views of those involved? What happened in the end, and what was the reasoning that contributed to the decision?

SUMMARY OF KEY ISSUES

- Personhood and potential for life
- Reproduction and medical intervention
- Genetic manipulation

- Community limits
- Abortion and autonomy.

SHORT NOTES

1   Collinson, *Fifty major philosophers*, p. 34.
2   Noonan, 'An almost absolute value in history'.
3   Tooley, 'Abortion and infanticide'.
4   Lockwood, 'When does a life begin?'
5   Warnock, 'Do human cells have rights?'
6   Warnock, *Making babies*.
7   See, for instance, Le Moncheck, 'Philosophy, gender politics, and in vitro fertilization'.
8   'Frozen embryos in legal limbo', *New York Times* article.
9   Haimes and Taylor, 'Fresh embryo donation'.
10 Hall, 'Bush OKs limited stem-cell funding'.
11 The President's Council on Bioethics, *Alternative sources of pluripotent stem cells*.
12 Johnston, 'Stem cell protocols'.
13 Robertson, 'Embryo stem cell research'.
14 The Secretary of Health and Human Services, Presidential Commission for the Study of Bioethical Issues, *Charter*, Washington DC 20201, 2010.
15 Plomer, 'Beyond the HFE Act 1990', p. 133.
16 Statutory Instrument 2001 No. 188, Human Fertilisation (Research Purposes) Regulations 2001.
17 Deckers, 'Why current UK legislation on embryo research is immoral'.
18 Stacey and Hunt, 'The UK stem cell bank'.
19 Robotham, 'Thigh gives heart a leg-up'.
20 Epstein and Parmacek, 'Recent advances in cardiac development'; Gong and Niklason, 'Use of human mesenchymal stem cells as an alternative source of smooth muscle cells'.
21 Naik, 'Patent ruling sets back EU stem-cell scientists'.
22 Morrow, 'When one body can save another'.
23 Jasny and Zahn, 'A celebration of the genome'.
24 UNESCO, 'Universal Declaration on the Human Genome and Human Rights'.
25 Otlowski, *Implications of genetic testing for Australian Insurance Law and Practice*.
26 Levitt, 'Let the consumer decide?'
27 Lovett and Liang, 'Direct-to-consumer cardiac screening'.
28 Suzuki and Knudtson, *Genethics*, pp. 345–6.
29 Beauchamp and Childress, *Principles of biomedical ethics*, 5th edn.
30 Hawkes and Rhodes, 'Human clones within two years'; 'Dolly's cloners say no to families', *Australian* article; Kuhse, 'Caution, not panic, on cloning'.
31 Pennisi and Williams, 'Will Dolly send in the clones?'
32 Hawkes, 'Arthritic Dolly is mutton dressed as lamb'; Smith, 'Cloning study points to early end for Dolly'; Schlink, 'Dolly dies of lung disease'.
33 Chong and Normile, 'How young Korean researchers helped unearth a scandal'.
34 Berg, 'Ethical aspects of early diagnosis of genetic diseases'.
35 MacLeod and Clarke, 'Forget cloning and pay attention to China'.

36   Qiu, 'Bioethics in an Asian context'.

37   *Roe v. Wade* (1973) 410 US 113; 'Abortion hero turns pro-life', *New York Times* article.

38   Annie Tummino et al v Frank M. Torti (Acting Commissioner of the Food and Drug Administration, US District Court for the Eastern District of New York, Brooklyn New York, Edward R. Korman, US District Judge, Judgment dated 23 March 2009; Memorandum and Order No 05-CV-366 (ERK) (VVP).)

39   Brooks, 'Commentary: RU-486'.

40   See <www.aph.gov.au/hansard> for both federal Senate and House of Representatives sittings in February 2006.

41   Tanne, 'South Dakota abortion ban encourages other states'.

42   Finnis, 'The rights and wrongs of abortion'; Thomson, 'A defense of abortion'.

43   Thomson, 'A defense of abortion', p. 48.

WHEN THE PATIENT IS YOUNG AND DEVELOPING

- Challenges to autonomy and informed decision making
- Who decides best interests?
- Ethically robust decisions
- Competence
- Information and comprehension
- Voluntariness
- Limiting what is asked

OBJECTIVES

Children in health care contexts bring into focus who is making health care decisions. In this chapter, the young and developing nature of the child is used to explore issues of autonomy and competency.

By now, you will have a basic understanding of many ethics concepts and terms, and these are relied on throughout this chapter. You may wish to review the glossary terms that have been added previously, particularly those in Chapter 4. Further terms that are added to the glossary are competence, comprehension, voluntariness, surrogate decision maker, and best interests.

CHALLENGES TO AUTONOMY AND INFORMED DECISION MAKING

As a health care worker, you can probably sense when your clients have limited autonomy. They may seem slightly or grossly incapacitated (mentally, physically, or both). By virtue of their (temporary or permanent) incapacity, it may be difficult for you to ascertain with precision what they want, and therefore to know what course they wish to pursue in their health care.

Sometimes there is no obvious incapacity. Rather, a limited understanding is just a product of the developmental stage of the client. Children are a large part of our population and a large proportion of the health care clientele. They also present some of the more perplexing autonomy dilemmas, as health care workers negotiate treatment with both the child and their parent or guardian. The themes in this chapter are also useful for thinking about declining or limited capabilities for active participation in decision making, which is discussed further in Chapters 8 and 9. Older people often lose part of their cognitive abilities. Any of us can, at some point, due to injury, sudden debilitating illness, or emotional or physical shock, be temporarily or permanently limited in our autonomy. At each of these times, we present health care workers with challenges as they go about the business of providing us with care.

In the face of these challenges, health care workers remain committed to the integrity of their clients. Sometimes it seems as if these challenges prompt an even greater effort in this regard. Human rights documents express a commitment to upholding the dignity and wishes of individuals, regardless of their current capacity or stage of development.[1] How that dignity can be maximised, and appropriate care instituted, is the real dilemma of caring for people with developing or diminishing autonomy.

EVERYDAY ETHICS

Think of a time when you had care and control of some children. Perhaps you are a parent, aunt, uncle, or much older brother or sister, or perhaps you were babysitting. In the course of the day, decisions need to be made. What to do? What to eat? How to clean up? How to negotiate disputes? How to deal with minor accidents and injuries? Think about how these decisions were made, and how much involvement the children had in them. You will probably find that this was different depending on the age of the children. Keep those everyday situations in mind as you think about children in health care contexts, remembering what children of different ages seem capable of in everyday contexts, and also distinguishing between when they are happy and when they are hurt, sick, or upset. You may also find that you had a tendency towards maximising the autonomy of the children, or of keeping control and acting paternalistically. Recognising your own bias in terms of autonomy and paternalism is useful for professional contexts in which you will deal with children.

WHO DECIDES BEST INTERESTS?

Our society recognises that a person with diminished autonomy may not be able to make all the necessary decisions for their own care. We rely on a parental obligation to children and a mechanism of guardianship for others with diminished capacity to make decisions in their interests if they cannot do so, after initially maximising their ability to make their own decisions. The common objective is to act in a way that is to their benefit and able to be judged by others to be in their **best interest**.

In the health care professions, where the autonomy of clients is a highly valued ethics principle and treatment decisions depend on rational and competent patients being partners in treatment plans, health care workers have additional protective obligations towards people with limited capacities.

Surrogate decision makers, who make a decision on behalf of another, may be used when the client's limited capacity to understand the nature of both the treatment and the illness at hand means that their autonomy cannot be upheld to a sufficient extent. While the client's family can help make decisions, they do not automatically become a surrogate decision maker for the client. Even a close family member will differ from the client in many ways, and therefore cannot replicate the values and personal choices of the patient. The best that can be hoped for is that an informed decision, based on the best interests and broad life-choices of the patient, will be made on their behalf.

There are limits to what these surrogate decision makers can decide. For example, the responsibility that parents have to make decisions on behalf of their children is, in effect, taken away when the procedures at issue are regarded as non-therapeutic and too risky. For instance, parents are limited in their capacity to consent to female circumcision and tattooing on behalf of their children.[2] Their power to make decisions on behalf of their children is also limited if it has been shown that they have acted against the child's best interest in the past. Society effectively reserves the right to intervene to ensure that the best interests of each child are upheld.[3] The ability of parents to give proxy consent for their children is, in essence, a safeguard to protect the well-being of children, and as such it may be limited if the child's best interests were not being served. Yet there is a dichotomy emerging worldwide, with trends in research guidelines promoting greater involvement of children in research participation decisions, and legal trends for children restricting choices and mandating the involvement of parents in certain decisions, such as for abortion in the USA. Intervention is generally more frequent for mature minors in mental health or personality disorders or life-threatening conditions, but it is not limited to these. Donna Dickenson argues that the agreement of the older child is needed for effective participation in treatment, so forcing treatment is problematic in a practical sense as well as ethically.[4]

Best interests
That which is judged to be to the maximal benefit of a person or persons in maintaining or furthering their health and welfare.

Surrogate decision maker
Person who makes decisions on behalf of another, acting as a proxy or substitute.

Guidelines and laws relating to substitute or assisted decisions are constantly evolving. The emphasis is on maximising the client's autonomy by assisting in the making of decisions and enhancing their comprehension. Once these steps have been followed, substituted decision making can occur if this is what is required.

So the guardians and substitute decision makers grapple with the concept of what is in the best interests of the client if the client cannot make that decision. The decision as to what is in the client's best interests is also informed by the professional opinion of the health care worker. The best interests of the client are, put simply, the primary interests of the client in maintaining and furthering their health and welfare.

On occasions, questions of best interests are decided by the courts. A process similar to the ethics analysis of gauging risks and determining limits to autonomy is used. A 10-year-old child was able to decide to donate bone marrow to an aunt of his who had leukaemia after the Family Court ruled that this was in his best interests. The risks to him were judged to be minimal, and the psychological benefits were weighed against these risks.[5] (Similar reasoning allows people to supply regenerative tissue for transplants to relatives.) Psychological benefit can include the exercise of one's own autonomy. The Family Court in this case assumed the role of guardian, as it does when there is a conflict of opinion over the best interests of a child. The crucial factor in a guardian's appraisal of the medical situation facing their charge is the value judgment involved in weighing the risks against the benefits.

ETHICALLY ROBUST DECISIONS

Ethically robust decisions are those that uphold autonomy. Further, the decision maker, in exercising their autonomy fully, has given consent that is fully informed and carefully considered. The basic elements of consent are achieved when the client:

- is competent (has the ability to understand what they are being asked to consent to)
- has the relevant information
- comprehends that information
- gives consent voluntarily.[6]

These elements are best achieved when someone has full autonomy and is allowed to exercise that autonomy. You will remember from Chapter 4 that autonomy means self-rule. If people internalise this abstract concept of autonomy, they are able to set their own course in life, and in health care, in a reasoned way that suits them best.

The following discussion of consent and autonomy in this chapter is divided into four areas: competence, information, comprehension, and voluntariness. It is designed to show how clients with a limited capacity for understanding complicate the issue of consent and pose challenges to the health care worker's duty to uphold autonomy. This section should be read in conjunction with Chapter 4.

The formal components of consent, outlined in the following paragraph, are set by law. This is one illustration of the way the law and ethics work together in setting acceptable standards with a legal emphasis of a minimum standard. The following discussion of consent demonstrates that ethics analysis can be similar to a legal analytical process in identifying elements and then exploring and testing those elements in a given situation, but remember that ethics ultimately emphasises the optimal, beyond the minimum required standard. Reflection on current standards and debate about possible improvements are essentially ethics discussions, and these can take place in your institution, within your profession, or in law reform or social policy forums.

COMPETENCE

Competence is a general term, relating to a person's ability and readiness to perform certain specified skills or tasks. In the area of informed decision making, this skill centres on the ability to analyse information and understand it meaningfully.

Competence
Ability to perform a specified task and readiness to do so.

A capacity to understand a proposed procedure, when considered in conjunction with age and maturity, and by implication the capacity to make a reasoned decision given that understanding, may demonstrate competence.

In the current ethical climate, the development of autonomy tends to be encouraged. For instance, children—particularly mature minors (usually children over 14 years)—can consent to minor procedures alone. With medical decisions, there is a tendency to adopt a midpoint, at 12 or 14 years, below which children are assumed to be incompetent, unless proven otherwise. Above the midpoints, children are encouraged to take more responsibility for medical decisions. These trends indicate the emergence of the view that children have a right to seek treatment autonomously. The United Nations Convention on the Rights of the Child supports due weight being given to children's views 'in accordance with the age and maturity of the child', which member countries strive to uphold.[7] This notion that the right of the child to autonomy should be upheld is also part of common law, the law that is built up through judgments handed down by courts, such as the one below.

> The common law can, and should, keep pace with the times ... the legal right of
> a parent to the custody of a child ends at the eighteenth birthday: and even up
> to then, it is a dwindling right which the courts will hesitate to enforce against
> the wishes of the child, and the more so the older he is. It starts with the right
> of control and ends with little more than advice.[8]

We recognise that a child's autonomy over their own lives and body develops continually. It would therefore make ethical sense as a child grows older to place, gradually, increasing reliance on their expressed wishes. This may mean relying on assent or agreement, even if these would not otherwise be sufficient to meet the criteria of consent.

In relation to mature clients, it is also possible to place reliance on particular indications of assent or agreement. This is similar to a maximisation of competence in the case of children; it allows appropriate decisions to be made by the client, given their capacity for reasoning and understanding of the likely risks and benefits.

There are ethical and legal grey areas in many aspects of children's maturity towards decision making. One quandary illustrates this. Imagine a minor who has not yet exercised a decision-making capacity for herself, but, by virtue of becoming pregnant and having a child, finds herself assuming decision-making responsibilities for her child. In a paper written with legal academic John Devereux, we argue that developing and supporting the minor is a high priority, as the minor's competence is crucial to ethically rigorous decision-making processes for herself and her child.[9]

EXERCISE 7.1 DEVELOPING AUTONOMY

As a tutorial exercise, map all the decisions you can think of that a pregnant girl of about 13 years of age will be asked to make in the few months leading up to the birth, and the few months afterwards.

Write a corresponding checklist of ethics concerns for each of those decisions.

INFORMATION AND COMPREHENSION

Information is essential in the consent process. The next step is for that information to be understood, or comprehended. The two steps rely on each other. To be fully informed you need to have access to good information, and also to appreciate its significance. The capability for understanding is competence. The capability is expressed in action by demonstrated **comprehension**.

Comprehension
Understanding, specific to issues under consideration.

You should ask whether your client is able to access relevant information, and then whether they are able to understand it. You may be able to assist in that process by presenting the information in a readily understandable fashion. The amount of information that clients are able to understand, the level of difficulty with which they can cope, and the effect of the way it is presented are all the subject of considerable research, even in relation to competent patients.[10] Of course, such issues become even more crucial when dealing with people of limited competence.

Some research on children's consent capabilities has shown that if information is presented in a personalised way children understand it much more readily. Rag dolls can be used to demonstrate how blood would be taken, for instance.[11] Other techniques that do not assume that the client has developed abstract cognitive abilities could also be used. To encourage them to elicit relevant information for themselves, children should be given ample opportunity to ask any questions they like.[12]

Health care teams constantly discuss how to resolve child and family best interests, particularly when there are conflicts with developing autonomy, lack of compliance with treatment regimes, and family rejection of treatment advice.[13] Developing a capability for decision making can be viewed as complicating already complex treatment issues, but is a necessary ethics process.

The gravity of such decisions makes a difference to whether a mature minor is deemed capable of making a competent decision. For instance, in the UK in 1999, a 15-year-old active girl became ill suddenly and required a heart transplant in order to survive. Her refusal of the transplant was overridden by a High Court judge, who deemed she was 'too overwhelmed' to make that informed decision. He approved the operation on grounds of best interests. This case is explored in Exercise 7.2.

EXERCISE 7.2 EXPRESSED WISHES AND CAPACITY

As a group exercise, discuss what you would do when faced with the girl's reported expressed wish: 'It's hard to take it all in. I feel selfish. If I had the transplant I wouldn't be happy. If I were to die my family would be sad. Death is final I know I can't change my mind. I don't want to die, but I would rather die than have the transplant, and have someone else's heart, I would rather die with 15 years of my own heart.'[14]

Once the legal ruling was explained to her, M gave her consent. The presiding judge, Johnson J, said in judgment, 'M will live with the consequences of my decision, in a very striking sense ... There is the risk too that she will carry with her for the rest of her life resentment about what has been done to her'.[15]

VOLUNTARINESS

Voluntariness is the final component of consent. People can feel coerced into agreeing, and this is particularly so for people with limited capacity because they tend to be dependent on others. Children can feel unable to disagree with the suggestions of their parents or health care workers.[16] Similarly, the aged and frail can have difficulty disagreeing with or questioning their practitioners or guardians.

Voluntariness
To decide own course of action with free and unconstrained will.

If you are ready for something even more complicated, try the next exercise. You should pay particular attention to the components of consent that you have now learnt about, and also the overall objective of maximising autonomous decision making. The exercise challenges you to consider the place of children in relation to their relatives who seek health care. In this case, a related child is present and available as an interpreter, a relatively common presentation in health care settings. Should the child be accepted as an interpreter though, and what are the ethical risks in terms of the child and the relative? You will need to consider the decision-making elements for both the relative and child to solve the puzzle. Bear in mind the following advice for professional interpreters who are part of medical consultations: to interpret the content, sense, and intent of what is said, and relay information in a neutral way, without withholding information or influencing decisions.[17]

An 84-year-old woman, Mrs M, comes to Casualty at 10 a.m. with her 9-year-old grandchild, Emi. They have arrived by taxi, and Emi has helped her grandmother to walk in and sit in the waiting area. Mrs M doesn't speak English, but Emi says that she can translate. Emi says her grandma hasn't felt well since last week, and has a pain in her chest and wheezing. Emi's parents are at work and won't be home until about 8.30 p.m.

You may like to read further on this topic in a jointly written article, which questions the ethical robustness of decisions made with a child as a link in the exchange of information between carers and patient. The article also questions the risk to the best interest of the child, who may feel an adult sense of responsibility and burden when placed in that position.[18]

LIMITING WHAT IS ASKED

In the context of research, we protect people with limited capacity, such as children and young people, by not including them unless the research is particularly relevant to them or people like them, and when research on other groups cannot answer the question specific to them—that is, their participation is indispensable.

As discussed in Chapter 12, there is a distinction between research that is for the benefit of the person or persons participating in the research (patients/clients) and that which is more for the general benefit of furthering knowledge. If the research is not therapeutic (that is, if it is not for the benefit of those participating), people with a diminished capacity are generally less likely to be included. This is particularly so in relation to children.[19]

Therapeutic research is much more ethically acceptable than non-therapeutic research, although how therapeutic benefit is defined is itself a matter of debate. As a general rule, the individual's position, and the likely outcome for that individual of whatever procedure is being contemplated, is the crucial consideration.[20]

There are equity issues regarding children's inclusion too, particularly if a social assessment of likely compliance with a trial treatment process is low given the parent's situation or lifestyle. For others, there is the burden of over-enrolment in serial trials if there is particularly good compliance with treatment protocols.[21]

The limits placed on the allowable risk to participants in non-therapeutic research highlights the way that responsibility is shouldered not only by society, but also by families in circumstances of limited capacity. The onus of deciding what treatment or procedures are justified is on health care workers and on substitute decision makers (those deciding on treatment plans on behalf of the patient).

In US research on healthy children, the concept of minimal additional risk over the risks of daily life has traditionally been relied on when no direct research benefit to the children is likely. A minor increase to this risk is acceptable only if those children have a disorder or condition, and the research is likely to benefit others from that group.[22] A more consistent notion of acceptable risk for children in research has been suggested by Nelson and Ross as the 'scrupulous parent' standard. This is a social construct about the level of risk a child should be exposed to.[23]

There are international instances of problems with non-therapeutic research, and with the consent process. One instance of apparent non-therapeutic research that received international attention—the storage of organs or tissues, without specific consent from relatives, of children who had died—raised tremendous ethics concerns. Though stored, they were neither examined nor used, nor had consent for their removal or storage been given. The inquiry into the practice at a UK hospital centred on a particular doctor, but during the course of the inquiry the practice was found to be more widespread than one site or one doctor. Stricter guidelines were recommended for the retention of organs, and it was recommended that consent for examination be mandatory. Many commentaries were written on the process of grief and bereavement for families, on discovering there was more of their child to be buried. Public trust in the hospital system and the veracity of treating doctors was also questioned.[24] Clearly consent, and the integrity of carrying out research processes that have been agreed to, underpins public trust in any process that is beyond the care for the individual.

Health care workers are constantly striving to improve health care and the treatments they make available to patients. Sometimes innovative research pushes the boundaries of current medical knowledge to its limits. When this research involves patients of limited capacity, and particularly children, there is unease among the community and the health professions. Community and ethics debate was heated when, in 1985, a newborn baby received a chimpanzee heart in an effort to keep her alive; she died shortly afterwards.[25] You are continually forced to examine what therapeutic benefit you hope to achieve and what the good is that you should and could aim for in the situation you are faced with. This is fundamental to our definition of health care, just as it is fundamental to the business of providing care (see Chapter 3). The belief that some good must be achieved is essential if a health care worker is to offer a potentially beneficial innovative treatment. This belief often takes the form of researchers championing the cause of the research, as is illustrated by a British researcher commenting on a ground-breaking living-donor transplant, performed on a 21-month-old child: 'We presented it to a large ethics committee and convinced them, although there was hostility at first.'[26]

The risks participants are facing are crucial to the assessment: Is someone about to die if not treated? Is their condition worsening rapidly? Do they face endemic risks? The latter was a consideration in early vaccine research in which children in institutions were participants. In the infamous 1970s Willowbrook experiments, vaccine trials for hepatitis were conducted on developmentally disabled children living under care in an institution called Willowbrook in the USA.[27] It was claimed that hepatitis was endemic there, and that therefore the children were likely to get it anyway; the side effects of the vaccine were therefore judged to be acceptable. This is a useful example for discussion of acceptable therapeutic boundaries. In my experience, the original research article, an account of a process that led to so much ethical and professional debate, fascinates health care students.

The Australian debate over vaccine research conducted in Australia in the 1950s and 1960s is mentioned in Chapter 10. In that research, orphan babies were given various vaccines, which had been altered to make them less toxic. The hope was that the babies would be protected from epidemics that were sweeping Australia.[28] So the same concepts of exposure to endemic and additional risk feature in academic commentary, as well as the discussion of who could or should agree to babies being included in such research, and who is best placed to consider the babies' best interests.

PAUSE & REFLECT	You may like to keep an eye on newspapers for discussions and critiques of health care or health research with children.
	When you read the pieces, note how the issue of autonomy is dealt with, and whether best interests features in the discussion.

SUMMARY OF KEY ISSUES

- Consent capability
- Enhancing decision making
- Competence to appreciate alternatives
- Information and packaging
- Comprehension
- Expression of choice
- Voluntariness
- Risk and best interests.

SHORT NOTES

1   United Nations, 'International Covenant on Civil and Political Rights'.
2   For instance, *Tattooing of Minors Act 1969* (UK) and *Female Circumcision Act 1985* (UK), both discussed in Dworkin, 'Law and medical experimentation', p. 193.
3   For instance, see Shawndra, 'State intervention in the family'.
4   Dickenson, 'Consent in children', p. 209.

5   *Re GWW and CMW*, Federal Law Court, unreported, 21 January 1997.

6   Similar components are described by Weeramantry and Giantomasso, *Consent to the medical treatment of minors*, p. 82. The components were established in *US v. Karl Brandt Nuremberg Code*, in *Trials of War Criminals before the Nuremberg Military Tribunals under Control Council Law*, no. 10, vol. 2, US Government Printing Office, Washington DC, 1949.

7   As in Article 12, 'The United Nations Convention on the Rights of the Child', 1989, was adopted by the General Assembly of the United Nations on 20 November 1989.

8   Lord Denning, in *Hewer v. Bryant* [1970] 2 QB 357 at 369.

9   Berglund and Devereux, 'Consent to medical treatment'.

10   Williams et al., 'Inadequate functional literacy'.

11   Berryman, 'Discussing the ethics of research on young children', p. 94.

12   Nicholson, *Medical research with children*, p. 144.

13   Harrison and Laxer, 'A bioethics program in pediatric rheumatology'.

14   Foster, 'Girl, 15, forced to have new heart'.

15   *R v M*, unreported, Royal Courts of Justice, Family Division, UK, 15 July 1999. Discussed in Forrester and Griffiths, *Essentials of law for health professionals*.

16   Grisso and Vierling, 'Minors' consent to treatment', p. 423.

17   Gietzelt and Jones, 'What language?', pp. 22, 23.

18   Berglund and Devereux, 'Consent to medical treatment'.

19   Berglund, 'Children in medical research'.

20   Ramsey, 'The enforcement of morals'.

21   Taylor and Kass, 'Attending to local justice'.

22   Department of Health and Human Services (US), 'Protections for children involved as subjects in research'; revised *Federal Register*, vol. 56, 1991, p. 28032, 45 CFR Part 46, Subpart D; Department of Health and Human Services, Food and Drug Administration, 'Additional safeguards for children in clinical investigations of FDA-regulated products'.

23   Nelson and Ross, 'In defense of a single standard of research risk for all children'.

24   For commentary and discussion of this issue, see Coombes, '"Paternalism" at the root of body parts nightmare'; Redfern et al., *The Royal Liverpool Children's Inquiry*.

25   Annas, 'Baby Fae', p. 15.

26   McBride, 'Living liver donor', p. 1418.

27   Krugman and Giles, 'Viral hepatitis', p. 1020.

28   Dow, 'Trials and terror'.

MID-LIFE AND HEALTH CARE CHALLENGES

8

- Patients/clients as consumers and community members
- Treatment in challenging situations
- Quality-of-life choices
- Non-compliant patients
- Pharmaceuticals and the development of new drugs

OBJECTIVES

Most of our lives are spent as adults, negotiating our own health challenges as they arise, and frequently taking on a role in the health care of our dependants. This chapter reinforces the earlier work you have done on the ethics of seeking and providing health care. The particular challenges posed for you as a carer by proactive or passive patients, differences in individuals' priorities concerning their health and health care, and urgent or challenging situations, are raised for your ongoing reflection.

PATIENTS/CLIENTS AS CONSUMERS AND COMMUNITY MEMBERS

The person who uses, or is likely to use, a health service is a consumer. More and more, consumers are regarded as active participants in health care. This is so in two senses: in the sense of being actively involved, as clients, in individual treatment decisions; and in the sense of having an impact on the design and operation of a health service. Their views on health care are valuable in alerting health care workers to the primary concerns and feelings of clients as they (the clients) negotiate the health care system.

A study of consumer perspectives on illness has been carried out in the Netherlands by de Ridder, Depla, Severens, and Malsch. These researchers used 'concept mapping' and discussion with consumers who had chronic disease. They found that consumers used two different dimensions to describe how they coped with illness: coping with the illness and coping with the health care system. In coping with the illness, autonomy and acceptance of the illness featured strongly. In coping with the health care system, a 'professional relationship with the physician based on mutual trust and respect between two equal partners' was emphasised.[1]

You will be familiar with the themes of client autonomy and the importance of a health worker–client relationship based on trust and respect, as you have encountered them earlier in this book. The theme of a person's acceptance of their ill health is new, and this varies significantly between people, as does their ability to cope with the challenges an illness presents in their lives. When a person falls ill, or has a need for a health service, he or she is coming to terms with that illness or need, and is at the same time entering a health service and seeking your help. This same study also makes a distinction between the modern consumer, who makes demands and is assertive, and the traditional model of the client, who feels powerless and relies heavily on trust.[2] There are different types of consumers. Some researchers question whether clients want to be involved in decision making. This is a separate issue from whether clients want to be informed.[3]

FROM THEORY TO PRACTICE

Consent and imbalance of power

Contributor: *Leanne Boase*

Think about what you now know about consent, and the active participation of both parties involved.

What could influence this active participation?

What relationships in health care could be affected by an imbalance of power?

If you heard a patient say 'I don't need to know anything, you know best, I trust you', when giving consent for a procedure, how would you ensure they were fully informed? Whose responsibility is this? Is there a role for advocacy?

Practise how you would approach the situation through role-play. Make sure you experience the roles of the client, the advocate, and the carer obtaining consent.

Consumers can be proactive in seeking not only what is available, but also the development or availability of further treatments or services. The section later in this chapter on the development of new drugs includes comments on consumer activists who, with an interest in the development of effective treatment for a particular condition, lobby and campaign governments and funding bodies to promote a research direction that may eventually result in a service being available to them.

Many consumers feel entitled to health care, as they are within a community that may offer it to them. If you accept a form of ethics that involves a sense of responsibility to others, then consumers also have a responsibility to society, ultimately, to seek only what is responsible and not to threaten the similar availability of resources to their fellow citizens.

But what of those who are so passive in terms of their own health and well-being that they make no use or scant use of the health care system for themselves? Is it also a responsibility of health care professionals to engage such people and encourage them to take advantage of health advice and health care? How far would that responsibility extend?

PAUSE & REFLECT	Take a few minutes to look back through the previous chapters. Try to identify all the theories and frameworks that you have already learnt about that would emphasise not only individual autonomy, but also put a limit to that autonomy because of a responsibility to be mindful of others in the community. See if you can construct an argument about responsibilities towards passive or non-attending patients.

Sometimes services are not so much pursued by consumers as promoted by society. For instance, consider a government immunisation program targeting basic diseases such as whooping cough, measles, and rubella. One quite complex ethics issue that needs to be planned for in the implementation of such programs is whether or not individuals should be able to decide to accept this service, that is, whether the program is compatible with allowing full autonomy. There is another layer of complexity in that such programs are usually carried out with very young children, and it is the parents who are effectively making the decision on behalf of their children and who have the responsibility to remember when a check-up and immunisation is due and to arrange a health visit for them. In one detailed paper which provided a précis of the debate, Michael Walsh argued that individuals should have a right to assess the benefits and risks of the immunisation program for themselves. The relatively small number of serious side-effects from vaccines may be more significant for some people than others, and poses a difficult dilemma for parents, as they try to balance their parental and societal responsibilities.[4] Can individuals make this choice themselves or has the choice been made at a societal level? Are the patients (or their parents) active consumers, or, by virtue of living in society, has immunising your child become a non-negotiable responsibility?

A former administrator of a children's hospital suggested in the midst of the debate that people who place others at risk by refusing such services should be denied other (non-health-related) state benefits: 'No parents have a right to deny a child's safety', and 'It's very simple. Nobody should receive child endowment or other benefits unless their child is fully immunised. If you accept the benefits of the State, you must accept your obligation to the community at large.'[5]

Rights and responsibilities are both featured in this statement. In accepting anything from our community, we are also reminded of our duties to others, who are collectively part of the community that has been able to care for us. This prompts a reflection on inherent responsibilities to others in our community and a reminder that in maintaining our health and that of our children, we are collectively contributing to a healthier society and population that may then be more self-sufficient and sustainable.

Immunisation can be effectively mandatory, in that unimmunised children can be excluded from state schools, during an outbreak, for their safety, and some federal government child care assistance has depended on up-to-date immunisation in Australia. There are widespread mandatory school immunisation requirements in the USA. A similar compulsory program operated for many years in the UK, with the allowance for conscientious exemption heard by a local magistrate. When concern increased over the safety of vaccination though, notably among UK parents, the compulsory nature of programs was revisited, and it is now presented as a vaccination program of 'choices' available through the National Health Service.[6] Italy and France have reduced their compulsory vaccination programs. If the perception of risks posed to individuals are seen to be serious, or imminent, they could outweigh the expectation that parents should immunise their children for the common good. There is a fine balance of autonomy and beneficence to be struck so as to maintain community good will and support in what is essentially a public health priority.

TREATMENT IN CHALLENGING SITUATIONS

As you have learnt previously, in deciding if someone can make an informed decision, the extent of their capacity and competence should be considered. Professionals keep in mind that exercising autonomy depends on the rational consciousness and reasoning ability at any particular time. When people are rushed into hospital and some particular treatment needs to be given urgently, a mini-mental test is sometimes used to see if that person is able to consent to the treatment. If they are found not to be competent at that time, a relative's permission may be sought or an appointed guardian may be contacted.

Paul Appelbaum and Thomas Grisso are eminent commentators on consent to medical treatment. They completed a study of patients' abilities to consent to medical treatment in two hospitals in Massachusetts and Pittsburgh, USA. Their sample included people who were hospitalised with acute, life-threatening conditions. Appelbaum and Grisso found that, like other patients, the acutely ill patients were able to give informed consent. Their judgment of ability to consent was made on the basis of the following four abilities:

- ability to communicate a choice
- ability to understand relevant information
- ability to appreciate the nature of the situation and its likely consequences
- ability to manipulate information rationally.

They used specific psychometric instruments (techniques developed to test psychology and cognition) to measure these abilities.[7] Their point is that even serious illness may not make people totally incompetent to consent. Their view would be that the ability to consent should be preserved and enhanced because of its fundamental importance in maintaining the integrity we derive from determining our own lives.

Bernat and Peterson have written on the issue of nominated surrogate decision makers, who may take over decision making for an incapacitated patient after surgical complications. While the patient may have consented to the actual surgery, once different post-operative decisions need to be made, the surrogate's decision comes under ethics scrutiny, particularly if it involves the refusal of further life-sustaining treatment. They argue that changed circumstances or complications make the surrogate's decisions more pertinent, and ostensibly different from the general consent to post-operative care that was given in a routine way by the patient prior to surgery. The expectation is that the patient's known views on incapacity and long-term disability would affect their surrogate's subsequent decisions in the circumstances of critical care. If they are not known, standards of best interests can apply first.[8]

Even if it is established that the client has limited capacity or competency, it may still be possible for them to make certain decisions. Social workers and residential carers whose clients are developmentally disabled advocate maximal autonomy for the client. There is a recognition that this is necessary not only because of the pursuit of autonomy, but also because exercising one's own life preferences supports physical well-being and social integration.[9] This recognition means that in the fields of social work and residential care, an awareness of the importance of autonomy and empowerment routinely accompanies training in ethics or philosophy.[10]

In many situations, health care workers think and act fast. Reflecting on potential dilemmas prepares you for how you might react, and what your options are. Taking on responsibility for treatment was discussed in Chapter 4. Emergency or critical situations make a decision to care quite crucial. What other help is available and the seriousness of the patient's condition make a difference in deciding whether a health care worker should attend and assist. The levels of duty to care can be debated in legal terms as well as in ethical terms. The commitment to help others (the good Samaritan principle) is recognised in such situations, and this means that even a practitioner who helps out without proper equipment and resources will, generally, be protected from being judged on the basis of professional standards that would otherwise apply. Some latitude is allowed the health care worker because of the immediacy of the situation.

Try resolving this dilemma. The essential elements of this vignette actually took place (but the story has been slightly altered).

A prisoner is booked in for a minor operation. On the day of the operation, the prisoner is transported from jail to the hospital in a prison van with two corrective services officers in attendance. The hospital is undergoing extensive renovations, and the parking close to the hospital is very tight. The prison van is parked a block away from the hospital, and the corrective services officers accompany the prisoner, soon to be patient, on foot to the hospital. At the corner of the hospital block, just after crossing a road, the prisoner attempts to escape. He runs away from the hospital, not back across the road, but down a side street. He is shot by one of the officers and is taken to the hospital.

· What should he be treated for?
· Do you think his consent to the original operation is still valid?
· Should he be treated for only the gunshot wound?
· What should the health care workers do?

You may like to canvass the interests at stake in terms of individual autonomy, the receipt of care and service, and the public's interests in efficient care provision. Is the fact that the patient is a prisoner relevant in health care ethics? Why or why not?

This should make for a lively discussion. Remember to listen with respect and attention to the views of others, especially if they diverge from your own.

FROM THEORY TO PRACTICE

Negotiating treatment

Contributors: *Erin Godecke* (speech pathologist), *Jacqui Ancliffe* (physiotherapist), and *Andrew Granger* (geriatrician, director of Stroke Rehabilitation Services)

A 28-year-old man was admitted to the neurology ward following an extended stay (70 days) in an intensive care unit with a severe hypoxic brain injury. He is fully dependent, has a permanent feeding tube in situ and a cuffed tracheostomy tube due to poor airway protection and multiple chest infections. He is MRSA +ve. He appears to have no meaningful communication system (i.e. no eye blink, yes/no response), but he responds to painful stimuli and to when he is moved.

It is now day 359 after his accident and his family are insisting that he be fed by mouth to increase his pleasure. He has had multiple failed attempts at oral feeding and decuffing

(Continued)

the tracheostomy tube, resulting in severe pneumonia. Clinically he has a very poor swallow, requiring suctioning to clear any oral bolus from his oral cavity post swallow. Microbiology have reported that further use of antibiotics for another chest infection is likely to be ineffective.

How would you negotiate further treatment/management of his oral +/- nutritional intake with the family?

Within the multidisciplinary team, who would you involve in the decision making for this patient? What role would each person have?

How would you ensure the patient wanted ongoing treatment? Who would make the decision on starting/ceasing further intervention for oral intake?

QUALITY-OF-LIFE CHOICES

Some professions work more with quality-of-life dilemmas than others. For example, rehabilitation counsellors engage a client in constructive discussion and organise social, emotional, and physical management plans to maximise the client's quality of life following an accident, illness, or physically demanding experience (such as drug addiction). What they are aiming for is to maximise the health and the life choices of their client. Quality of life is a value-laden term. It raises issues of what you should aim for with your patients—what you should allow or facilitate your clients to aim for. This is addressed in Chapter 4.

Quality of life is a key part of an ethics model proposed by Jonsen, Siegler, and Winslade. They stress that quality of life is not just a summation of medical indications and what the future has in store for someone physically. They argue that the value a person places on certain aspects of their well-being and life is part of their experience of the quality of living.[11] It is intertwined with an individual's perception and life preferences. Trying to assess this for someone else is, therefore, inherently difficult, and possibly fatally ethically flawed. The perspective that is used in determining quality of life is crucial: is it that of the sufferer or the health planner? Some commentators have been particularly concerned that the self-interest of health care workers may skew the quality-of-life measurements made in relation to their clients.[12]

Quality-of-life measurement and quality-adjusted life years (QALY) are measures of life expectancy, adjusted for disability and pain. They reduce complex social and well-being factors to a single score. Increasingly, narrative is being suggested as a better way of understanding such complex qualitative concepts.[13] The narrative approach to ethics examines stories told by patients or professionals, or experiences recorded in published material, to understand what issues are prominent from those particular perspectives. When QALYs are used to point to the relative successes of some treatments (and so to justify funding certain health programs at the expense of others) this generates debates about ethics. The use of QALYs was one highly controversial aspect of the Oregon cost program that was mentioned in Chapter 3. There is also a concern that formulas developed for determining increases in QALYs in relation to a particular condition may lead to a false expectation of real benefit for all sufferers of that condition.[14]

When the outlook for a client is poor, there may at some point be a debate on whether treatment should continue. When children are involved, this debate can be particularly heart-wrenching. The pain and suffering inherent in the child's condition, as key features of their quality of life, and in the proposed treatment, should be weighed against their expected life-span. The extent of the potential benefit is ethically crucial in deciding whether to continue with aggressive treatment (treatment that involves, for example, painful invasive surgery or other procedures causing pain and disruption to a child's life). The benefits should be weighed against the risks. For instance, prolonging life for a short time may not be a benefit that justifies as much risk as would the benefit of providing a potential cure.[15] Adults may choose a time when, for them, engagement in active health care just doesn't seem worthwhile.

NON-COMPLIANT PATIENTS

Non-compliant patients are part of routine health care work. You do your best to assess people, and then give them advice. If they don't follow your advice they can reduce their chances of effective recovery or improvement in their health. Shapiro et al. have described a skills-based approach for student learning reflection techniques so that they are 'able to work through emotional responses of anger, frustration, defensiveness and detachment towards patients and others'. The emphasis of the training was on being aware of one's own emotional reaction if patients 'did not seem to listen' to advice or 'apparently did not care about their health, and remaining ready to care when the patient was "ready" to engage with the care they could offer'.[16] Non-compliant patients test your commitment to putting further energy into their care. Think about the following situation, imagining you are in the role of the health carer.

PAUSE & REFLECT

A client regularly appears at the walk-in, no appointment necessary clinic, usually when unwell and wanting a medical certificate that states he is unfit for work that day. Frequent advice is documented in the notes about the need to eat more healthily and to exercise, so as to build an immune system that is more resilient to common infections, and for a follow-up visit so that any underlying cause of being sick so often can be looked into. With each appointment, a common response is 'I don't have the time' or 'I am only here for a certificate', sometimes said in a hostile manner.

What is your reaction to this? Could you use any reflective techniques to avoid an immediately emotional response towards him?

EXERCISE 8.2 ACCEPTANCE OF ADVICE

If you were working in a rehabilitation team, consider what assistance you would like to be able to deal with the following case.

You work in a rehabilitation team. A young man, Mr Y, aged 19 years, has come to see you. Mr Y's medical record shows that he has multiple health issues. He is slightly intellectually impaired, is on anti-epileptic medication, and has occasional rage outbursts. Recently he was in a car with three friends and was involved in an accident. At the time of the accident, one of his friends was riding on the roof of the car, and another was on the boot. The car was speeding on a dirt road, and rolled. Mr Y was inside the car, in the front passenger seat. He broke his leg so badly he needed surgery to have plates inserted. He is still on crutches. Mr Y's parents have rung you before the appointment. Apart from the lack of Mr Y's compliance with the physiotherapy suggested, they are worried about his risky behaviours and want you to convince him to find new friends. Mr Y asks for your help in getting more independence from his family.

In identifying the issues, take the time to flick back through past chapters of this book to refresh your memory on professional skill, resources and allocation, meeting and working with patients, developing and diminishing capacities, and so on. The scenario is quite a bit more complex than it seems on the surface.

Try to solve a couple of the ethical issues that arise in treating this young adult, preferably with the benefit of group discussion.

For the case-specific issue, role-play a process of consultation between the relevant parties (after deciding who is relevant), and suggest a compromise between them.

PAUSE & REFLECT

Now would be a good time to look back at the cases that were presented in Chapter 1. What can you now add to your reflection on those cases, given your developing understanding of the complexity of the issues in those situations?

FROM THEORY TO PRACTICE

Consent

Contributors: *Erin Godecke* (speech pathologist), *Jacqui Ancliffe* (physiotherapist), and *Andrew Granger* (geriatrician, director of Stroke Rehabilitation Services)

An 82-year-old woman was admitted to an acute care hospital with a large left middle cerebral artery stroke.

She was previously fit, very active, and independent with all activities of daily living. On formal testing and assessment, she presented with severe expressive and receptive aphasia characterised by inconsistent single word and short phrase utterances. She inconsistently understood single words but appeared to understand within a supported contextual environment with pictures, gesture, and extra time to process information.

She is refusing to eat and drink and participate in physiotherapy, occupational therapy and speech pathology each day. She frequently says 'let me die', 'leave me alone' and 'I don't want to be here'. Every day she has pulled out her nasogastric tube and intravenous fluid bung. Her family want her to have all intervention and want her transferred to a rehabilitation facility. She cries if she is taken to therapy areas and is clearly distressed by her current status. The medical team are planning to prescribe antidepressants and place a PEG feeding tube in for transfer to a nursing home as she is not participating in therapy.

How would you communicate with her to determine if she understood that she is likely to improve with rehabilitation if she participated?

How would you determine if she gave consent for therapy?

How would you determine if she gave consent for antidepressants?

How would you determine if she gave consent for placement of a feeding tube?

After revision of the earlier chapters, and particularly the information in Chapters 3 and 4, while considering the patient as an active consumer of services, try the following exercise with a group of fellow health workers, or with a group of students.

EXERCISE 8.3 DEVELOPMENT OF A SERVICE

Pick a good that your profession offers and trace its development and availability. This will make you revisit what your profession sees as a good, and how the potential for achieving that good is balanced against, on the one hand, possible harms, and on the other, the need to gather and deploy the resources necessary to aid its development and accessibility. As you find out about your good, think about what it means for your commitment, as a health care professional, to the principles of caring, doing no harm, respecting autonomy, and fair distribution. You may find that the relative emphasis you place on each of these will change. As you complete this exercise, take the time to look through the glossary terms you have already encountered in the earlier chapters. You should feel confident in your developing understanding of the process of ethics analysis, particularly in thinking about trained and skilled professionals ready to provide care in health care contexts, responding to consumer requests and needs.

PHARMACEUTICALS AND THE DEVELOPMENT OF NEW DRUGS

When you treat people, you look at what you can do, and you look at what is available as a resource to use in that management process or treatment process. Because new approaches and new treatments are constantly being developed, you need to keep up to date with professional literature to be able to make an informed assessment. This section looks at the development of new drugs. It is about the potential availability of a particular 'good', so it will serve as a further revision of some of the justice discussion in Chapter 3.

The development of new drugs is of tremendous ethical and social importance. It is fuelled by a need to find better ways of helping people with health problems, from niggling problems to minor episodic illnesses and chronic illnesses, and right through to serious and life-threatening conditions. The development of new drugs involves a massive human-resources commitment and substantial financial investment. It relies on government policy to provide both incentives and restraints (the latter for ethical purposes). More and more, the development of new drugs is being scrutinised and lobbied by patient advocates, and is increasingly attracting the scrutiny of social scientists and ethicists.

Given the political, economic, and social forces involved in drug development, it is not surprising that the policy objectives and guidelines surrounding this issue change from time to time. Australia provides us with a clear example of this, particularly in relation to regulations for the evaluation of new drugs. The regulations seek to provide a balance between benefit and risk, with the latter including the health risks posed to participants in any trial of the drug prior to its release. The resources available to support the development of the drug, and its eventual availability, are considered, as is the worth of the project. In its consideration of all these factors, drug evaluation illustrates many of the key features of resources and justice debates.

The information that the health department has typically sought in its evaluations has been extremely wide ranging, and includes pharmaceutical, chemical, animal, pharmacological, and toxicological data (as well as clinical experience). In other words, they tend to ask for basic scientific information and information on the drug's application in the clinical context. The department relies heavily on skilled scientists to assess the information. This system has developed gradually, taking shape from 1970 when Commonwealth legislation was revised to give the minister for health the power to issue permits for the importation of drugs (based on an analysis of the drug's quality, efficacy, and safety). Before that, the focus of the legislation was predominantly on the quality of manufacture of the drug, and on ruling out the likelihood that it posed severe and life-threatening risks.[17]

The realisation that thalidomide, an apparently harmless and effective morning-sickness drug, was linked to physical deformities in the children of mothers who took the drug resulted in tighter drug-evaluation systems in Australia and all around the world. However, in the quest for timely availability of new drugs, the drug evaluation system started to change again in the 1990s. Groups lobbying on behalf of AIDS patients conducted effective campaigns for a drug regulation system that 'maximises the safety and efficacy of treatments, while at the same time expedites access to those treatments'.[18] Summary data to support the drug being registered is now permitted, and human research ethics committees are relied on for the assessment of research proposals for drug trials in humans. Ethics committees must ask: does the proposed benefit justify the risk, and, if so, how much risk? Further, they need to consider whether it is acceptable to expose human participants to this risk, and other potential risks, before it is known whether the treatment will in fact work.

The decision process in human research ethics committees is the subject of further discussion in Chapter 12. The main job of these committees is to consider the ethics of research. They do so under the mandate of, but independently from, the institution in which the research is to be conducted, and they are guided by national guidelines.[19] The committees rarely have basic scientists—such as chemists, physicists, biologists, or pharmacologists—on board, and some committee members feel uncertain about their role in considering drugs and drug trials with human participants. The ethical challenge now may be to provide these committees with the support and expert advice they need to make a reasonable risk–benefit assessment of drugs, and to continue to protect the safety and welfare of human participants in research.

Drug production is a business, conducted by companies who need to turn a profit to sustain their business and investment. There is tremendous pressure for drugs to be provided cheaply once they are proven effective. Whether the pharmaceutical industry can be a medicine provider, particularly in less developed countries, is a matter of debate. The business invests large amounts of money years in advance of any anticipated return on new drugs. Many generic drugs are produced cheaply once patents expire, and governments support subsidies of essential drugs in their own countries. The issue has been heatedly debated in the African context of high morbidity rates and the impoverishment of large affected communities.[20]

Drug companies routinely conduct large research projects in developing countries, with treatment groups receiving treatments at no cost. The WHO issues guidelines on drug research from time to time, to apply across national boundaries so that research trials are of a high safety standard, even when countries do not have their own requirements. It is aimed at a basic protection, regardless of country, as is consistent with the WHO's universal view of health promotion, which was explained in Chapter 3.

Perhaps the challenge of bioethics in the applied research fields and the current age of globalisation is to transcend national and cultural boundaries, and to identify standards for research and development which are transparent, and acceptable to those affected by the research. The debate on the acceptable balance between risk and potential benefit in developing new drugs continues in Australia and is likely to continue worldwide as well. This debate is at the heart of research (research is discussed further in Chapter 12). The key questions are: What are the risks entailed? What risk is reasonable in the quest for new or better ways of providing health care? Which portions of the community should be asked to bear that risk? Further, what are the possible expected benefits? Which portions of the community should expect to receive those benefits, if they are proven? These are fundamental justice considerations regarding the definition of goods, harms, the pursuit of goods in the face of possible risks, the distribution of resulting benefit, and the bearing of burden.

This debate is in some ways also a debate about autonomy and beneficence. It is recognised that where no proven treatments are available, there is a place for the exercise of patient choice to undertake greater risk, and drugs and drug trials can be fast-tracked to allow that choice. However, there is an underlying limit to the amount of risk that people can choose to expose themselves to, and that limit is the willingness of professionals to help them. It is increasingly recognised that there is a limit to the amount of resources that can be committed to trying unproven treatments. Each proposal for increased patient participation and choice in drug trials is debated on the grounds of appropriate choice and appropriate risk.

The trend towards patient choice may have been carried to extremes, especially in the case of a serious, infectious, and life-threatening condition such as HIV and the resulting AIDS-defining conditions (illnesses indicating that a patient's HIV has progressed to AIDS). Towards the mid-1990s, the pendulum of professional opinion slowly swung back to again limit client choice to undertake risk, and a greater emphasis began to be placed on safety and reliable results.

Drug regulation illustrates how fluid the debate is over acceptable risk and objective benefit. The debate can swing depending on the context, perceived threat, and available resources. It is also constructed differently by different groups. To groups lobbying on behalf of those with seemingly incurable conditions, more risk in trying unproven treatments may be acceptable. To health professionals, a conservative risk would be preferable. If our society had virtually limitless funds, or if our society trusted entirely that individuals could choose their own best path in medical treatment, there is no doubt that the balance between, on the one hand, personal choice, and on the other, safety and reliability, would be quite different.[21]

Every now and then, a trial of a new medicine in humans brings about unexpected harm. When this happens, the need for protective mechanisms, and considered weighing of risks against benefits, is highlighted. Drugs are tested on healthy volunteers in the early phase of clinical trials. Catastrophic immune responses can and do occasionally occur in such trials, such as in one trial in the UK in 2006. Remarkably, all of the six volunteers survived, with one requiring months of hospitalisation and all facing serious long-term ill health. Calls for tighter restrictions on potential risks posed to participants predictably followed, as well as vigorous discussion of consent protocols for such trials.[22] Consent in research is discussed further in Chapter 12.

SUMMARY OF KEY ISSUES

- Challenges in balancing autonomy and justice
- Critical decisions and urgent contexts
- Perspective in deciding priority and quality of life
- Balancing risks and benefits for clients and others.

SHORT NOTES

1   De Ridder et al., 'Beliefs on coping with illness'.
2   Ibid., p. 557.
3   Deber et al., 'What role do patients wish to play?'
4   Walsh, *The National Childhood Immunisation Campaign*.
5   Joel, 'The man who cares for kids'.
6   Salmon et al., 'Compulsory vaccination'. For UK vaccination program choices, see <www.nhs.uk/Planners/vaccinations>.
7   Appelbaum and Grisso, 'Capacities of hospitalized, medically ill patients to consent to treatment'.
8   Bernat and Peterson, 'Patient-centered informed consent in surgical practice'.
9   Newton et al., 'Focusing on values and lifestyle outcomes'.
10 Henry et al., 'Attitudes of community-living staff members towards persons with mental retardation, mental illness and dual diagnosis'.
11 Jonsen et al., *Clinical ethics*, p. 151.
12 Richardson, 'The importance of perspective'
13 Edgar, 'A discourse approach to quality of life measurement in the measurement of quality adjusted life years'.
14 Fryback and Lawrence, 'Dollars may not buy as many QALYs as we think'.
15 Leiken, 'A proposal concerning decisions to forgo life-sustaining treatment for young people', p. 19.
16 Shapiro et al., 'Teaching the art of doctoring'.
17 *Therapeutic Goods Act 1966–73* (Cwlth), particularly section 29(1), *Therapeutic Goods Amendment Act 1991* (Cwlth), section 4.
18 Australian Federation of AIDS Organisations, *Submission to the Baume Review*, p. 4.
19 For instance, National Health and Medical Research Council, Australian Research Council, Australian Vice-Chancellors' Committee, *National statement on ethical conduct in research involving humans*.
20 Henry and Lexchin, 'The pharmaceutical industry as a medicines provider'; Lee, 'What is past is prologue'.
21 Berglund, 'Bioethics'.
22 'Urgent changes needed for authorisation of phase I trials', editorial, *Lancet*.

DECLINING PHASES OF LIFE AND END-OF-LIFE CHALLENGES

- – Decision-making components in action
- – Declining phases and end of life
- – Suicide
- – Euthanasia

OBJECTIVES

Declining capabilities are a routine part of a lifespan. At some stage, frequently in old age, we can all expect to diminish in our capacities and health, and decline towards a natural death. This is not a dramatic ethics dilemma in itself, but it does raise ethics issues in terms of decision making for care throughout that phase of life. The consideration of this practical aspect of care integrates your earlier reading on autonomy and consent, with particular emphasis on competence.

The more dramatic ethics issues that arise when death is actively pursued by an individual or is hastened by others are also considered in this chapter. The classic ethics positions in the debate on the acceptability of such personal and professional behaviour are provided. Deontological positions are prominent in the critical reflection on the ethics of suicide and euthanasia, and you will notice that the consideration of the autonomy of the person who is demonstrating or stating a choice to end their life is also a constant theme in the discussions. The terms advance directive and slippery-slope argument are added to the glossary.

DECISION-MAKING COMPONENTS IN ACTION

An assessment of the client's competence (their ability to understand the treatment on offer) is routinely made in health care, and particularly in aged care. A question about competence is often asked by nurses, medical practitioners, relatives, or other visitors. Each is monitoring whether the patient understands their situation and the options available. Despite the fact that the assessment of competence is routinely carried out and is a vital skill, it has been the subject of few practical guides. One helpful list of issues to consider has been formulated by a team of clinicians and ethicists, which you can pose as questions as you consider the circumstances of each patient:

- conducive environment and conducive frame of mind for decision making
- extent of cognitive function and stability over time
- adequate information available to the patient, which has been given and understood
- view of health professional
- additional factors relating to social situation and family.[1]

These questions clearly go beyond a simple 'mini-mental examination' of the patient, which focuses on the patient's orientation to time and place (and awareness of environment), to the environmental constraints on competence and decision making.

The rule of thumb is that it is rare for people to be incompetent for all decisions they must make. The competency of any particular client should be assessed with respect to their current circumstances and the specific decision that faces them—consent is consent to a specific treatment.

This routine assessment of competence is ethically critical. Without competence, a person cannot give valid consent. If their competence is limited, then there are limits to what a person can consent to. Generally the limits are that only minimally risky and minimally invasive procedures can be consented to. That is because someone must be capable of making a decision before they can be judged to have made it. Try the next exercise as a review of the issues of competency and decision making. You may like to look back to earlier chapters, particularly Chapter 7, as you consider the elements of consent, and ponder on furthering autonomy and the assessment of competency.

EXERCISE 9.1 DIMINISHING COMPETENCY

Now, as a review of the competency issues, think about a case story about Lisa and Martin, two people with dementia, who live in an aged care home.[2] Lisa's husband has died, but Martin's wife is alive and visits him regularly. Lisa and Martin spend most of their time together, and appear to believe that they are married, even wanting to sleep together at night. They appear very happy, apart from when they are separated into their own rooms by staff. Lisa and Martin's children have been asked about their views, and they have asked

(Continued)

for the two to be separated at night. The staff feel they have to protect Martin's wife, and try to make sure Lisa and Martin are not together when she arrives.

Think about what issues this situation raises for Lisa, Martin, their families, and staff. Concentrate on competence, choices permitted, and veracity.

With declining capacity to make sensible decisions for one's own safety and welfare, others begin to step in and assume the day-to-day aspects of care, safety, and comfort. Ensuring a safe environment for patients is difficult, particularly in contexts which are inherently dangerous if a person is prone to wander or fall.

Nursing professionals routinely face the ethically complex issue of how to ensure a patient remains in a safe environment if the patient's own capacities for avoiding danger are impaired. Ethics tools can help with this consideration, as a paper by Ann Gallagher demonstrates. Different restraint techniques, including psychological and technical (physical) options for stroke care patients, were analysed with reference to Jonsen's model. You will remember this model from Chapters 4 and 8.[3] Written from a practical nursing perspective, Gallagher argues for restraint only as a last resort, after consideration of alternatives and the impact of such a choice, given the medical indications, patient preferences, quality of life, and contextual features that are part of the situation under consideration.[4]

DECLINING PHASES AND END OF LIFE

When patients suffer a cardiac event, this is sometimes unexpected, but most often it is an expected part of the previous decline of an elderly or seriously ill patient, and marks the natural end of their last phase of life.

Nevertheless, a choice must often be made about whether or not to resuscitate a patient. Some commentators lament the fact that cardiopulmonary resuscitation (CPR) is being increasingly used in all hospital deaths, so much so that people are not being allowed to die. Intervention could be seen as prolonging suffering and doing harm in what often seem to be inevitable deaths. Laws are sometimes passed in some jurisdictions to excuse health care workers from the obligation to resuscitate patients who are classified as 'Do Not Resuscitate' (DNR).[5] In general, these reforms stipulate that where a patient has rapidly diminishing lung or heart functions, care and comfort may be given instead of CPR (or other resuscitation techniques). This is ethically important. The imminent death of a patient does not excuse health care workers from offering help, but the goal of this help may not be saving life.

In an ideal situation, anticipating the end of life allows the patient and carers to be comfortable about the 'plan' ahead when the inevitable does occur. Ethics reflection can be helpful in exploring the path ahead for both patients and carers. Consider the compelling description of the collaborative application of Beauchamp and Childress's principles in a Californian intensive care unit, when a young woman became ill ten months after her lung transplant and subsequently died. You will remember the explanation of Beauchamp and Childress's principles of beneficence, non-maleficence, autonomy, and justice in Chapter 2.[6] The process of her coming to terms with the imminent death, and the role of the clinical team in 'creating a warm and open environment', is described as a collaborative and ethically aware engagement, with frequent open discussion of quality of life and end-of-life issues, and limits to options in care. The patient herself made the decision on the timing to remove her intubation tube and stated her final wishes by writing letters to her family and fiancé.[7]

An **advance directive**, which means advance indication of the decisions a patient has made about guiding their future treatment and care, is increasingly being sought from patients whose condition makes it likely that they will lapse into a critical situation. Their autonomy continues to be important, and what they would wish in particular clinical circumstances is taken into account. Just as is the case with consent, however, their expression of choice needs to be specific. Advance directives can be difficult to accept because, although a patient may express what they would like to happen given a particular situation, the unpredictability of their symptoms means that they may not be able to grasp the true nature of what it would be like for them if that situation did come about. This means that the validity of carrying out their wishes can seem questionable to those evaluating the directives in the context of the emerging situation.

The practice of patients providing advance directives relies on the assumption that a competent patient is able to choose whether or not to undergo further treatment, including life-sustaining treatment. 'Living wills' mandate which treatments patients do or do not want, and are prepared ahead of time to be used if the patient becomes 'incompetent'.[8] Their practical use as the only expression of an autonomous care decision is limited by the fact that, routinely, decision-making power may be retained by many more people (that is, family) than was anticipated. When no specific advance directive has been given by the patient, clinical judgment and the 'guardian process' are routinely used. As you will remember reading in relation to children in Chapter 7, such a decision that is made for others is based on grounds of best interests, effectively upholding beneficence, rather than the autonomy of the patient.

Advance directive
A directive given by a patient in advance that represents their autonomous wishes and is intended by them to guide their treatment and care in the future.

FROM THEORY TO PRACTICE

Aged care perspective

Contributor: *Tracy Edwards*

Providing ethical care in an aged care setting requires special consideration. Many clients will have dementia or other cognitive impairment. Others do not, but still may or may not

(Continued)

be able to communicate their thoughts. The degree of impairment varies hugely between clients and often even within the one person. Cognitive impairment can fluctuate with acute illness, time of day, and certainly over a longer period. A diagnosis of dementia does not necessarily mean a lack of capacity for consent. Deciding as a health care professional how to gain consent can be a complex business and yet this is crucial to a person's dignity at a time when other control over even basic functions is diminishing.

It is a mistake for the health professional to feel that their experience will always guide them in the best choice of treatment for a particular person.

Consider the case of Eve, now aged 93 years. Eve has advanced dementia and lives in a nursing home where she now requires help with changing position, toileting, and eating. She spends her days in a bed or comfortable float chair. It would be very easy for the professionals looking after Eve to make decisions about any health issues in a unilateral way—in fact, that would often be the most time-efficient. However, if the same professionals were to get together and discuss what they would want for themselves in the same situation, we would find that as individuals they might have quite different views.

What if the patient developed rectal bleeding, a possible sign of cancer? Who would want to investigate to find out? If the decision is not to pursue active treatment, who would still want the test? What if the test was invasive or uncomfortable?

What if the patient got a chest infection? Who would want to be transferred to hospital if oral antibiotics failed? Who would want any antibiotics at all? Who would just prefer to be kept comfortable, even if that meant possible sedation or increased chance of death?

What if they could no longer swallow well, were not eating, and were losing weight. Who would want to be tube-fed?

What if they, like Eve, had dementia but it had not yet progressed very far and they could still walk and talk to people in a meaningful way and recognise family? Would their thoughts be different?

What if they had a major family event looming like the birth of a baby or a wedding?

Having worked in aged care for a number of years, I find that perhaps the biggest fear most clients voice is being powerless in a system that continues to treat and test in the face of increasing disability. Most fear this more than death. Every presenting problem presents choices. The only way we will know we are acting in the client's best interests is to talk to them early about the things in life that they value and the care they want, or if they lack capacity, to honour their previously expressed wishes. Previously appointed guardians or their family or people responsible may know their previous thoughts and wishes better than us, and to honour a person's autonomy is to talk to those designated people.

The choices may extend beyond care around death, as the background to the following exercise shows.

EXERCISE 9.2 TRAGEDY AND FURTHER CHOICES

An interesting combination of ethics issues has been debated in various countries when married men die from sudden illness or traumatic injury, and their wives seek to obtain semen from them before they die so that they can store the semen in an IVF facility and use the semen to conceive a child at a later date. See if you can list what sorts of ethics issues the following scenario raises.

In 1995, Mary's husband became suddenly ill from meningitis and died aged 30 years. Mary said they planned to have children, and asked doctors to extract and store his semen, which they did. Later, Mary was denied permission to use the semen in the UK but subsequently won a High Court case to take the semen to Europe and use it there, in an agreeable IVF facility. There, she conceived a first child in 1998, and a second, four years later, in 2002. The birth certificate did not initially list a father's name.[9]

Think about choices and how they are made and expressed, and the process of reproductive assistance involved.

In the Netherlands, there are also explicit guidelines for withholding or withdrawing intensive care from newborns who are 'nonviable' or dying. These are justified on the grounds of consequent suffering, futility of treatment, and quality of life, and are in some contrast to the approach in other countries of 'saving' babies born at progressively earlier weeks of pregnancy. The Dutch argument is that this results in tremendous morbidity, meaning ongoing disability and health issues, due to poor health outcomes for extremely pre-term infants of below 26 weeks of a normal 42-week gestation.[10] Since the information on complications of a premature birth that is routinely presented to an expectant mother is limited, and many premature infants are delivered in an emergency admission, there may be scant time to prepare the parents for being involved in treatment decisions on their newborn. This presents an ethical difficulty for their optimal involvement in decisions on the infant's treatment, particularly in the earliest decisions on giving intensive treatment.[11]

PAUSE & REFLECT

Thinking about two prospective parents in this situation, look back to the decision-making components that you read about earlier in this chapter. Which of those components is readily achievable as the parents prepare to make decisions on behalf of their newborn?

Can you guess which parent often becomes the primary decision maker in this situation? Why?

Try and identify the parent who is most likely to satisfy more of the decision-making components for an ethically robust decision-making process at the time of an emergency admission.

(Continued)

You will probably realise that maximising the information available in readiness for any such decision depends on both parents having had access to professional advice and information throughout the pregnancy, and also, ideally, on the couple sharing the information each had received separately during the preparation leading up to the birth. This would maximise their autonomy of course, but it would also increase the quality of their direct input into best-interests decisions for their newborn.

FROM THEORY TO PRACTICE

Ethical dilemmas in health care settings

Contributor: *Jade Cartwright* (speech pathologist)

While ethics is an intrinsic part of everyday practice as a health professional, there are certain contexts where ethical dilemmas can arise more frequently. I experienced this working as part of a multidisciplinary team managing clients with complex neurodegenerative conditions including Huntington's disease and dementia. As a speech pathologist my key role was to support my clients and their families to optimise communication and swallowing functions and improve quality of life. Over the years, my colleagues and I worked through a range of ethical dilemmas including non-compliance with recommendations, barriers to best practice, and, inevitably, end-of-life issues. A woman with advanced dementia who was living in a residential aged care facility remains fresh in my mind. Her husband had cared for her at home for many years and was still very involved in her physical and emotional care. I would visit the facility regularly to review her swallowing and give support and education to her husband, who visited her every day and still expressed the same degree of love and admiration for her as the day they married. As lifelong partners she was his life and I watched as he sat with her, held her hand, and gently assisted with her meals. When she was approaching the end of her life and struggled to finish each mouthful of food or drink that her husband gave her, he clearly cherished every moment that he got to spend with his wife. As her dysphagia or swallowing difficulties worsened the inevitable recommendation came that she was no longer able to eat or drink safely, with attempts causing her increasing distress. Her husband expressed to the team a strong desire for a feeding tube to be placed. His wife could no longer communicate, care for herself, or mobilise independently, but her husband clearly stated that he was 'not ready to say goodbye' to the woman he loved. While he honestly felt that she would not have chosen the feeding tube or her current situation for herself, he felt that he could still bring quality to her life and a connection that was worth fighting for. She did not have an advance health directive and he was her enduring guardian. Much time was spent working through this end-of-life decision with staff at the facility and the visiting GP, and a feeding tube was eventually placed to meet the husband's wishes.

This is a complex scenario. You are not expected to reflect on whether the outcome was right or wrong, rather:

- Identify which ethical principles apply.
- What are the qualities of a 'professional carer' that are needed to deal with this scenario?
- Are there any questions that you would like to ask the team or the client's husband?
- What responsibilities does a health professional have to their client, their employer, their colleagues, and themselves in this scenario?

SUICIDE

Suicide is the killing of oneself. Arguments about whether or not suicide is a legitimate action tend to centre on whether a person should interfere with their own life. Arguments against the legitimacy of suicide often rely on the 'God-given' sanctity of life; those supporting its legitimacy often rest on the principle that ending one's own life is a natural extension of autonomy.[12] Both sides seem to agree that suicide attempts by 'incompetent' people, who by definition are not acting autonomously, should be thwarted. Depressive symptoms, for instance, can often be seen in people who attempt suicide. Health care workers whose clients manifest suicidal tendencies often intervene to treat or refer the client for their depression, to ensure their safety and help them to return to competent decision making.

EXERCISE 9.3 FINAL PLANS

You may like to ponder the following dilemma. It was written as part of a study about ethics in a general practice setting. The vignettes in the study were constructed in response to the ethics concerns of general practitioners and consumers (these concerns were determined from a survey).[13]

A 52-year-old woman has breast cancer with bony secondaries (the spread of cancer to the bones). She is not currently in pain, and could, with treatment, have a good quality of life for two or more years. She tells her GP that she will not take the medication and that after getting her affairs in order she is going to kill herself. The GP discusses this with her, and suggests that she seek counselling, but she refuses.

Some six months later she is found dead in bed, having overdosed on medication prescribed for a recent hip fracture.

Even if suicide is not illegal, aiding suicide still could be. Do you think the doctor did aid the suicide? Is the choice the woman's alone?

A Swiss hospital has reportedly decided to allow patients with the intention of committing suicide to use their beds, with the explicit help of assisted suicide groups. The patient must have an incurable disease, be of sound mind, have expressed a persistent wish to die, and carry out the final act themselves. The hospital has been reported to state their overriding principle of respecting the patient's wishes as determining their decision.[14] The debate on suicide is explored further in the next section on the subject of euthanasia. Physician-assisted suicide is seen as one type of active, voluntary euthanasia.

EUTHANASIA

Euthanasia literally means an 'easy death', or a 'good death'. It has been hotly debated, particularly in the Australian context of the debate over the Northern Territory law giving people a right to a physician-assisted death (*Rights of the Terminally Ill Act 1995* [NT]). The passing of this Act was followed by the lengthy development of protective guidelines before a handful of people used it to gain medical assistance to die. Subsequently, a private member's Bill, known as the Andrews Bill, designed to overturn this legislation, was introduced into the Commonwealth Parliament. Eventually the *Euthanasia Laws Act 1997* (Cwlth) overturned the Northern Territory law in the Commonwealth Parliament. This Act made euthanasia equivalent to murder or manslaughter. The initial Northern Territory Act and the process involved in both its inception and its eventual defeat involved people at all levels of the community in active debate about euthanasia.

As in any medical decision involving an ethical or moral element, the practitioner may decide not to participate in the process. As is the case with abortion, if the practitioner does not wish to assist in the process, they would be obliged to refer the patient to someone who would be prepared to discuss or investigate the issue. This discretion is part of the notion of professional caring. It is up to each professional to decide what type of care they are prepared and willing to offer; in other words, to define beneficence in their own terms (this was discussed in some detail in Chapter 4). Beyond this initial decision on the part of the practitioner, the extent of the illness and what can be done for the patient is a key consideration, as is the reasoned and informed nature of the decision-making process. Much of the debate over the Northern Territory legislation was about whether fewer patients would be asking to die if more could be done to offer dying patients effective care and comfort in palliative care. Even apart from the question of the adequacy of palliative care, patient autonomy and patient perception of the extent and significance of their illness is a crucial consideration, whether as a safeguard that the decision to die is voluntary, or as the primary reason to allow physician-assisted suicide. These issues assume varying degrees of significance in the various euthanasia debates, depending on how much autonomy is valued in its own right.

EXERCISE 9.4 PRINCIPLES IN REGULATIONS

The process proposed in the Northern Territory Act is represented in the flowchart below.[15]

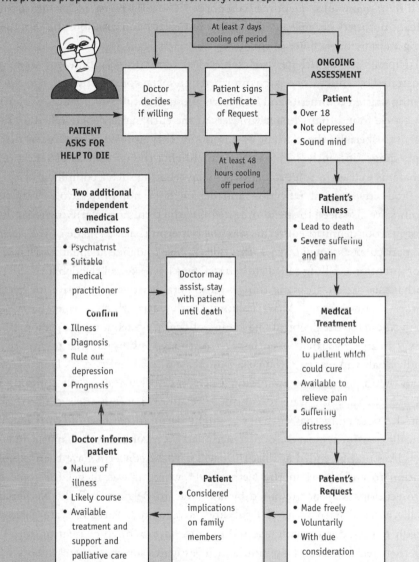

There is a sense in the Act of the importance of establishing that the patient's illness is terminal, that it is the patient, and not some other party, who is seeking the 'treatment', and that there has been considered and slow reflection (on the part of both the doctor and the patient) in reaching what is, in effect, the final decision of a person's life. As an exercise in identifying the nature of the key ethical issues in the process (and the Northern Territory legislation's response to these), try tagging the boxes in the flowchart with the principles of beneficence, non-maleficence, autonomy, or justice. The competent and autonomous nature of the decision is a crucial link in each step.

The death of the first person to make use of the provisions under the Act was reported in the media. Although the first media report on his situation stated that he wished to remain anonymous, his name was revealed and his explanatory letter referred to in many subsequent media reports.[16] The GP who cared for him assumed significant notoriety because he was willing to explain and promote the rationale of allowing an individual choice of this sort.[17]

Participants in the debate used key ethical terms in very different ways, as is demonstrated by a piece of research informed by a social constructivist perspective. By examining written comments and interviews about the issue in Australia, the authors of this article found that while key players in the euthanasia debate relied on moral arguments, especially the concept of autonomy, they applied these arguments and concepts quite differently.[18] This analysis highlights the usefulness of reflection on the debate, as well as the importance of actually debating such a complex and emotive issue. Productive ethical reflection and debate does not only involve canvassing viewpoints: we also need to spend time defining the terms and clarifying what we are discussing. Poor definition of terms was one criticism that was made of the Andrews Bill. In particular, as noted by Cica, this Bill's failure to define adequately what is 'the form of intentional killing called euthanasia' may have skewed the debate.[19]

Euthanasia can mean many things; most notably, it can be 'active' or 'passive', 'voluntary' or 'involuntary'. Active, voluntary euthanasia, which is what the debate is currently about, is 'the deliberate hastening of death, on request by a person, to ease distress'.[20] In an early article on euthanasia, Anthony Flew argues that the will of even one individual who wants euthanasia can create a legal right to it. This argument relies on the importance of upholding a person's liberty and on the suffering that would occur if their life were to continue.[21] Caution is often advised to safeguard against the possibility that euthanasia might occur in connection with less than extreme illnesses, or against the occurrence of active, involuntary euthanasia, in which people's lives may be ended against their will.[22] These concerns have been expressed in relation to euthanasia in the Netherlands, where it was illegal for some time but prosecutions were not required by law. Now, in Belgium and the Netherlands, medically assisted euthanasia is legal, and is regulated. Patients state their wish repeatedly to their doctor, with whom they must have an ongoing relationship. Their doctor then seeks a second opinion and investigates alternative treatments which may provide potential improvement in the patient's condition, and notifies the review committee of the patient's request. Each case is subject to a review process before final plans are proceeded with.[23] The **'slippery-slope' argument**—an argument that relies on the notion that allowing something in one situation opens the way for the same action to be used unacceptably in different situations—is often used in debates over euthanasia.

The form of euthanasia that seems to be implied by the Northern Territory Act can be called suicide. The procedure involved the patient initiating the process by pressing computer responses to confirm that he or she wished the fatal medication to be

Slippery-slope argument
An argument that small 'slips' in standards will lead to larger 'downwards slides' and a degradation of standards, so that any small slips should be vigorously guarded against.

administered. The doctor had of course aided the process by setting up the equipment and preparing the fatal compound. The first documented physician-assisted suicide in the USA in the 1990s by a former physician was with an Alzheimer's patient who travelled across America to seek his help to die. The article that first reported this suicide is a useful starting point for discussion. The picture in the article shows the suicide 'device': three intravenous bottles connected up to a drip. The process is set up by the physician, then the drip is started by the patient pushing a button. The process begins with a harmless saline solution. This solution is then increasingly infused with two drugs to induce unconsciousness, and finally, heart-cessation and death. This article reports that the former physician, 'a long-time advocate of euthanasia, said he took the action partly to force the medical establishment to consider his ideas. He said he knew he might face arrest.'[24]

EXERCISE 9.5 ADVICE FOR PROFESSIONALS ON ASSISTING WITH FINAL PLANS

Whether patients are entitled to ask for this help, and whether doctors or other health care workers should provide it, are crucial questions. Examining ethics-related codes can help you to identify the controversial points in the euthanasia debate. Take one professional code and one consumer code of rights and responsibilities, such as is set out in the Queensland *Health Rights Commission Act* (or in an Act of any other state),[25] and try to identify points of possible support or opposition to the action that the former physician reportedly undertook. This exercise highlights the emphasis, in both consumer and professional codes, on patient autonomy. It also underlines the importance, in the context of euthanasia, of assessing how ill someone is, and whether treatment options are available or have been tried. One medical association code of ethics states the following in relation to the dying patient: 'Remember the obligation to preserve life, but where death is deemed to be imminent and where curative or life-prolonging treatment appears to be futile, try to ensure that death occurs with dignity and comfort.'[26] There is a fine balance between allowing and promoting patient choices (and patient life-wishes) and bringing harm to patients. You will most likely discover that there are some principles that can be interpreted as being in favour of professional assistance in euthanasia, and others that can be interpreted as being strongly opposed.

Circumstances where the client is too young to express a choice, or is otherwise incapable of doing so, can generate debate that runs for decades. This happened in a case in the early 1980s in which a newborn infant with Down's syndrome received only nursing care and painkillers, under medical instructions. The doctor was acquitted of attempted murder, and a debate began over issues of personhood, disability, treatment decisions, and, more broadly, euthanasia. The case is the basis of Raanon Gillon's classic book *Philosophical medical ethics*.[27]

It is perhaps not surprising that a debate over euthanasia polarises people's viewpoints according to their preferred ethics frameworks. Neil Brown has suggested that the debate is characterised by a split between utilitarians, who may consider actions that, although concerning or even harmful, will result in a desired end, and deontologists, who will always act to preserve rules such as the integrity and sanctity of life.[28]

> **PAUSE & REFLECT**
>
> You might like to reconsider which ethics theories and frameworks you feel assist your reasoning on issues that have been raised in this chapter.
>
> Remember to think back to the everyday issues of decline as well as the more dramatic aspects of end of life.

SUMMARY OF KEY ISSUES

- Diminishing competency and autonomy
- Sudden, planned, or foreseen end of life.

SHORT NOTES

1   Finucane et al., '"Is she fit to sign, doctor?"', p. 402.
2   Parker and Dickenson, *The Cambridge medical ethics workbook*, p. 144.
3   Jonsen et al., *Clinical ethics*.
4   Gallagher, 'Ethical issues in patient restraint'.
5   Lederberg, 'The psychological repercussions of New York State's do-not-resuscitate law'.
6   Beauchamp and Childress, *Principles of biomedical ethics*, 5th edn.
7   Stecher, 'Ethics at the end of life in transplant recipients'.
8   Devereux, *Medical law*, 2nd edn, pp. 322–3.
9   Based on Schlink, 'New baby from dead husband', p. 46.
10   Dutch Pediatric Association, *To treat or not to treat?*
11   Schroeder, 'Ethical issues for parents of extremely premature infants'.
12   Honderich (ed.), *The Oxford companion to philosophy*, p. 859.
13   Berglund et al., 'The formation of professional and consumer solutions'.
14   Chapman, 'Swiss hospital lets terminally ill patients commit suicide in its beds'.
15   The key points in this flowchart are from 'Death with dignity', *CCH Australian Health and Medical Law Reporter*, CCH, Sydney, updated regularly, sections 22–268.
16   Alcom, 'Mercy death world first'.
17   Slaytor and Lesjak, 'Euthanasia seminar'.
18   Oosterhof et al., 'The interpretation of morality'.
19   Cica, 'The euthanasia debate in Australia', p. 3.
20   Baume, 'Voluntary euthanasia and law reform'.
21   Flew, 'The principle of euthanasia'.
22   Murphy, 'Physician-assisted suicide and the slippery slope'.

23   Smets et al., 'The medical practice of euthanasia in Belgium and the Netherlands'.
24   'Doctor helped woman commit suicide', *New York Times* article.
25   *Health Rights Commission Act 1991* (Qld).
26   Australian Medical Association, *AMA Code of Ethics 2004*.
27   Gillon, *Philosophical medical ethics*.
28   Brown, 'The "harm" in euthanasia'.

10

CARING IN AN INSTITUTIONAL AND SOCIAL CONTEXT

- Community input into acceptable limits
- Institutional limits
- Religion and health care

OBJECTIVES

All care is influenced, in some way, by the institution and society in which it is made available. This chapter explores the opportunities for institutional and societal influence, and discusses the ways in which different philosophical standpoints identify different types of influences. Community consultation as a process of ethics debate is described. Guidance by moral or religious orders in the application of health care is used as a case study of the community and cultural influences on the ethics of health care. Particular choices made by professionals and clients in given institutional and societal positions are discussed in terms of ethics. The expectations of society are discussed and given prominence.

Concepts that are added to the glossary include: culture, community, consultation, religion, conviction, and the ethics theory of proportionism.

COMMUNITY INPUT INTO ACCEPTABLE LIMITS

Community views are becoming essential to bioethics. It is no longer sufficient for professionals to define ethics problems, or ethical solutions, alone. Community views are being sought on particular ethics issues, and communities themselves are demanding to be heard on many ethics issues. Communities are able to decide how much they support existing health care, and contemplated changes to health care.

The **community** voice is not present in the jargon of either health care workers or ethicists, but it can be heard if you listen. Hearing community views is important in many of the key ethical theories, or at least is compatible with them. In liberalism, in which there is little role for cohesive community control over individual actions, there is nevertheless a sense of a general community consensus on the limits to autonomy. Libertarianism also implicitly assumes that there is some kind of community agreement and that there are obligations to endure certain burdens for the good of the society to which we belong. Within the framework of libertarianism, only a majority community view—the general will—would be the acceptable basis of a limit on liberty.[1]

A strong sense of community limits—self-defined by the community—is essential to communitarianism, a form of ethics that is gaining popularity in Europe.[2] In deontological theory there is, at the very least, a minimum ethical standard that one would expect to be shared among members of the community, below which these community members would not go. In Kant's work there is a sense that we should respect others and that there should be a limit to how much we interfere or harm them, so that each person can develop their own moral self.[3] The concept of consultation is also compatible with specified principlism, which holds that principles can be identified but that their meaning and application should be defined with reference to cultural norms or standards.[4]

Whichever your preferred ethics theory, it would quite obviously enlighten you as a health care worker to know what the community you serve regards as acceptable; to know, in other words, how much a client could ask for, and how much others could offer them or ask them to undertake, and still be regarded by the community as an ethical citizen. Further, if you regard the process of defining acceptable practices as a joint responsibility of professionals and the community, there needs to be a means of expressing views from the community, and you need to hear those views and communicate your stance to the community.

In routine health care you may not be able to assume that you know the type of health care, or manner of delivery of that care, that is appropriate for particular communities. In some cultures, such as South-East Asian cultures, there are strong beliefs about hot and cold water, and running and still water, particularly in the context of women in labour and immediately post-partum. These beliefs are very different from Western notions, and so we might expect very different attitudes to the use of labour-floor facilities. One research project on the attitudes of midwives to their patients found that the midwives who were surveyed thought that some Asian women were '"bad patients" who lacked compliance; made a fuss about nothing; and did not have normal maternal instincts'. The judgment made about the patients by these midwives was probably due to a lack of cultural understanding. Anthropological research is now

Community
Group of people defined by shared social engagement.

bringing a greater understanding of cultural differences in the context of health care.[5] If prospective patients do not view a health care service as culturally safe, they may delay seeking effective care.

Feminist research is similar in that it focuses on aspects of culture and power that define expectations and possible ethical behaviours, in the context of the doctor-nurse relationship or the health professional–client relationship. Culturally informed research may well be a useful model for other professionals too. Until we communicate and listen to community voices, we won't know if our current system of health and health care practices is acceptable. In the case study mentioned above, acceptable cleansing facilities were simply not available until the Asian women were listened to.

EXERCISE 10.1 CLIENT AND COMMUNITY VIEWS ON PRACTICES

Try this exercise. Think about how you might hear your client's views on a vexing issue, something that seems to be at the heart of your health practice. Pick an everyday instance, such as queues to see you, waiting lists, or what you usually do first in a consultation. How could you find out the client's view?

In some communities, even asking for someone's name has cultural and ethical significance. In the context of drug-using communities, health professionals sometimes forgo 'real' names so that they can provide care to people who would otherwise be fearful of attending a health care service. It is reportedly quite common to see 'Mickey Mouse' or other fictitious names on records. This only became possible when that particular community's fear of the use and recording of real names was acknowledged.

FROM THEORY TO PRACTICE

Ethnic perspective and ethics

Contributor: *Jenneke Foottit*

Form student groups that have students from different ethnic backgrounds in each, and argue issues of consent to be ethical but from an ethnic perspective.

Consultation with the community is routine and is expected for health departments in the Western world. Patient representatives or community representatives are routinely included as members of key committees that develop standards for health and/or research practice. Human research ethics committees (HRECs), which consider the ethics of research at the institutional level in Australia, include laypeople. Institutional review boards (IRBs) in the USA must include at least one non-institutional member, and in the UK the comparable committee must have laypeople as at least half of its members, and these should additionally reflect the diversity of public opinion.[6] Those people are assumed to be a link to the community. They, along with the other non-clinical members of the committee, try to comment on research from the perspective of the research participants and the community.

Have a look at the composition of the governing board of the health care institution you work for. You will no doubt find that there are some community representatives there. They have a say in setting the operating objectives and priorities (prioritising objectives is addressed in Chapter 3). They also play an important part in scrutinising the extent to which institutions succeed in meeting their stated objectives.

The National Health Service in the UK has built a process of consumer and patient involvement into the design and delivery of regional health services, and involves patients in rating the services they have received as part of an improvement process. Community comments can also be made on an interactive website.[7] In the USA, the Consumers Union produces information and guides on health care costs and access issues, and publishes the magazine *Consumer Reports*. All over the world, local organisations undertake advocacy and education in their own states and countries. There can be elections for community representatives to some committees and health care bodies at a local level.

During a process of law reform it is now common to undertake large-scale community consultation. There are frequently public advertisements calling for submissions, and also the active recruitment of people through surveys to hear their views on certain reforms that are being considered. In early stages of research in specific communities, such as Aboriginal communities, it is common for wide consultation to be undertaken, as the research process itself is a collaboration and must be in tune with cultural and community expectations.[8] Government policy making is increasingly incorporating community participation in different sectors.[9]

Given the value placed on community expressions of its point of view, there is an expectation that a representative view is heard. This expectation has been expressed repeatedly in relation to contentious issues. For example, in 1990 community views on AIDS research were formalised by the AIDS Clinical Trials Group (ACTG) in the USA (the decisions made by ACTG had effect nationwide).[10] These viewpoints, called 'ACTG community positions', were subject to particular scrutiny, given the power that AIDS activists had to influence the availability and accessibility of treatments.[11] People began questioning whether the views of the gay (predominantly) white male members of AIDS activist groups also spoke for other sections of the community. So the process of consultation is itself also the subject of ethical scrutiny.

Throughout this book, there is a theme of encouraging communication between professionals and the community on preferred ethical standards for the practice of health care, and this theme is explored further in Chapter 12, in the context of health care research. An opportunity for such consultation exists through the mass media.

The popular press reports on health issues, treatment, policy, and research, providing a source of health information for the general public, and an opportunity for the community to comment on existing or proposed health practices or research. Media reporting on health issues can be seen as communication between, on the one hand, interested and accessible community members and professionals, and on the other, other political actors.[12] The main job of the media is to reflect the state of society by reporting on current issues, which obviously include community concerns over health treatment and health research.

Indeed, there is such potential for the press to be successfully used by professionals in sending out particular health information that one research council has issued the following warning: 'The job of journalism is not public relations for the health messages of the day. It is to question and probe and analyse.'[13] The danger is that the more successful the health or scientific community is in using the media, the less open the media may be to contrary views, or the less able it may be, by virtue of limited space, to report other key community insights.

Some inquiries can be prompted by media reports, such as on the immunisation trials on orphans in the 1950s and 1960s, which featured in the media a few years ago. The issue of the use of wards of the state for the research was of particular concern to both the public and the orphans (who were unaware that they had been part of the research).[14]

In that instance, concern over the particular issue was expressed, and the issue was opened up for debate. It was then reflected on over time. Professionals, researchers, the patients, and the community were all involved in the debate. The process of reflection can often be traced in later media reports.

Current newspaper clippings can be very useful as triggers for learning about ethics. They raise interest in the ethics of current issues. Students often feel they know something about the issues and can talk about them, and they often raise the question of who should comment on ethics. This can lead to role-playing on which sectors of the community might have which particular concerns. Newspaper articles frequently concentrate on individual cases, and can thus be used as vignettes in classroom settings, allowing the class to consider particular health problems and their associated dilemmas. The internet also increasingly acts as a source of health information and as a source of comment on health care matters. So, you could easily do a similar exercise using internet-sourced clippings and items of comment.

The community view in an ethics debate is usually termed 'community input' or 'community consultation' because it is not seen as mandating professional behaviour. Community views could, however, guide your professional behaviour by informing you of what may and may not be acceptable to any given client group; given two morally similar (to you) choices, you might choose the path that is culturally sensitive and ethically preferable in the eyes of the community you serve.

Seeking community input is part of the dynamic nature of ethics. Standards, and the situations to which we apply them, can change. Re-examination of ethics issues, at times in partnership with the key parties affected, is likely to be an enduring theme of modern health care ethics. Community concerns highlight how we work and live in a complex society. We need to communicate with each other so that our standards are appropriate. We need to use the benefits that stem from pooling our ideas and resources, and, as we each seek to use what we need from the societal pool, we need to be careful not to infringe on the dignity and self-respect of individual members of society.

The cultural and community context of treatment and ethics decisions is highlighted in a training program with the acronym CARE for systematic personal ethics consideration for trainee physicians. C is for the physician's core beliefs, A is for action in similar situations in the past, R is for reasoned opinions of others, and E is for experience of others in similar situations in the past. Each item is critiqued as part of the ethics reflection, so the model is shorthand to prompt reflection on reasonable options.[15] Notice that the model explicitly acknowledges the personal beliefs of the carer as well as the community context in which that care is applied.

The public, through their governments and international alliances, can express active social support for research directions, especially in the face of threats or risks, and provide money for research initiatives. For instance, an unprecedented sum of money (around US$2 billion) was made available to the United Nations by member nations to investigate and contain bird flu (H5N1).[16] At times other than crises, research is driven more by gradual refinement of existing techniques and innovation rather than urgent social need. Community **consultation** can be integrated into that process. When dramatic new technology is available, or new procedures are tried that have implications for a **culture**, there is often media coverage.

Transplantation of hands is a new procedure in this century, demonstrating how complex procedures are now undertaken with advances in transplantation medicine, and in the precision of surgical technology. There are implicit cultural tolerances of body parts beyond organs being 'harvested' and used for others. Our tolerance of external body features is even being tested with the trial of facial transplantation for people who have experienced devastating facial disfigurement. In England, The Royal College of Surgeons considered the matter. The College discouraged full face transplants due to an anticipated inability to assess the physical or psychological safety of the process. In view of the difficulty in assessing the risks, they concluded that there would be a less than satisfactory consent process.[17] Consent, you will remember from Chapter 4, depends on the availability of good-quality information on both the risks and likely benefits. In a different country, the view of surgeons differed. The first partial face transplant was performed in France in 2005, for a woman with severe disfigurement from dog bite wounds. The surgical team were reported to have waited for ethical reasons, but had been technically confident and

Consultation
Active process of facilitating the expression of opinions, taking advice, and cooperative deliberation.

Culture
Social expectations and norms of a particular community or civilisation.

ready for some time. The donor had agreed to be an organ donor, but the donor's family's permission for face transplant was additionally sought, and granted.[18] Compliance with anti-rejection medication regimes after surgery is receiving as much attention as the clinical complexity of the procedures, because the post-care process is long term and intensive.[19]

EXERCISE 10.2 NEW FRONTIERS AND PERSONAL VIEWS

Try this exercise to think about what you, and those working with you, would accept. If you are facilitating the group discussion, expect to hear different views and encourage people to express those different views.

As a group, try to describe differences in what each of you would accept in terms of different types of organ, tissue, and body part transplantation.

Identify cultural, religious, and personal limits to what each person would accept.

Community support for potential advances should not be assumed, as eminent ethics commentators, such as Hans Jonas, have been noting for some time.[20] In early and ancient history, there is poignant evidence of community input into professional standards. For instance, the Roman public rejected most experimental treatment on people who were seriously ill, and publicly castigated practitioners who carried out unacceptable experimental treatments, whether or not the experiments succeeded or failed.[21]

Many contemporary third-world cultures reject the notion of progress as it is understood in Western medicine.[22] Western communities may also strongly disagree with new medical technologies and treatments on cultural or religious grounds. One example is the German community's opposition to experimentation on human embryos. The community objected to such an extent that public discussion of this and related issues (such as euthanasia and organ transplantation) was stifled in the 1990s, when philosopher Peter Singer visited. According to one commentator on the heated community protests that accompanied Singer's tour, the community's distrust of such research may stem from the Nazi abuse of civilians during the Second World War in eugenically motivated experiments on humans.[23] Eugenics is the altering of the characteristics of a population through a wide variety of methods. In this example, the public reacted by stifling the debate. The protests may well have been motivated by the hope that, without sufficient debate, human-embryo research would not go ahead. Public reactions involving attempts to stifle discussion are as important an expression of a community as extensive debate on the issues. The wishes of the community should be seriously considered by researchers if a social definition of justice is to be accepted. Under such a definition, community advice must be sought so that the benefits and burdens (of specific advances in health care) to individuals and the community are acceptable. As Douglas states, '[t]he public reception of any policy for risks will depend on standardized public ideas about justice'.[24] Frankel similarly considers that limits to professional choices, particularly in research, should be provided through social policy so that individuals are better protected from harms that are regarded as unacceptable by society.[25]

At an individual level, as treatment progresses, circumstances and achievable outcomes change. A pragmatic approach such as **proportionism** looks for an acceptable resolution of difficult ethical dilemmas, rather than the 'right' thing to do. This relies on gauging your own confidence in certain decisions. If a variety of ethics theories and reasoning would support a certain decision, your confidence would increase. If there is divergent opinion on what is best to do, your confidence would decrease but you could still choose a 'best' answer from among the alternatives, based on the weight of the reasons. Canvassing divergent options and divergent views from stakeholders or interested parties is the hallmark of pragmatism and proportionism, because a resolution is chosen while still recognising that not all people will view it as 'right' or 'best'. A user-friendly process for decision making in paediatric critical care nursing has been described by Daniel Wueste. This takes into account the developing nature of the medical indications and social circumstances of each case, and that views of stakeholders on what is best to do can themselves change over time, given what is at stake. At each decision point—such as whether to operate to correct serious birth defects, whether to offer transplantation, and what to do when parents become less than compliant with management, perhaps due to social difficulties—resolution is aimed for not only with the greatest convergence, but also with confidence in an overriding argument if there is divergence.[26]

Proportionism acknowledges that individuals and communities will have different perspectives on the most acceptable course of action.

Community views on, or expectations of, research in general have been explored more actively in the last 50 years.[27] Before that, there was a sense that research ought not to be pushed too far as it might disquiet the community, and there was a general consensus that there was a limit to how ethically risky research could be before the community would find it unethical. Community consultation surveys have been carried out which demonstrate that respondents are able to draw a line of acceptability and distinguish some research as unacceptable to them. In a way, this gives research above their line of acceptability a community mandate, and research below this line a community caution or even injunction.[28]

Attitudes to controversial research are specifically canvassed from time to time, such as that using embryonic stem cells (see Chapter 6). Some research shows disparate findings, with just over half of those surveyed supporting the research, although just over half of those surveyed opposed public funding for the research.[29] Community views can change, and such surveys quickly become historical data on what the community view was at a certain time.

Proportionism
An ethics theory in which rules and values can be used as guides, but their application takes into account the practical alternatives in a given situation, with allowance for human nature.

Willingness to participate in actual research as a subject is a slightly different matter. It relies not only on agreement with the research process, but also on trust in the research process and the researchers. In America, the Tuskegee Study of Untreated Syphilis (1932–72) led to a profound distrust of medical research among African-American people. The injustice of leaving people untreated to 'observe' the progress of the condition, thereby allowing exposure to risk to their families, is still thought to detrimentally affect participation rates in research today, despite a presidential apology in 1997 for the government's past conduct.[30]

Chalmers and Silverman favour 'public consideration' of formal and informal medical research as a type of risk assessment, not so much as a community judgment of acceptable risk but more because they believe that the community should take responsibility for the reality that progress involves some risk. They caution against the idealistic double standard of wanting the benefits of research without the inevitable risk of harm that accompanies research. They would prefer the community to acknowledge that acceptable means for the ends of research must include risk.[31]

Two key safeguards appear to have the backing of the community. The first is the opportunity for community consideration of acceptable benefits and burdens in research. The second is informed consent on the part of each research participant. As discussed earlier in this section, the safeguard of community input is partially fulfilled by the inclusion of lay members in research ethics committees. The capability of community members to consider research acceptability is now assumed, and is an invaluable part of a research ethics discussion. Community consultation may be more obvious when medicine is pushing its own bounds. Remember though, it is just as ethically important to seek community comment and input on routine aspects of health care as it is to consult in more dramatic areas, such as cutting-edge research and challenging areas of practice.

INSTITUTIONAL LIMITS

Institutional goals and service expectations are discussed in Chapters 2 and 3, and will not be repeated here. Some specific professional responsibilities and limits, whatever the institutional context, are also covered in Chapter 11. Every institution has its own culture that continually shapes the professional work done within its ambit. The culture of peers also moulds ethical aspirations and standards.

Quality-assurance processes and peer review provide opportunities for institutions to refine their written protocols for service delivery and the limits within which professionals work. Increasingly, institutions are encouraging staff to report positive events as well as adverse events. In terms of ethics, what works and what doesn't work in a system are just as important as how good or bad the people working within that system are. There is continual institutional reflection on the safe and ethical limits within which their members operate.

In addition, institutions operate under a state or national umbrella. Comprehensive operating guidelines and expectations are provided by government health departments. Some examples of guidelines and limits on the prioritisation of patients for admission into public hospitals are discussed in Chapter 3. Chapter 4 includes a discussion of safeguards in relation to medical records.

Operating guidelines have ethical assumptions built into them. These assumptions relate to appropriate levels of training and skill for particular jobs, what care to offer and how to deliver it, social expectations of what would be a priority in particular situations, and availability of care.

Debates at institutional levels are also important, as upper-level policy guidelines can guide, but not give prescriptive answers for every specific situation. Guidance documents from reputable councils are plentiful. For instance, a UK council aims to stimulate debate and assist policy makers and practitioners with general guidance as they explore issues in biology and medicine. The Nuffield Council on Bioethics is highly regarded internationally. The UK Clinical Ethics Network advises on reflective processes in clinical ethics committees. The US Office of Research Integrity can assist institutions if they are considering best practice issues, or potential misconduct by their research staff or affiliates. As these organisations provide their advisory documents free on public access websites,[32] institutions can use them no matter where they are situated in the world.

Even with such a wealth of guidance available readily as resource documents on the internet, worldwide, each institution has ultimately to decide if it is meeting a need adequately, and if its employees are playing a proper part. If the work of an employee is falling short of existing standards, an institution may prefer to dismiss that employee rather than allowing them to risk either the work of the institution or the public's trust that the institution will provide adequate care.

RELIGION AND HEALTH CARE

Early Western writings on ethics were more obviously intertwined with religious philosophy and theology than is the case today. These writings struggled with the power of God, and the nature of man as related to the world and to God. Western philosophers transformed and challenged the Church, particularly throughout the Reformation. Doctrines about man's manipulation of life emerged.[33]

The religious philosophies of non-Western cultures are currently receiving attention in the context of health care ethics. Robert Veatch has written extensively on this matter.[34] Given the multicultural nature of many modern Western societies, it is increasingly common to find summaries of the implications that different non-Western philosophies have for health care included in textbooks. Some non-Western philosophies and **religions** give specific guidance on how medical practitioners should treat their patients. For instance, under Chinese medical ethics, which have

Religion
System of faith and belief according to recognised sacred teachings.

Confucian, Buddhist, and Taoist affiliations, modesty and hard work are valued. Under the teachings of Islam, a practitioner should treat the person's body and mind, should encourage what is good, and should restrain people from doing what is bad. Virtue and equal treatment of rich and poor is emphasised, and certain rules are laid down, such as not procuring abortion.[35]

If you are religious, your religion can, and probably does, affect your work as a health care worker. It is one of the things that forms your values and how you try to relate to others. It would be artificial to try to have two moral or ethical standards—one religious standard for purely religious life, and one professional standard for work. In Chapter 2, religion was noted as one of the influences that goes towards defining you as an individual.

EVERYDAY ETHICS

For many people there are some cultural taboos and religious prohibitions that guide everyday life. Try to list as many as you can for yourself, then next to each one list medical interventions that you have heard of that would not be acceptable to you.

In some ethics theories, reaching agreement on what is 'right' or 'ethical' may not be crucial. Some theories, such as proportionism, emphasise acknowledging difficult situations, diverse views, and guiding values and rules, and then simply doing the best you can in the sense of finding a path that is practical in a given context, and allowing for the fallibility of human nature. It is a pragmatic approach, and is ideally chosen with a knowledge of the ethical choices, including rules and values, balancing those with what is practically achievable.

There are times when a religion we may adhere to prompts us to examine our place in current health practices, either as providers or as consumers of services. Abortion, euthanasia, and blood transfusion are perhaps the most often cited examples (abortion is discussed in Chapter 6, euthanasia in Chapter 9).

Commenting on euthanasia from a Singaporean perspective, Kamaljit Singh and Goh Lee Gan state that the vast majority of the Singaporean population is religious. The population, therefore, would react on religious grounds to euthanasia, or any other issue. These authors summarise the key religious views held by Singaporeans, as follows:

- Christians and Buddhists tend to value both life and non-interference with life affirmatively (Christians, because they believe life has divine origin; Buddhists, because they believe life has spiritual destiny).
- Muslims tend to view suffering as a mitigation of suffering in the hereafter, in accordance with Islamic law.
- Jews tend to hold the sanctity of life to be infinite, in accordance with Jewish laws.[36]

FROM THEORY TO PRACTICE

Cultural aspects of ethics and health care

Contributor: *Jade Cartwright* (speech pathologist)

Early in my speech pathology career I packed my bags for London, for a working holiday that many allied health professionals set their sights on. My longest and most memorable stint was working for a health care trust in East London, described as one of the most culturally diverse and deprived areas in England. Cultural diversity can present unique challenges to health care providers, but this was one of the most enriching and rewarding posts of my career to date. What I learnt about the entwined nature of client-centred, ethically sound, and culturally sensitive practice helped shape the health professional that I am today. I was working on a community stroke team and much of my day was spent visiting clients in their homes soon after discharge from hospital to provide rehabilitation services. Many of my clients were of Bangladeshi origin and Muslim faith. As such, one of the most prevailing values that they held in regard to their health care was that of 'God's will'. This allowed many of my clients to accept their stroke as part of God's 'plan' or 'test' for them and sought God's guidance and help in their recovery.

This challenged my own health care beliefs as many of these people who had survived life-changing strokes had excellent rehabilitation potential. My personal view was that the harder you worked and engaged in an evidence-based treatment plan the more functional recovery you could expect to see. However, for many of my clients with strong religious beliefs, they did not have any sense of control over their rehabilitation. Their recovery was in the hands of God and some said that they had no right to interfere with God's will. Ultimately, their value system determined what health care actions should be taken, instead of turning to the research or evidence base, as more Western cultures tend to do.

This work taught me to embrace and celebrate diversity, to step back from my own belief system and to ensure that my clients and their unique needs were always at the centre of care. I needed to continue treating all of my clients in the same way, never judging, never stereotyping. It was also important to provide information that would allow them to make an informed decision about their care, while working collaboratively and negotiating treatment goals within their own value system. During this period I reflected at length on my role as a health professional and my own beliefs, which is the cornerstone of ethical practice. It is often through such ethical challenges and reflection that we learn and grow most, both professionally and personally.

How does this scenario sit with your own values and beliefs about health care and ethical practice?

Any practices that challenge religious convictions can raise dilemmas for individuals holding those particular **convictions**. Any part of practice that challenges religious convictions is also ethically suspect for individuals who adhere to those

Conviction
Firmly held belief.

faiths. For instance, Jehovah's Witnesses believe that it is wrong to place foreign blood matter into a person's body. Thus, for strict Jehovah's Witnesses, any part in a process that aims to place blood or blood-derived products into people poses a dilemma. Therefore problematic medical practices include not only blood transfusion but any collection or use of blood products.

EXERCISE 10.3 RELIGIOUS CONVICTION AND ACTIONS

Consider the following example, which was discussed in the Australian mass media in 1990.

A taxi driver was allegedly called to pick up a package from the Red Cross and deliver it to a hospital. The package contained blood. The blood was urgently needed for an operation, but it never arrived. It was allegedly found abandoned near the driver's taxi depot, with the packets pierced and unusable.

What do you think?

If the driver did in fact dump the blood, and tamper with it, did he have a right to act on what seems to have been his religious convictions that use of blood was fundamentally wrong?

Conversely, did those who gave it to him have an obligation to ensure that he was agreeable to delivering the blood before they entrusted it to him?

This perplexing hypothetical works well as a group exercise. It stimulates discussion of what the bounds of acceptable behaviour are, who determines these bounds, and whether it is community expectations or moral and religious conviction that should prevail. Bear in mind that the taxi driver is not a health professional. He has not sworn to abide by a code of ethics. He has not agreed with the charter of the hospital. Yet he, like many other non-health professionals, is involved in the delivery of health care services. Like the millions of hospital support staff (and ancillary staff) around the world, he is one of the people who makes the system, and the current set of health services, succeed or fail.

People can express their professional autonomy by non-performance of certain procedures. Perhaps the taxi driver's alleged action was an example of this: an expression of his choice not to be party to something he regarded as unacceptable. Is that any different from the fact that Catholic health care institutions do not provide abortions? You may like to think about the difference between not being party to something and actively stopping such procedures from happening under someone else's purview.

Religious groups routinely adopt, and act on, positions on health issues. Consider, for instance, the following Roman Catholic Church position on AIDS health-education. The extract, from the *St Vincent's Bioethics Newsletter*, comments on a workshop on AIDS held by the St Vincent's Bioethics Centre, in Melbourne:

> The plenary sessions highlighted the urgent need for the Catholic community to respond to the inadequacy of the 'safe sex' approach to AIDS education, its need to integrate its services with those already existing in the wider community, its role as a witness to personal compassion as a remedy to the fear incipient in such a public health crisis and its leadership as the largest religious grouping in Australia.[37]

There clearly is a difference between condoning an action and providing compassionate care for people affected by that action or at risk from it. This is similar to the difference between the obligation to provide care and the obligation (in cases where clients have done something that we find abhorrent, or where we have ethical objections to the treatment they desire) to pass the responsibility for care on to others.

Health care workers occasionally come face to face with this difference. For instance, at the time of the Port Arthur massacre in Tasmania, the injured victims and the alleged gunman were brought for hospital treatment to the same emergency department. Workers dealt with the injured victims as well as the alleged perpetrator, all of whom were entitled to the best available care on offer. Those who felt that, if confronted with the responsibility of dealing with the alleged gunman, they could not place the best interests of the patient first excluded themselves from the job of caring for him. A challenge to your willingness to care may be posed by your cultural as well as your moral sense of good, as is discussed by Olsen in relation to nursing.[38]

SUMMARY OF KEY ISSUES

- Community consultation and community expectations
- Institutional standards
- Beliefs and religion as an overlay.

SHORT NOTES

1   Mill, 'On liberty'.
2   Zwart, 'Rationing in the Netherlands'.
3   Sullivan, *Immanuel Kant's moral theory*.
4   De Grazia, 'Moving forward in bioethical theory', p. 525.
5   See, for example, Mulhall, 'Anthropology, nursing and midwifery'.
6   For Australia, see National Health and Medical Research Council, Australian Research Council, and Australian Vice-Chancellors' Committee, *National statement on ethical conduct in research involving humans*, 2009, s5.1.30, p. 85. For UK, see Department of Health, *Governance arrangements for research ethics committees*, s4.2.3, p. 20. For USA, see Department

of Health and Human Services, Office for Human Research Subject Protections, *Protecting human research subjects: Institutional Review Board Guidebook.*

7   National Health Service, *Patient and public involvement in the NHS*, 1999; surveys at <www.nhssurveys.org>; comments made at <www.nhs.uk/patientsvoice>.

8   Dunne, 'Consultation, rapport, and collaboration'.

9   Peel, 'Community participation in decision making and service delivery'.

10   Institute of Medicine, *The AIDS research program of the National Institutes of Health*, pp. 44, 45.

11   Gilmore, 'The impact of AIDS on drug availability and access'.

12   As proposed by Price and Roberts, 'Public opinion processes', pp. 784, 788.

13   National Health and Medical Research Council, *The media and public health*, p. 11.

14   Walker et al., 'Wooldridge backs inquiry on guinea-pig'; Dow, 'Trials and terror'.

15   Schneider and Snell, 'C.A.R.E.'.

16   Parry, 'Funding of bird flu initiative exceeds expectations'.

17   Royal College of Surgeons of England, *Facial transplantation*.

18   Spurgeon, 'Surgeons pleased with patient's progress after face transplantation'.

19   'Troubled transplant man throws in bad hand', *Australian*, article.

20   Jonas, 'Philosophical reflections on experimenting with human subjects', p. 245.

21   Ferngren, 'Roman lay attitudes towards medical experimentation', p. 496.

22   Dickens, 'Issues in preparing ethical guidelines for epidemiological studies', p. 183.

23   Nicholson, 'Bioethics attacked in Germany', p. 22.

24   Douglas, 'Risk acceptability according to the social sciences', p. 5.

25   Frankel, 'The development of policy guidelines governing human experimentation in the United States', p. 46.

26   Wueste, 'A philosophical yet user-friendly framework for ethical decision making in critical care nursing'.

27   Lovell, 'Ethics at the growing edge of medicine'.

28   Berglund, 'A survey of Sydney adults about the conduct of medical research'.

29   As cited in Weed, 'Ethics, regulation, and biomedical research'.

30   Baker et al., 'Effects of untreated syphilis in the negro male'.

31   Chalmers and Silverman, 'Professional and public double standards on clinical experimentation', pp. 390–1.

32   For the Nuffield Council on Bioethics, see <www.nuffieldbioethics.org>, for the UK Clinical Ethics Network, see <www.ethics-network.org.uk>, for the Office of Research Integrity in the USA, see <www.od.nih.gov>.

33   Honderich (ed.), *The Oxford companion to philosophy*, p. 761.

34   Veatch, *Cross cultural perspectives in medical ethics*.

35   Devereux, *Medical law*, pp. 14–23.

36   Singh and Gan, 'An Asian perspective on euthanasia', p. 40.

37   *St Vincent's Bioethics Newsletter*, 6(4), 1988, p. 12.

38   Olsen, 'Populations vulnerable to the ethics of caring'.

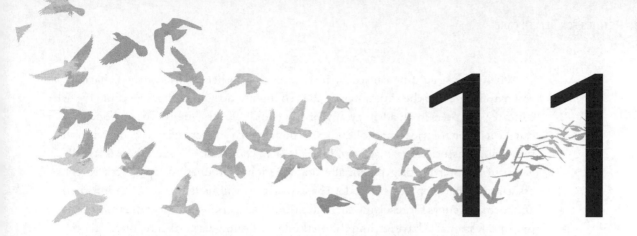

11

MONITORING AND EDUCATION

- Peer standards and implementation
- Institutional standards and implementation
- Legal standards and ethics
- Self-reflection

OBJECTIVES

This chapter concentrates on the way in which ethics standards come to be voiced in practice, and how ethics education occurs in the professional world. The process of individual, professional, and external reflection on practice is examined. The workings of ethics committees are used as a case study of how ethics is debated in particular forums. Readers are alerted to ways of keeping up to date with the often regularly changing standards that might affect them. The terms character, insight, and conflict of interest are added to the glossary.

PEER STANDARDS AND IMPLEMENTATION

It is vital to be aware of proper professional conduct in professional practice, and of limits that should not be exceeded. You need to be vigilant in respect to both your own behaviour and the behaviour of others around you. You have a responsibility to work ethically, and to think about the broader ethics of the organisation for which you work. The themes, outlined in Chapter 2, of goals and duties, aspiring to the highest practical standards of behaviour, and abiding by rules are key factors in peer standards.

When harm could be caused by institutional or other professionals' behaviour, you may decide that the situation is serious enough to do something. You could try to educate your peers in an advisory way, or you could refer the matter to someone who can. Professional advice from colleagues, or bodies such as peer review committees and professional associations, may help. Take a look at your code of ethics; there is usually a clause about reporting potentially unprofessional or unethical practices to the association that prepared the code. The association will usually have both informal and formal avenues for resolving such situations. Obligations to report unethical and/ or unprofessional behaviour, and the methods for dealing with such reports, have the ultimate dual aims of protecting the public and protecting the profession's reputation.

EVERYDAY ETHICS

Think of a job you have or have had in the past. Try to identify the reporting and oversight mechanisms for that job. Who did you report to? Who made sure your tasks were conducted properly? Who corrected you if there was a need to? As you gained experience, how did the reporting mechanisms work? What would have got you sacked? Did you cooperate with the line of reporting, or did you subvert the system of accountability?

Mentoring and continuing education programs are an everyday part of professional life. Professional conferences and journals keep you up to date with standards and developing expectations, and with better ways of delivering services to match client expectations.

While professionals strive for excellence in care, mistakes sometimes occur and they can be serious. Treatment errors can cause disruptions to care and recovery, and sometimes even death. A constructive discussion of adverse events and the development of a culture of open reporting to enable that discussion may be more effective in reducing future mistakes than a culture of blaming and shaming individuals. However, open discussion and the gathering of information is constrained by the realities of legal process.[1]

There are registration systems for professions that require registration in order to be deemed to meet certain standards to be able to fulfil their roles properly. These are established along with disciplinary provisions for professionals who subsequently do not uphold those standards. The standards set are backed by the legal requirements of the profession. Peer reviewers express the expected professional standards, and also their disapproval if a practitioner departs from them. Disciplinary sanctions can range from educational programs and mentoring for continued professional development to restrictions on practice, and even deregistration if the matter has been heard by the upper level tribunal or a judicial hearing.

The professional standards committees of the health professional councils or registration boards may investigate professional conduct. The complaints that prompt these inquiries can be made by anyone: the client, another member of the public, a fellow professional, or administrative staff. The powers of such committees are often set by the committees themselves, and once set are enshrined in law; these laws are best understood with reference to a legal text.[2]

The following matters would be typical of registration board inquiries: failure to attend in an emergency; lack of adequate knowledge, skill, judgment, or care; and cases where a practitioner's ability to provide care is impaired in some way. The treatment itself is a prominent source of complaint—for example, a complaint about an incorrect diagnosis or inappropriate treatment plan. The manner and politeness of the practitioner is also of great concern to many complainants. The types of complaints made against practitioners are commonly documented in the annual reports of registration bodies. Complaints can range from concerns over competence (misdiagnosis, incorrect clinical advice, complications following procedures), to those about conduct (inappropriate prescribing, medical records, medical reports and certificates), and from concerns about communication to those about practice administration.[3] Each complaint needs to be assessed, and investigations can be carried out by a complaints commission.

Language proficiency is defined as part of professional competence, along with sufficient physical and mental capacity and professional skill.[4] Assessment of competence in English is routinely part of a screening process for suitability for registration of overseas practitioners, as a safeguard for safe and effective teamwork and communication with patients.

In Australia, the national system of registration of those who are suitably qualified by AHPRA, combined with inquiry powers at state level into performance and conduct, together provide a system of professional regulation. There are mandatory reporting requirements for fellow practitioners to make their concerns about others' health or capacity to practise known, and members of the public can make complaints.

The emphasis of such monitoring or standards panels is to protect the public and to maintain public trust in professional services. Public interest may be served by reprimanding the practitioner, educating the practitioner, and/or providing mentoring. The safety of the public is paramount.

The **character** and conduct of a professional are open to scrutiny in such inquiries. That means that the general motivation and character of the person can be assessed, particularly if conduct has been alleged to be against a patient's best interest or against the interests of the profession. You will remember from Chapter 2 that the ideal profession aims to provide care and act in the interest of others.

Character
Moral qualities of a person.

Committees and tribunals can take the opportunity to pass their findings on to the relevant professional associations, colleges, health departments, and hospitals, so that the lowered professional standards can be rectified and further unsatisfactory practice guarded against.

A professional's disciplinary record, in terms of conditions of registration and possible deregistration, can be requested by potential employers. There is some debate about whether it should be available to potential patients, on the grounds of privacy.

The practitioner may not be obliged to disclose matters that have not been completed, partly on grounds that only completed adverse findings against them should strictly speaking be recorded as matters against their professional standing.

Professional councils are involved in proactive education, increased peer discussion forums for information exchange, monitoring of performance, and support for higher risk practitioners, such as impaired practitioners, to contribute to maintaining and improving standards. Impairment programs that are offered by many professional councils support impaired practitioners when they remain in practice. The programs necessarily include an element of treatment being provided for the practitioner, and possibly practice limits applied, so that the risk to the public is minimised. These programs can be applied at any time in a professional's career, for reasons of physical or psychological impairment. They rely to a great extent on the **insight** of the practitioner that further help is needed should a crisis or a change in their condition occur, and a willingness of the practitioner to practise within safe limits. There may be an additional fundamental problem in applying these to students or professionals in periods of rapid learning and the application of new skills. These people are in the process of acquiring skills rather than maintaining them. The challenge is to support the individual but anticipate when these periods of stress will be too much, so that patients remain safe at all times. For those practitioners, effective and alert mentors and supervisors are vital.

There are inbuilt systems of accountability and monitoring within hospitals and health care organisations that aim to recognise and remediate professional care that is substandard. Generally, the role falls to immediate supervisors and clinical directors if planned intervention or re-education is warranted.

Some complainants from within the health care system find that official institutional or professional avenues are not sufficient to halt unsafe and/or unethical practices. Such complainants may face the uneasy dilemma of deciding whether to go outside the health care system and alert others to the practice. This is called whistleblowing. To 'blow a whistle' has had many colloquial meanings in the past. It has meant, variously, the whistle to stop work for a break (or smoko), the sounding of an alarm, or an alert to danger. Nowadays, whistleblowing has taken on the last of these meanings—an alert to danger. It is an alert by a particular person to the fact that an organisation, or someone within an organisation, is engaging in dangerous behaviour (or behaviour that is potentially dangerous). By definition, whistleblowing occurs when other internal alerts have failed. It is an alert to the world outside the organisation, a signal that an insider feels that public discussion is needed. The alert is made in the public interest. One definition of whistleblowing, relied on by Vinten, goes as follows: 'the unauthorised disclosure of information that an employee reasonably believes evidences the contravention of any law, rule or regulation, code of practice, or professional statement, or that invokes mismanagement, corruption, abuse of authority, or danger to public or worker health and safety'.[5]

It may take some time before the public becomes aware of a matter that a whistleblower is concerned about, as the example described by Irene Blonder on cervical cancer

Insight
A reflective process of examining own behaviour and motives, and recognising deficiencies.

research in New Zealand shows.[6] In that research, women with early-stage abnormalities of the cervix were examined over time, and no intervention was carried out for some who subsequently progressed to stages of cervical cancer. When the colposcopist tried to raise his concerns within the medical profession, he encountered resistance, and at some later point he decided to publish his concerns to promote discussion. Journalists pursued the matter and subsequently there was much discussion of it in both the popular and medical press. Finally, a government inquiry into the research was held. This research is discussed further in Chapter 12. Similarly, when a UK anaesthetist tried to raise the issue of higher than normal mortality rates for children's heart surgery in one particular unit, and the lack of provision of those statistics to parents contemplating the surgery for their children, he encountered antagonism. Eventually, professional and public inquiries were convened, and his concerns were supported, but he nevertheless moved to another country, feeling there would be limited career opportunities for him afterwards. He has told his story in a paper that is recommended tutorial reading on the process of professional concerns and speaking out, and it should ideally be read along with subsequent commentaries and the Bristol inquiry report.[7]

EXERCISE 11.1 PROFESSIONAL CONCERNS AND TRYING TO BE HEARD

As a group, source the article and read what the anaesthetist says about his concerns and the process of trying to make his concerns heard.

- Summarise the steps he went through to voice his concerns.
- Note the different levels of recourse in his organisation and profession that he had available to him.
- Can you suggest anything else that he could have tried?
- This case was in the UK. Are there any differences in your own country?
- What do you think of his eventual course of action in whistleblowing?

Many whistleblowers report that going outside their organisation and peer structure generated considerable resistance from their profession and caused them personal hardship.[8] It is a difficult decision to make, and it should be considered carefully in respect of, first and foremost, the likely effect such an alert will have, and second, whether or not the problem might be constructively tackled at the peer or institution level, where the problem is occurring and where it impacts on clients.[9]

The crucial decisions in whistleblowing are:

- Is there an opportunity to make an internal report, rather than taking the complaint outside the profession or institution?
- Would whistleblowing educate the profession and the public about the problem?
- What are the risks involved?
- Is the harm sufficiently serious to warrant whistleblowing?

- What values are at stake?
- How timely would the alert be?
- What is the likely outcome of, on the one hand, pursuing the complaint internally, or on the other hand, whistleblowing?

FROM THEORY TO PRACTICE

Using newspapers as triggers for discussion

Contributor: *Jenneke Foottit*

Use news items of ethical or unethical behaviour. Ask students to identify the ethical issue and discuss how they would resolve it.

INSTITUTIONAL STANDARDS AND IMPLEMENTATION

Informal peer monitoring is continual within institutions, as colleagues take the time to bounce ideas back and forth and to discuss both past events and planned management options. Formal institutional peer review is usually termed 'quality improvement' or 'quality assurance', or simply 'QI' or 'QA'. Different hospitals set up different systems of QA, which although varying in process share two basic elements: a process of overview and a process whereby the relevant bodies are alerted to potential problems in standards of practice. Senior or junior members of staff can be called on to present their recent cases, and the cases are open for reflection and discussion. The aim is not to criticise individuals but to ensure that high standards of care are maintained, and that all staff learn, from each other, ways to maintain that standard. Sometimes guidelines are developed from patterns of care that seem appropriate for particular conditions or types of clients.

There is a firmly held assumption that health care workers are striving to achieve the best for their clients and are placing their clients' interests first. The ultimate goal of institutional standards is to streamline and clarify care so that the institutional team delivers the best care to the client.

As research ethics committees developed, they were increasingly asked to consider clinical (treatment) ethics issues in addition to their established role of considering research ethics. Some institutions have set up separate clinical ethics committees. More routinely, professionals resolve ethics issues within their own practice with team and peer assistance, but sometimes they seek assistance from an ethics committee, particularly when there is a complex issue involving a large team or conflicting views between carers and family. Committee involvement is more common in the USA, where ethics consultants are employed in large hospitals. They can have beepers and are on call for urgent consideration of ethics issues. In the UK, committees have developed fairly recently, and individual consideration of cases is possible.[10] Outside the USA, ethics committees seem to concentrate more on policy formation in order to guide clinicians in complex cases in the future, rather than to facilitate individual case decisions.[11] These are not necessarily dramatic issues. They could be as seemingly simple as when to allow care of a child to proceed without accompanying parents or guardians, or when to suggest a child be offered the opportunity to speak with their carer on their own. Or, how to ensure specific groups of clients make best use of the available services, given cultural or physical limitations.

EXERCISE 11.2 FROM CASE DECISIONS TO POLICY

Look back to the exercise that you worked on in Chapter 8, about the young man who liked to take risks and his friends who also liked to ride around in cars.

Looking back at the case, try to identify issues that are case-specific, and ones that could usefully be the subject of general policy.

For the case-specific issue, role-play a process of consultation between the relevant parties (after deciding who is relevant) and suggest a compromise between them.

Once you have re-familiarised yourself with the case issues think further about policy issues, and how your institution could develop a guideline that would help practitioners facing similar case issues in the future.

Draft a guiding principle.

Be sure to justify your guidance with appropriate ethics theory.

Research projects involving humans as research subjects need formal ethics committee approval before they can proceed. The subjects can be patients or healthy volunteers. The review is to assess the ethical acceptability of the research. This means that the risks and benefits of the research are assessed in terms of burdens and benefits. The process of the research is assessed, with such aspects as the free and informed consent of volunteers scrutinised. More on the process of assessing the ethics of research is included in Chapter 12.

In Australia, research ethics are considered at the institutional level by the human research ethics committee or HREC. The concerns and workings of these committees are described in more detail in Chapter 12. All Australian institutions that wish to be eligible for Commonwealth funds must review the ethics of proposed research. In doing so, they refer to the principles expressed in the joint Statement by the National Health and Medical Research Council, the Australian Research Council, and the Australian Vice-Chancellors' Committee, the *National statement on ethical conduct in research involving humans*. Under somewhat relaxed provisions of the usual ethics review by the full HREC, all research must still be reviewed for ethical acceptability under the joint Statement, but that involving a 'low risk to participants' can be reviewed by a panel or delegate. Research of more than low risk must be reviewed by a HREC. HRECs are composed of at least eight members, with a required minimum composition of a chairperson, one layman, one laywoman, one person who performs a pastoral care role in the community (such as a minister), one lawyer (not engaged by the institution), at least two members with knowledge of and experience in the types of research considered regularly, and at least one member who has knowledge and experience in the professional care and treatment of people. The other provision is that at least a third of the committee is made up of members external to the organisation. HRECs do not, strictly speaking, express institutional standards because they remain independent from the institution and their members are not for the most part employees of the institution; but each committee sets the benchmark that must be applied in the institution that they serve. HRECs do not often monitor research directly, and monitoring is more broadly an institutional responsibility. However, they do receive regular reports from researchers on their projects and on any adverse events that have accompanied this research. They can inspect research sites or records, or interview participants if they wish, either randomly or in response to concerns about research process or risks.[12]

Professional associations are simply not resourced to monitor research directly. However, the strong professional responsibility enshrined in many professional codes effectively requires each professional to monitor the practice and behavioural standards of other professionals. Professionals have an obligation to report suspected unethical behaviour to their professional association.

Very similar systems operate in many countries. In the UK, research ethics committees (RECs) are the committees that review research at an institutional level. The committees are overseen by a health department authority and there are required governance arrangements, including the composition of committees to include at least half lay members, reflecting the diversity of public opinion, and expert members to assist with the understanding of technical aspects of research method and clinical care.[13] The procedures are increasingly streamlined, including standard application forms, information sheets for participants, and committee decision making and documentation processes. There are additional guidelines available, issued by research councils, to assist research ethics reflection by researchers and deliberations undertaken by committees.[14] This streamlining and loss of some autonomy for institutional-level committees initially prompted some criticism, with the fear that the committee members' consideration may be overwhelmed by administrative requirements.[15]

In the USA, institutional review boards are the equivalent committee. IRBs have a mix of institutional and non-institutional members, including community representatives. They must have at least five members, with varying backgrounds and experience, expertise to review research activities, diverse racial and cultural heritage, sensitivity to community attitudes, and knowledge of acceptability in terms of regulations and laws. The IRB may not be entirely composed of one profession, and must have at least one primarily scientific and one primarily non-scientific member, and at least one member not affiliated with the institution. The Office for Human Research Protections provides oversight for research funded by the Department of Health and Human Services, since IRBs must conform to federal regulations if that research is to be validly funded.[16] There have been concerns about the consistency and depth of research considerations, with some calls for further oversight over all human research,[17] and ongoing revision and refinement of the rules and regulations are likely.

In New Zealand, health and disability ethics committees (HDECs) and institutional ethics committees (IECs) and their operation are regulated by the National Ethics Advisory Committee and the Ministry of Health. Their role is not limited to ethics approval for research but extends to treatment ethics issues in an advisory capacity. The New Zealand system of streamlining ethics considerations was in large part initiated 20 years or so ago, after the inquiry into the cervical cancer research. There has been a concern about ensuring diverse committee representation and transparent decision-making processes. The ethics committee membership is diverse in terms of culture, gender, and disability; at least half is laypeople who have not been registered health practitioners, officers employed in health boards or authorities, or health researchers. Additionally, HDEC committees have two health researchers, a pharmacologist, a biostatistician, two health practitioners, and half male and female composition is regarded as optimal. IECs require research, Maori, and ethics experts, and ideally a lawyer, among their expertise members.[18]

The common requirement of committees having laypeople not affiliated with the institution, or involved with research or health care, is to minimise potential conflict of interests. The purpose of the lay member is to have someone independent from the institution and the production of research, who can provide an independent view and also ensure that those with affiliations to the institution act in a transparent and accountable manner. So if the lay members were also employed by the institution, in the present or even in the past, they might be seen to have a special loyalty to the institution. That loyalty would be termed an 'interest', and would be at odds with the interest in maximising accountability and carrying out an impartial review. The interests could be in conflict, hence the term '**conflict of interest**'. Conflict of interest occurs when someone is making a decision in which they have a vested interest. This is not helpful when an objective decision is needed. So it is routine for committee members to declare conflict about certain matters that are before a committee, for instance, that they are employed by the institution that seeks x, y, or z, or that as a researcher they are affiliated with the research team seeking approval. In that instance, a member would remove themselves from making a decision about that particular proposal. The perception of potential conflict of interest attracts as much criticism as actual conflict of interest, so it is something that is guarded against quite strictly.

Conflict of interest
A situation in which two potentially opposing and incompatible interests exist.

LEGAL STANDARDS AND ETHICS

A sense of both the lower limits and the optimal levels (or ideals) of acceptable behaviour was introduced to you early in this book, in Chapter 2. Many people would regard the minimum standard as being represented by the law, and the upper, or optimal, level represented by ethics. In short, the law provides a minimum standard, while ethics acknowledges a minimum standard (which is not always the same as law) but strives for the maximal standard.[19] Both standards are fluid. The law is simply a reflection of what we regard as fair play and fair burden in our society.

Jeremy Bentham is an example of a philosopher who has promoted a particular view of how ethics and law are related. An early utilitarian, Bentham espoused the principle of achieving the greatest good for the greatest number. The utility he concentrated on was felicity, or happiness. The means to pursue it, Bentham thought, were reason and law. In brief, he thought that the stability of law would provide for a structure within which happiness could be achieved. He felt that this fundamental aim of felicity should be recognised in law, and he set about suggesting legal and societal constructions that would ensure it. His concern was at a societal, and particularly a governmental, level.[20] This was a grand plan to express societal goals and limits in a legal system. We in fact do use law to express societal expectations of professional behaviour.

The law is an empowering force in health care ethics. We use laws to give professions authority and mandate over their skill and the trade in that skill. Yet we also use the law to constrain professionals if the standard is not met. As described previously, a complaints mechanism is available under legislation to anyone who feels that health care service standards, of whatever health profession, are not met. Complaints commissions commonly investigate complaints, and then decide whether to refer the matter to the relevant professional panel or tribunal for consideration of whether the complaint is proven, and for a decision on penalties.

Laws relating to professional standards cover not only skill and competence, but also the manner in which service is provided and the character of the practitioner; in essence, they cover the way that practitioners are ethical in their conduct of their work. These components of professional work were suggested to you in Chapter 2. The intertwining of professional skill and proper conduct is recognised at law. Together, skill and ethics make an acceptable health care worker.

Broader societal expectations and standards are applied by law. This law is not limited to legislation passed by Parliament and applied by either professional panels or tribunals. The laws governing such expectations and standards also come from the criminal and civil jurisdictions. In the criminal jurisdiction, laws about particular actions can limit what practitioners can become involved in. The most obvious examples are laws relating to abortion and those relating to the legality of euthanasia. Such laws are expressions of the lower limits of behaviour that society will tolerate. These limits are constantly debated by politicians, and can change. For instance, euthanasia was legal in the Northern Territory for a short time until a debate in the Commonwealth Parliament resulted in the law being overturned. Abortion and euthanasia are discussed more fully in Chapters 6 and 9.

The community, through the judiciary, can challenge the professions to change their ethics standards so that the professions stay in touch with community expectations. Judges are, broadly speaking, obliged by legal doctrine to follow previous decisions, called precedents. But they can, with reasoned legal arguments, come to a different conclusion and therefore a different decision if the context for application of the law is significantly different from that in which the previous decision was applied. So the law is constantly evolving. The law acts as a safeguard for injured or 'wronged' clients, and as a message to other professionals that unless they apply certain standards in caring for their clients, they risk being sued.

Some systems virtually exclude civil action for damages, most notably in New Zealand where there is a no-fault compensation scheme for injury, including medical injury. Since negligence law is the dominant societal process in most Western countries, however, professionals need to be either up to date with the law or find an avenue for being briefed on the latest developments in law. Further, ignorance of criminal legal standards is not generally seen as an excuse for illegal behaviour.

SELF-REFLECTION

As you have worked your way through this book, you have been encouraged to practise self-reflection. You have been encouraged to reflect on what is important to you (and why), on what you should try to do (and why), on what you should not do, and on what you could do better.

In Chapter 2 you were asked to identify your own virtues, values, and important goals in your health care work. You were asked to acknowledge your skill limits, and the consequences if you were to overstep those bounds. You may be your own best safeguard in aspiring towards virtues and goals, and in not letting your standards drop too low. This process should continue throughout your professional life.

Take the time now to look back over all the reflective exercises you have done in previous chapters. As you browse through, consider how integral reflection is to the development of your skill and ethics, and in the application of your skill in an ethical manner.

SUMMARY OF KEY ISSUES

- Continuing development and reflection
- Accountability to peers and society
- Law as an arbiter of societal limits.

SHORT NOTES

1   Liang, 'The adverse event of unaddressed medical error', p. 351.

2   Devereux, *Medical law*, 3rd edn.

3   NSW Medical Board, *2004 Annual Report*, p. 17.

4   *Health Practitioner National Law (2010)*, at section 55.

5   Vinten, 'Whistle while you work in the health related professions?'

6   Blonder, 'Blowing the whistle'.

7   Bolsin, 'Professional misconduct: the Bristol case'; English et al., 'Would you "blow the whistle"?'; British Royal Infirmary Inquiry, *Learning from Bristol*.

8   Lennane, 'Whistleblowing'.

9   This is further discussed in Berglund, 'Thoughts before whistling'.

10   Hope and Slowther, 'Clinical ethics committee in the UK'.

11   Doyal, 'Clinical ethics committees and the formulation of health care policies'.

12   National Health and Medical Research Council, Australian Research Council, and Australian Vice-Chancellors' Committee, *National statement on ethical conduct in research involving humans*, 2009, Chapter 5.1, p. 81.

13   Department of Health, *Governance arrangements for research ethics committees*.

14   Economic and Social Research Council, *Revised framework for research ethics*.

15   Kerrison and Pollock, 'The reform of UK research ethics committees'.

16   Department of Health and Human Services (US), Office for Human Research Subject Protections, *Protecting human research subjects: Institutional Review Board Guidebook*.

17   Emanuel et al., 'Oversight of human participants research'.

18   Health Research Council of New Zealand, *HRC guidelines for ethics committee accreditation*, pp. 6–7, 13; New Zealand Ministry of Health and National Ethics Advisory Committee, *Operational standard for ethics committees*.

19   See Annas, *Judging medicine*.

20   Honderich (ed.), *The Oxford companion to philosophy*, p. 85.

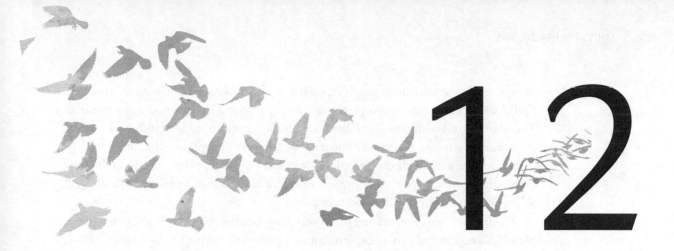

12

AND SO TO RESEARCH

- Being a researcher and a carer
- The patient as a research subject
- Prominent ethics concerns in research
- The Belmont principles
- Research ethics committees and submitting an ethics proposal
- Writing up

OBJECTIVES

Professional health care workers are likely at some stage to undertake health research. This chapter is a practical guide to the important ethical choices to be made in research. A checklist of prominent ethics concerns for major types of research projects is outlined. Readers are encouraged to express further ethics concerns themselves.

This chapter relies on many glossary terms that have been previously defined, such as risk and benefit, and the principles of beneficence, respect for persons, and justice. You may like to revisit these terms as you work your way through the chapter. A new glossary term of transparency is added.

BEING A RESEARCHER AND A CARER

The general duty to do good and minimise harm applies to health research, just as it does to health care. While the benefits that research may achieve for the population are important, the first duty is to the client or research subject. Being a researcher and a carer is a delicate balance between ensuring ongoing trust in care relationships, and not exposing clients to unnecessary risks. Professional colleagues can give advice on appropriate professional conduct; each association's code of ethics can provide a useful reference on values and principles to keep in mind in the conduct of research. Those who are both researchers and carers must come to understand their clients' conditions better at the same time as they are testing options that may lead to better care for a wider class of people. As you will note below, there are guidelines for separating out the research recruitment from the carer, in case a patient feels 'obliged' to participate if their doctor asks them to.

The importance of separating out research and caring roles was highlighted in the New Zealand cervical cancer experiments, discussed widely in the late 1980s.[1] (This case was noted, in Chapter 11, as an instance of whistleblowing.) In this research, women presented regularly for what they believed were thorough check-ups. They believed that they would be treated for any gynaecological conditions diagnosed during these check-ups. They assumed that if they were not treated, then nothing was wrong with them. The research was, in fact, to observe the development of pre-cancerous cervical cells. Many of the women progressed to cancer and died while they were participating in the research. The research prompted debate about the institutional review standards that were applied when the hospital was considering the ethics of the research. This debate led to changes in the legal requirements laid down for the constitutions of New Zealand ethics committees.[2] Australia checked its own standards as a result, and research institutions engaged in reflection on their own ethics safeguards.[3]

This long-term observation of the development of a condition is somewhat similar to the Tuskegee experiments, in which black American men were observed as their syphilis progressed without treatment. The observations continued even after treatment with penicillin became available.[4] Being a researcher brings with it a responsibility to co-researchers (to ensure the integrity of the research) and funding bodies. Care should be taken to declare potential conflicts of interests to supporting agencies. Divided loyalties to, on the one hand, a business that is funding the research, and on the other hand, being employed by caring institutions and caring for patients, can be perceived by colleagues and the public as an unacceptable conflict of interest.

There can be other potential conflicts too, such as that of a researcher and financial beneficiary from a biotechnology or pharmaceutical company. Potential conflict of interest rules have come into effect in many countries, but most notably in the USA in recent times, at the National Institutes of Health (NIH). All NIH researchers were initially banned from consulting with biotechnology or pharmaceutical companies, or owning shares in them, although this was subsequently limited to leading investigators, NIH officials, and their families.[5] The intention is to preclude a conflict between the interest in conducting research impartially and the interest in finding results favourable to a company that is also an employer.

THE PATIENT AS A RESEARCH SUBJECT

There are occasions when patients themselves push the bounds of treatment to a point where it effectively becomes research. They might have heard about a new treatment that they want to try, or there might be no known cure or treatment for their illness and they are willing to try anything. This often happens when patients have a terminal condition, or a condition for which researchers and clinicians cannot offer an effective cure. There is well-established evidence that HIV/AIDS patients, for instance, consistently sought new and unproven treatments in the 1980s.[6] In effect, they also forced their carers to become researchers. As there was a serious risk facing them, many people with HIV/AIDS might have decided that there was little distinction between research and treatment. As one AIDS community slogan stated: 'A research trial is treatment too'.[7] The challenge posed to the drug-regulation system by making experimental drugs available was discussed in Chapter 8.

There is considerable responsibility placed on the individual health care worker in situations such as these. They still need to protect their patients from further harm, but when all available options have been tried, there is generally a willingness to let patients pursue more risky but as yet unproven treatments.[8] These treatments of 'last resort' do not have the same strict rules of drug regulation applied, so they need not always be used in the context of a clinical trial if terminally ill patients wish to try them. A number of significant advances in cancer treatment have been developed as a result of aggressive treatments being tried by very ill people. Occasionally, world attention is focused on patients who choose radically new treatments—for example, in the mid-1990s the so-called 'Baboon man' asked for baboon-marrow transplants to be given to him as a possible immune system boost. He was suffering from HIV/AIDS. At the time, the health care practitioner involved said that the only surprise was that the experimental treatment went so well. It did not make him better, but then it did not make him worse either.[9]

At other times, carers will actually want their patients to try a new research protocol. The autonomous nature of the patient's decision is so important ethically that it is routine for another health care researcher to recruit subjects. That is because patients can feel obliged to be participants if asked by their own carers. This feeling of obligation is termed 'dependency'.

PROMINENT ETHICS CONCERNS IN RESEARCH

When you conduct research with people, you are researching human participants. The following list is of some possible methods of researching health in human participants:

- accessing medical records
- asking questions in an interview or questionnaire

- doing a physical examination
- performing a blood test or taking a tissue sample
- giving an experimental treatment
- doing an experimental operation.

You may be able to think of more types of research. If you can, note them down. You may notice that the methods above are expressed in terms of what you do with the participants. That reflects the key ethics concern in research: what are research subjects being asked to do? This is where ethical reflection on research should start. You may also notice that as the list progresses, the level of invasiveness increases. Research subjects, health care workers, and the community are particularly concerned with how invasive or intrusive are the procedures research subjects are being asked to consent to.

EVERYDAY ETHICS

Have you ever been asked to take part in research? A phone survey perhaps? A questionnaire at the doctor's? A focus group at university? What were you asked to do, and did you feel inclined to participate? Some people are generally more willing than others to take part in research. Everyone should be able to decline.

You may be surprised that all of these methods are thought of as involving human participants. Even looking at medical records or analysing blood and tissue samples are thought of as researching people. The people do not have to be right in front of the researcher for the research to be thought of as having human participants.

A few general questions should start you on the way to ethical reflection on research that you may have conducted. If you participated, think about the research from the perspective of the researcher.

– What was your research about?
– Were you skilled enough to undertake the research?
– Where did your research subjects come from?
– What did you ask your research subjects to do?
– How did the participants consent to the research?
– How was your research used?
– Was the process worth it, given the results?

You could answer these questions for any research project that you undertake in the future or that you have observed.

The answer to each question has ethical significance, as is explained below.

WHAT IS THE RESEARCH ABOUT, AND ARE YOU SKILLED ENOUGH TO UNDERTAKE IT?

Research should have a purpose, a reason sufficient to justify the inconvenience or risk posed to the research participants. Researchers have a responsibility to care for research subjects, which includes being skilled enough to maximise care and minimise risk.

HOW ARE RESEARCH SUBJECTS TO BE RECRUITED, AND WHAT ARE THEY BEING ASKED TO DO?

The recruitment of research subjects involves questions of acceptable burden and free choice, on the part of subjects, in their decision to participate. What research subjects are asked to do can determine the ethics of the research: an ethical limit to the burden or risk to be borne by participants is always considered, but this limit can change depending on the importance of the research, and the endemic risks faced by the potential participant.

HOW ARE THE RESEARCH SUBJECTS BEING ASKED TO CONSENT?

The consent of research subjects is paramount, particularly as research is, by definition, not necessarily for their benefit—there is little room to justify paternalism.

FOR WHAT PURPOSES WILL THE RESEARCH BE USED AND WAS THE RESEARCH WORTHWHILE?

The likely use of the research determines both its importance to the public and the benefit for individual participants. Research can change how we think about the best available treatment or assess health, or it can consolidate what we already know. Practical use of research indicates that putting research subjects through the research has been worth it. Only once the process is understood, and the results are known, can we really decide whether the research has been justified. The difficulty in terms of ethics is that this question has to be answered hypothetically before the research begins.

EXERCISE 12.1 ETHICS ANALYSIS OF RESEARCH

As an exercise in applying these questions, take the time to look through a professional journal that is relevant to your profession. Many libraries have their recent journal copies displayed on reading shelves, and you can easily skim through a few to find a research article. Back copies are normally located in bound volumes on the library shelves. You could try visiting a university, hospital, or community library, which should all have a selection of health-related journals. Try to visit a library if you can, rather than accessing professional journals through the internet, so you take some time to browse through a range of professional resources.

A research article is one that explains the result of a research process, including the background of the research, its method, what was found, and the researchers' interpretation of the findings.

When you answer each of the questions, make some notes on what you think the ethical significance of each issue is. Then discuss your views with a friend or colleague.

All the issues mentioned in relation to the above questions are interrelated. For instance, if a method is inappropriate because it does not fit the research purpose or produces erroneous results, the research could be seen as unethical because (since no advancement in knowledge will occur) the inconvenience to the subjects is for no purpose. If the subjects were drawn from a vulnerable or dependent population, and the research was used to improve health care for the affluent only, we may decide that the research is unethical because it is unjust. More connections between these issues are explored below, within the context of a principlist examination.

THE BELMONT PRINCIPLES

The Belmont principles—beneficence, respect for persons, and justice—are used as tools here to identify and examine further key ethics concerns in research. As is suggested earlier in this book, the principles are useful as a shorthand way of checking that the relevant moral concerns are taken into account. The principle of respect for persons is a variation of the principle of autonomy, with a primary concern of ensuring that free and uncoerced decisions to participate are made by participants. The principle of beneficence, when used as a Belmont principle, encompasses non-maleficence; it is about maximising benefit and care, and minimising harms or risks. You should feel free to add your own specific ethics concerns to these principles.

Issues involving the assessment of the risks and benefits to individuals can be thought of as coming under the principle of beneficence; issues surrounding personal autonomy can be viewed as being under the principle of respect for persons; and issues relating to the benefits and burdens to society in general may be considered as coming under the principle of justice. This categorisation of issues is consistent with the Belmont Report's suggestions for the use of these principles.[10] The principles should all be considered in any research situation. That is because some issues relate to more than one principle—there can be conflicting ethics concerns in research practice, as in any health practice.

BENEFICENCE

The maxim 'do no harm', a major element of beneficence, is critical in research. This is because it is not always possible to achieve the other element of beneficence—the injunction to 'do good'—for each research participant. This is in spite of the future benefits to others, benefits that are frequently claimed as a justification for research.

An honest appraisal is needed of what, and how much, benefit is likely from the research. This benefit constitutes both the private and public interest in conducting the research, because some benefit may be to the individual participant, either during the course of the research or shortly thereafter, and some benefit may be to the community in the future. You can ask yourself this question: What purpose does this research serve?

A risk assessment is a crucial first step in avoiding harm. The amount of risk that is acceptable (and by whom), and how that risk is assessed, is of ethical concern. Even though some studies suggest that the risk to research participants is low in most cases, any risk potentially violates the maxim 'do no harm'.[11] That means that all risk, even if minimal, should be explicitly acknowledged and documented.

After acknowledging risk, the next step is to assess whether that risk is acceptable. If the participant is already facing some sort of risk because, for example, they are suffering from an illness, this can make a difference to the ethical acceptability of research. If the proposal aims ultimately to reduce that risk, then this affects the risk–benefit assessment. The World Medical Association's (WMA) Declaration of Helsinki makes use of the distinction between therapeutic and non-therapeutic research in assessing acceptable risk (this distinction and its implications for consent were discussed in Chapter 7). Risk is weighed against the potential foreseeable benefits to the participants and others. The benefits and harms of a potential therapeutic treatment are generally weighed against the benefits and harms of treatments that are already available.[12] The level of acceptable risk is lower in non-therapeutic research. Under the Declaration of Helsinki, research must be discontinued if harm may be caused to the participant.[13] An obligation to benefit and to do no harm is important in both therapeutic and non-therapeutic research. As the researcher's ability to fulfil the 'do good' maxim diminishes, their responsibility to fulfil the 'do no harm' maxim increases correspondingly. Ethics committees increasingly weigh up the 'value' of proposed research and the risk it entails.[14]

Risk can, of course, be difficult to assess, especially in procedures that have not been used before. In assessing risk in such situations, it may be useful to rely on similar research conducted previously on animals or very early approximations to human use (for example, in vitro examination of blood or tissue response). A high level of clinical and scientific judgment is needed to make this risk assessment. The acceptability of risk is necessarily a value judgment. As a researcher, you decide what you are prepared to ask people to undertake. Ethics committees make a similar judgment before research proceeds. Participants decide whether they are prepared to participate, and they take on those risks, for potential benefit to themselves and/or others.

The concern in all research is that some invasive procedure, whether physical or non-physical, may be performed on a participant. In medical research this invasion is likely to be to the physical integrity of the person, but in non-medical research it is more likely to be to their psychological integrity. Both physical and psychological integrity are essential to the well-being of the individual and must be protected. Consistent with that concern is a commitment by the researcher to stop the research if the risk to this integrity becomes too great.

RESPECT FOR PERSONS

The principle of 'respect for persons' seeks to ensure that an individual's wishes are respected, even if they differ from those of the researcher, or from those expected of the individual by the researcher. Each potential participant should be given the opportunity to express their wishes both before being included in the research and throughout the research process itself. Broadly, the principle implies respect for the rights, wishes, and individuality of the participant. Ensuring informed consent to research and maintaining the confidentiality of the data are processes that uphold the dignity and individuality of research participants.

The fundamental ethical standard in research is that people should take part of their own free will. This is supported in several human rights statements, such as the United Nations Covenant on Civil and Political Rights, and in UNESCO's Universal Declaration on Bioethics and Human Rights, which states: 'Scientific research should only be carried out with the prior, free, express and informed consent of the person concerned.'[15] This is echoed in all research ethics codes. In order to uphold the integrity of the consent process, individuals who have the capacity to make decisions about research participation should be allowed to do so. They should also be free to withdraw at any time.

Apart from the competency to make decisions, the capacity for autonomous decision making also requires an environment that is free of coercion. If the environment is not free of coercion, a request for participation may not be ethical. This means that a refusal to consent should not lead to any detriment (other than the agreed-upon risks of the research) or loss of standing for the patient. A non-coercive environment also means that there should be no such implied threat either. Informed consent as a health care process is examined in Chapter 4.

Control over personal information is a fundamental extension of the principle of 'respect for persons'. It means giving an individual control over information about themselves—not just control over their own physical self, which is often protected by consent. Confidentiality of information implies that personal information should be held in confidence and should not be included in any further research or made available for other purposes, unless the individual whom the information is about gives consent. Confidentiality obligations are tested in research that uses information that is already stored for another purpose (such as medical records) and in research that involves collecting information that may be useful for another purpose. The use of personal information for purposes other than those consented to requires that there is sufficient public interest in those further purposes, and this decision often falls to the ethics committees in the case of research.

Ideally, research participants should be aware of the research process as it progresses from start to finish. This includes being informed of the results of the research, so that they may learn from it and can maximise the benefits or minimise the potential harm of the research for their own lives. To use people as subjects but not inform them of the results (if they wish to know the results) could seem exploitative.

A further area in which there is potential for exploitation is payment. The question of how much, if at all, to pay research subjects is difficult to resolve, and it depends ultimately on the population from which the research subjects will be chosen. Some compensation for participation is preferable, but it should not be so large as to amount to coercion to participate. Many researchers use a model of 'compensation for time'—in the form of issuing taxi vouchers and providing lunch vouchers for the day of the research—rather than monetary payment, which could induce low-income earners or unemployed people to take part in risky research for the money. This would effectively exploit that less affluent section of the population for the benefit of the whole population.

JUSTICE

The principle of justice involves considering the fair distribution of the benefits and burdens of research within society. To achieve that, the duty of professionals to conduct research and to advance knowledge so that society may benefit needs to be acknowledged. However, the advancement of knowledge cannot be at the expense of the individual patient or research subject, so, effectively, concerns of beneficence and respect for persons take precedence. Research should not be regarded as ethical, no matter how great the community benefit, if individuals suffer too greatly in the conduct of that research. This concern over the suffering of research subjects is at the heart of criticisms of experiments conducted by the Nazis during the Second World War, and is a constant concern when underprivileged or institutionalised participants are used for research that is designed for the benefit of privileged or non-institutionalised persons.

You should note that, in theoretical terms, placing beneficence and respect for persons over justice makes explicit the distinction between the good for the individual and the common good. This distinction is often a source of confusion when applying the principles of beneficence and justice.[16] Economic writers may challenge the primacy of other principles over justice, preferring to set societal objectives (such as economic growth), which can be used to implement beneficence and respect for persons.[17]

On a practical level, you need to assess what the social benefits and burdens of the research will be, who will bear the burden of research, and who will potentially benefit from it. Only then can you make a decision on the acceptability of the research.

The sharing of knowledge and the dissemination of information gained from research is an element of the duty to society to distribute the benefits and burdens more knowledgeably and fairly within that society. If you are conducting research, you should write up and present your results accurately, noting its pitfalls as well as its successes. Your findings and your description of the research should be made publicly available—for example, at conferences, in professional forums, or in professional journals. It is also advisable to make this information available in a form that can be accessed by the community.

The dissemination of knowledge saves the same burden of risk being placed needlessly on future prospective research participants. It maximises the potential benefits of research: disseminating the knowledge gained allows others to move further on the basis of your results, instead of repeating the research (or failing to offer the best available treatment) because they are not aware of your results.

In summary, the key ethics considerations for researchers are the following:

- beneficence
- assessment of the benefits of the research
- assessment of the risks of the research
- weighing risks against benefits
- respect for persons
- informed consent from research subjects
- research subjects being free to withdraw from the research
- confidentiality
- informing research subjects of results
- paying/compensating research subjects
- justice
- advancement of knowledge for the benefit of society
- assessment of the distribution of benefits
- assessment of the distribution of burdens
- fair balance of benefit and burden
- sharing of knowledge and dissemination of results.

RESEARCH ETHICS COMMITTEES AND SUBMITTING AN ETHICS PROPOSAL

Ethics committees provide an opportunity for professional, institutional, and community concerns about clinical and research practice to be discussed and decided upon. The committees are essential for researchers, who need their approval before they can conduct research, and they provide a useful referral process for clinicians. More on institutional-level review and ethics committees was included in Chapter 11.

There can be some confusion about how to refer to ethics committees that consider the ethical acceptability of research protocols before they are allowed to proceed. The committees are called research ethics committees in the UK, health and disability ethics committees or institutional ethics committees in New Zealand, and institutional review boards in the USA. In Australia, committees that consider research ethics are called human research ethics committees, but before 1999 they were called institutional ethics committees. In Australia, committees that consider clinical treatment ethics are called clinical ethics committees, but they are called institutional ethics committees in the USA. This section is headed 'research ethics committees' because the term 'research' denotes the function of the committees. Researchers and committees plan and decide under relevant national ethics guidelines. These guidelines are important as standards because all researchers and HRECs are obliged to consider research in the light of the principles they promote, sometimes due to funding provisos, and otherwise due to institutional or professional expectations. You can access the relevant guidelines on the internet, from particular research councils, or as linked by your research office website at your base institution or professional association, and you should do so if you are planning to conduct any research. They are usually organised around the basic values of respect for human beings, research merit and integrity, justice, and beneficence; and the 'design, review and conduct of research must reflect these values'.[18] You will remember that some examples of these guidelines were noted in earlier chapters when membership of the committees was discussed.

The similarity between statements is not surprising given their common purpose of protecting human subjects and maintaining the progress of understanding through medical research. The statements are designed to ensure that unethical research, such as that examined in the Nuremberg trials, does not occur again. The Nuremberg trials examined, among other war crimes, medical research conducted on Nazi-held prisoners of war. Those responsible for the experiments were put on trial and were ultimately convicted of having committed crimes against humanity. The experiments included sterilisations, placing people in freezing conditions to observe the effect on their body, infecting people with typhus to observe the reaction, and even killing so that the body could be dissected as a specimen. The resulting Nuremberg Code, setting out principles of how to deal with research subjects with respect and preserving their dignity, forms a vivid historical backdrop to many subsequent discussions of the ethics of research with human participants.[19]

The World Medical Association's Declaration of Helsinki is the base document of many research guidelines that have been developed. This is routinely discussed and updated at assembly meetings, but retains its name of Helsinki because that was the city where the meeting was held that approved the earliest version of the Declaration. You can find the latest revision of the Declaration and also potential revisions that are under discussion on the WMA website (www.wma.net). The conduct of research in different contexts such as the developing world was a topic under intense discussion over the last decade. The background to this is that when new treatments are being trialled, there is usually a comparison group, which does not receive the new treatment. This is so that the effects of the trial treatment on the research participants can be compared and evaluated against others with similar conditions, and not just against changes in the condition of the human participants who are receiving the treatment. This forms a more reliable comparison, and is the standard approach in quantitative research studies.[20] Traditionally, placebo groups were the comparison, and those in the placebo group did not receive treatment of any kind. Now, however, the norm is that the best proven and most available treatment is given to those in the comparison group, so they are no worse off than if they were not in a research trial. The effect of the new treatment can also be compared to how people progress if they received the standard treatment of the day. In the developing world the difficulty is that the best proven treatment simply may not be affordable or available to people. It is a difficult ethics quandary for researchers, who want to help and fulfil their duty to take part in improving medical care and treatment, and to decide what their responsibilities are to research subjects in countries where the basic care is not as good or lacks many choices available to similar research subjects in the developed world. The WMA requirement (clarified in 2004) was changed so that the best available treatment for the participants, both during and after the conclusion of the trial, needed to be identified for the ethics committee's consideration. There is ongoing discussion about the merits of this standard.[21] Comparison with a placebo when a current proven intervention exists is not acceptable.

So reference to professional codes, national guidelines, and international standards should be routine for researchers who are planning research. These are designed to help researchers conduct research ethically, and should be referred to by professionals in addition to seeking peer deliberation and discussion of issues. Ethics committees have an educative function, as well as a gate-keeping role. They can be asked for advice when researchers face difficult issues.

If you are preparing to submit your research proposal, first contact your ethics committee and ask them the following questions:

- Is there a pro-forma for submission?
- When does the committee meet?
- What is the deadline for your submission to be included in the agenda for the next meeting?

It is common practice for proposal deadlines to be one or two weeks before the meeting date. This allows time for agendas to be prepared, for the committee to identify and ask for any information missing from the proposal, and to make copies of the proposal and distribute these to the committee members. The members read the proposals before they meet, and they are expected to give each proposal due consideration.

As a researcher, you need to be aware of that review and reflection process, and give it the time it deserves. There may be administrative requirements particular to your ethics committee—for example, your committee may require you to submit multiple copies of the proposal. Find out these administrative details early on, preferably well ahead of the deadline for proposal submission, so that you do not miss the deadline for the meeting. Committees may only meet four times a year. You need to be careful that you do not unduly delay the granting of ethics committee approval.

EXERCISE 12.2 A PROPOSAL FOR CONSIDERATION

Try this group discussion exercise. Allocate roles to people along the lines of ethics committee composition. These were noted in Chapter 11. You will remember that Australian committees have, as a minimum, a chairperson, two laypeople, a person with a pastoral care role in the community, a lawyer, two researchers in relevant fields, and a health carer from any of a variety of health professions. Various ages are commonly sought for this membership. You may prefer to construct a UK-, NZ- or USA-style committee to consider the proposal.

A community health fund has promised funding for a trial of a new treatment of eye infections, in a remote area populated largely by Indigenous people. The researchers plan to provide refrigeration equipment for the duration of the trial, which is needed for the medicine and preparations, as this is routinely lacking in the area. The research will extend over a two-year period. People of all ages who attend the monthly community health clinic, and who are diagnosed by the community health nurse as having a particular type of eye infection, will be offered the chance to take part in the research. Half (randomly assigned on the basis of random numbers allocated for the sequence in which they attend) will be asked to follow the routine advice given, and the other half will be offered the new treatment regime. Researchers will follow up all patients at monthly intervals, and a serious deterioration in any participant will trigger a new assessment of treatment requirements. This assessment would take place in a community base hospital. Transport for the assessment would be arranged by the research team. Any subsequent change in treatment advice and treatment arrangements, if they needed to withdraw from the research, would be the responsibility of the individual and community.

As a committee, consider the proposal. Be guided by a national statement on ethical conduct in human research, and a general ethics guideline, such as your profession's code of ethics.

Once research is under way, the responsibility for monitoring the ethical conduct is shared: the researcher continues to reflect on the ethical dimensions of the process, as do their peers, the institution, the ethics committee, the funders, the participants, and the community. Ethics committees can actively monitor and audit all research within their institutions, regardless of the funding source, and in some countries government-funded offices undertake this responsibility for publicly funded research. For instance, public offices, such as the US Office of Research Integrity, set guidelines for research conduct, assess alleged research misconduct in publicly funded research, and support institutions responding to allegations of misconduct by their members.[22] Information can be given to them by any complainant. Routine random audits can also be carried out to check for study teams who disregard discrepant data, or data that does not 'fit' their hoped-for outcome, and they can generally check the integrity of data files and patient records. The Office publishes misconduct findings on its website.

EXERCISE 12.3 MONITORING AND INVESTIGATION

Try this tutorial exercise. Imagine that you have to investigate an allegation about research misconduct, made by a research participant, Patient B.

A new treatment is being trialled for the control of a chronic and debilitating condition, and Patient A is a close friend of Patient B. Although random allocations are meant to occur, Patient A apparently asked to be assigned to the treatment group after realising that the medication she had been assigned was no different from that which she had been taking for some time in the context of routine treatment. She had taken the medication she was given for the research trial to an independent lab and asked that it be analysed. It was three weeks after the trial had started, but she managed to change groups, and all of her data was allegedly transferred to the 'treatment' group for inclusion in that analysis. Patient B is disgruntled that she may be on the comparison group treatment, and has been told she cannot be informed which group she is in and, in any case, cannot change groups.

Alternatively, consider an allegation made by a junior member of a research team, in a large multi-institutional trial, that the published findings differ from that in the research records.

Consider what sort of evidence would need to be collected in order to investigate the allegations.

If proven, what action, if any, do you think should be taken in regards to:

• the participants
• the investigators
• the institution?

Look up the Office of Research Integrity website (www.ori.hhs.gov) to see if its summaries of investigations into allegations of scientific misconduct match your proposed process of investigation. Its 'evidence' records may help too. The basic process is to check facts, assuming there is a consent from research participants for the records to be available for audit, and to interpret them with the assistance of knowledgeable peers.

WRITING UP

The reporting of research is an important step in ensuring that the results are known, and that the effort and resources that went into the research have some tangible result. Knowledge is furthered, even if results are null or not as expected, if you share what you have learnt by engaging in the research process.

The participants may wish to know the results of the research as well, particularly if the findings are of personal relevance. In social research, it is common to expect to discuss the findings, as a courtesy to the participants and communities who made the research possible. When writing up results, there is an obligation to report the findings accurately, and be publicly accountable for those published findings. This is a question of researcher integrity. Knowingly falsifying results is regarded as research misconduct.

Journal editors require authors to sign their explicit responsibility and public accountability for the research and the results as published. To be justified in claiming authorship, authors must have made a substantial contribution to the design, data collection or analysis and interpretation, and to drafting and approval of the final version of the reporting of results.[23]

Journals will require documentation that a project has been approved by an ethics committee. This is to ensure that they do not publish research that has not been ethically reviewed.

Most journals now require conflicts of interests in the research, such as receiving sponsorship from commercial companies with an interest in the results, to be disclosed and published alongside the results in the interests of **transparency** and accountability. Readers can then judge the potential bias of the research report accordingly.

Transparency
Being candid and open to scrutiny.

You may have noticed 'scandals' from time to time in the media. If you see an article about a research project that is portrayed as a scandal, think about whether the researcher's integrity or potential conflict of interests are at issue. Happily, most research is conducted without such ethical pitfalls, with researchers being in the main driven by a genuine desire to help others and make a difference to people's health and welfare.

SUMMARY OF KEY ISSUES

- Responsibilities to care and to advance knowledge
- Ethics as a part of research design
- Ethics as a part of research process
- Administrative requirements
- Regulations.

SHORT NOTES

1   Coney, *The unfortunate experiment*.
2   Gillett, 'The new ethical committees'.
3   McNeill, 'The implications for Australia of the New Zealand Report of the Cervical Cancer Inquiry'.
4   Jones, *Bad blood*.
5   Flynn, 'The NIH ethics crackdown'.
6   Levine et al., 'Building a new consensus'.
7   Annas, 'The changing landscape of human experimentation'.
8   For instance, Oliver and Webb, 'Sildenafil for "blue babies"'.
9   Associated Press, 'Baboon man out of hospital'; 'Baboon marrow fails to boost AIDS patient', *Australian*, article.

10   US Department of Health, Education, and Welfare, *Ethical principles and guidelines for the protection of human subjects of research* (the Belmont Report).

11   Levine, *Ethics and regulation of clinical research*, p. 39.

12   World Medical Association, 'Ethical principles for medical research involving human subjects', revised 2008, Paragraph 32.

13   Ibid., Paragraph 20.

14   Cassarett et al., 'A taxonomy of value in clinical research'.

15   United Nations, 'International Covenant on Civil and Political Rights'; UNESCO, 'Universal Declaration on Bioethics and Human Rights'.

16   Veatch, 'Justice in health care', p. 277.

17   Mooney et al., *Choices for health care*, pp. 48, 49, 55.

18   National Health and Medical Research Council, Australian Research Council and Australian Vice-Chancellors' Committee, *National statement on ethical conduct in human research*, Section 1, p. 5. For current guidelines, in Australia, see <www.nhmrc.gov.au>; for UK, see <www.dh.gov.uk>; for USA, see <www.hhs.gov/ohrp>; for New Zealand, see <www.hrc.govt.nz>.

19   Spicker et al. (eds), *The use of human beings in research*.

20   Berglund (ed.), *Health research*.

21   Blackmer and Haddad, 'The Declaration of Helsinki: an update on paragraph 30'.

22   Department of Health and Human Services (US), Office of Research Integrity, 'Sample policy and procedures for responding to allegations of research misconduct'.

23   International Committee of Medical Journal Editors, *Uniform requirements for manuscripts submitted to biomedical Journals*.

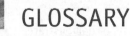

GLOSSARY

Absolutism

An ethics theory in which a rule or rules are identified as fundamentally important, and of unvarying significance.

Accountability

Process of being open to scrutiny for assessment of conduct of responsibilities.

Advance directive

A directive given by a patient in advance that represents their autonomous wishes and is intended by them to guide their treatment and care in the future.

Autonomy

The principle of allowing and promoting self-rule, of people making decisions about their lives.

Beneficence

The principle of doing good and providing care for others.

Benefit

Positive effect or outcome.

Best interests

That which is judged to be to the maximal benefit of a person or persons in maintaining or furthering their health and welfare.

Bioethics

Reflective ethics process applied to the health care context and life sciences.

Casuistry

Ethics theory in which previous decisions are analysed in terms of values, and factual and cultural contexts, and used to guide future decisions.

Character

Moral qualities of a person.

Claim

Implicit or explicit demand to receive a good, as one's due.

Client

Person or organisation investigating or receiving service.

Communitarianism

An ethics theory in which the relationship of a person to a specific community is identified, and the interests and needs of that community as a whole take priority over individual interests and needs.

Community

Group of people defined by shared social engagement.

Comparative justice

Justice model of need in which goods are distributed on the basis of demonstrated most need, compared with the demonstrated needs of other community members.

Competence

Ability to perform a specified task and readiness to do so.

Comprehension

Understanding, specific to issues under consideration.

Compulsory

Required action for all, with enforcement provisions.

Confidentiality

Limited distribution of another's personal information, due to respect for privacy.

Conflict of interest

A situation in which two potentially opposing and incompatible interests exist.

Consent

Agreement.

Consequentialism

An ethics theory in which the consequences of actions are the focus, both on the actor and on others affected by the action.

Consultation

Active process of facilitating the expression of opinions, taking advice, and cooperative deliberation.

Conviction

Firmly held belief.

Cost–benefit analysis

A calculation of the cost of delivering a service with demonstrated and calculated financial benefits.

Cost-effectiveness analysis

A comparative assessment of costs in achieving an agreed objective or beneficial outcome.

Cultural safety

Acknowledging and abiding by the social expectations and norms of a specific community.

Culture

Social expectations and norms of a particular community or civilisation.

Deontology

An ethics theory in which the process and components of actual or proposed action is the focus, with reference to agreed values and rules.

Dignity

Quality of worthiness.

Distributive justice

Justice model of need and entitlement, in which goods are distributed based on demonstrated and comparative interest and entitlement to receive community benefits and the expectation or capacity to bear burdens.

Doctrine

Tenet or lesson held out or taught as a true guiding rule.

Doctrine of double effect

Ethics doctrine in which the intention of likely positive effects is considered to morally excuse certain foreseen negative effects.

Duties

Obligations and specific tasks that one is bound to fulfil, or actions from which one is bound to refrain.

Duty of care

An obligation to take reasonable care in dealings with a person, once there is an undertaking to provide care or advice, or contribute to such specific benefit for a specific person.

Entitlement

Recognised need to create community obligation to fulfil interest or claim.

Ethics

Reflective process of analysing and examining moral issues and problems.

Goals

Ideals and objectives aimed towards.

Good

A desirable end or object.

Health

State of physical, mental, and social well-being.

Health care

The provision of care with the objective of maintaining, restoring, or improving health or comfort.

Health care professionals

Those trained in recognised and registered professions to be providers of health care.

Human rights

Fundamental assertions and expectations of basic rights, thought to be due to all human beings.

Ideals

A standard or concept of excellence which is aimed to be met.

Information

Details specific to issue under consideration.

Informed consent

Agreement given contingent on information and understanding of the proposed process, significance of decision, and potential benefits or risks entailed.

Informed decision making

Alternative term for informed consent, also encompassing the active participation of both parties in determining options to be potentially agreed to, and in identifying significant material risks and benefits to be explored.

Insight

A reflective process of examining own behaviour and motives, and recognising deficiencies.

Interest

That which is to one's advantage or benefit.

Justice

The principle of fair allocation of community resources and burdens.

Justice as fairness

Justice model of equality, in which goods are distributed with the aim that community members are restored to equivalent levels.

Law

System of basic rules and regulations of interactions in a specific community, binding on members as expressed in that community's government-enacted rules, or derived from its judicial decisions.

Libertarianism

An ethics theory that aims for the greatest good for the greatest number, with good defined by each person pursuing their own defined wishes and liberties.

Liberty

Freedom of will, as expressed in choice of thought or action.

Mandatory

Required action, contingent on being under certain command and corresponding enforceable obligations.

Medical ethics

Specific term for ethics in the medical and biomedical context.

Morals

Significant lessons prompting reflection to identify a virtuous, right, or acceptable course of conduct.

Need

Demonstrated interest in receiving a good.

Non-maleficence

The principle of not harming others, and of minimising harm to them.

Norms

Accepted standards, which can be used to judge conduct.

Obligation

Something one is bound to fulfil or perform.

Paternalism

Decision-making framework in which care and control of another is undertaken.

Patient

Person receiving care.

Person

Live human being, or live human being in development, with essential and recognised qualities of intrinsic capacity or function.

Personal morality

Significant lessons prompting reflection to identify a virtuous, right, or acceptable course of conduct of an individual, largely affecting that individual.

Personhood

Quality of being a person.

Potentiality

Capacity to develop in a certain way, given the opportunity and suitable development conditions.

Principle

A fundamental proposition, from which specific goals or duties can be derived.

Privacy

State of secrecy or concealment.

Private interest

Issues of importance and significance to an individual, defined on an individual basis to be in that person's best interest.

Professional code of ethics

Expression of principles, rules, ideals, and values of a specific professional group, creating responsibility to strive for states, ideals, and goals, and to uphold certain rules, in each member professional's conduct.

Proportionism

An ethics theory in which rules and values can be used as guides, but their application takes into account the practical alternatives in a given situation, with allowance for human nature.

Public health

Field of health care concerned with assessing and improving health and preventing illness or disease on a population basis.

Public interest

Issues of importance and significance to the structure of a community, and to the general benefit of a significant group of a community's members.

Reflection

A process of thought and analysis on past, present, or future issues, applying deep and serious consideration.

Relativism

An ethics theory in which divergent perspectives are canvassed, with a view to establishing courses of action that are acceptable to those perspectives in their given context.

Religion

System of faith and belief according to recognised sacred teachings.

Respect

Hold in high regard and esteem, and to refrain from interference with a respected person.

Respect for persons

Principle of upholding autonomy, generally used for research participants.

Responsibility

Obligation and duty to fulfil certain tasks or series of tasks.

Right

Claim that is recognised as imposing obligations on others to fulfil it.

Risk

Chance of negative effect or outcome.

Rules

Derived and specific expression of fundamental principles or ideals that are agreed to have moral force, so as to obligate subscribers to that moral stance to abide by them.

Skill

Level of competence in a specific task or series of tasks.

Slippery-slope argument

An argument that small 'slips' in standards will lead to larger 'downwards slides' and a degradation of standards, so that any small slips should be vigorously guarded against.

Social morality

Significant lessons prompting reflection to identify a virtuous, right, or acceptable course of conduct of individuals, with significant implications for the choices then available to others in society.

Surrogate decision maker

Person who makes decisions on behalf of another, acting as a proxy or substitute.

Transparency

Being candid and open to scrutiny.

Trust

Confidence in another person, or persons within an organisation, to act in an expected manner.

Utilitarianism

An ethics theory in which the outcome of actual or proposed action is the focus, and the acceptable course of action is that in which the greatest good for the greatest number is achieved.

Utility

Quality of usefulness for a desired purpose or outcome.

Values

Concepts given worth or importance in life and interactions, making up a value-system.

Veracity

Truthfulness, accuracy, and completeness in information relied on by others.

Virtue

Worth or quality of particular moral excellence.

Voluntariness

To decide own course of action with free and unconstrained will.

Wishes

Desired states, thoughts, or actions that would bring happiness if attained or realised.

A GUIDE TO FURTHER READING

You may like to read further on ethics. Some of the classic books listed below are geared to particular ethics theories. Most are written for clinical contexts. Some of the books on the list are compilations of the work of different philosophers.

Annas, G. J., *Judging medicine*, Humana Press, Clifton, NJ, 1988.

Beauchamp, T. L. and Childress, J. F., *Principles of biomedical ethics*, 6th edn, Oxford University Press, New York, 2008.

Campbell, A., Charlesworth, M., Gillett, G., and Jones, G., *Medical ethics*, 2nd edn, Oxford University Press, Auckland, 1997.

Charlesworth, M., *Bioethics in a liberal society*, Cambridge University Press, Cambridge, 1993.

Gillon, R., *Philosophical medical ethics*, John Wiley & Sons, Chichester, UK, 1986.

——, (ed.), *Principles of health care ethics*, John Wiley & Sons, Chichester, UK, 1994.

Honderich, T. (ed.), *The Oxford companion to philosophy*, Oxford University Press, Oxford, 1995.

Jonas, H., *The imperative of responsibility: In search of an ethics for the technological age*, University of Chicago Press, Chicago, 1984.

Jonsen, A. R., Siegler, M., and Winslade, W. J., *Clinical ethics: A practical approach to ethical decisions in clinical medicine*, 4th edn, McGraw Hill, New York, 1998.

Kuhse, H. and Singer, P. (eds), *Bioethics: An anthology*, Blackwell, Malden, Massachusetts, 2006.

Mill, J. S., *Three essays*, Oxford University Press, London, 1975.

Moreno, J. D., *Deciding together: Bioethics and moral consensus*, Oxford University Press, New York, 1995.

Nicholson, R. H., *Medical research with children: Ethics, law, and practice*, Oxford University Press, Oxford, 1986.

Parker, M. and Dickenson, D., *Cambridge medical ethics workbook: Case studies, commentaries and activities*, Cambridge University Press, Cambridge, 2001.

Pellegrino, E. D. and Thomasma, D. C., *For the patient's good: The restoration of beneficence in health care*, Oxford University Press, New York, 1988.

Singer, P., *Practical ethics*, Cambridge University Press, Cambridge, 1979.

Sullivan, R. J., *Immanuel Kant's moral theory*, Cambridge University Press, Cambridge, 1989.

Warnock, M., *Making babies: Is there a right to have children?*, Oxford University Press, Oxford, 2002.

BIBLIOGRAPHY

'Abortion hero turns pro-life', *Sydney Morning Herald* (reprinted from *New York Times*), 12 August 1995, p. 17.

Acute and Co-ordinated Care Branch, Commonwealth Department of Health and Ageing, 'Primary care initiatives: Further co-ordinated care trials', <www.health.gov.au/hsdd/primcare/acoorcar/abtrials.htm>.

Aiken, L. H., Clarke, S. P., Sloane, D. M., Sochalski, J., and Silber, J. H., 'Hospital nurse staffing and patient mortality, nurse burnout, and job dissatisfaction', *Journal of the American Medical Association*, 288(16), 2002, pp. 1987–93.

Alcorn, G., 'Mercy death world first: Cancer sufferer first to die under Northern Territory euthanasia law', *Sydney Morning Herald*, 26 September 1996, p. 1.

Alexandra, A. and Woodruff, A., 'A code of ethics for the nursing profession', in M. Coady and S. Bloch (eds), *Codes of ethics and the professions*, Melbourne University Press, Melbourne, 1996, pp. 226–43.

American Health Information Management Association, 'AHIMA Code of Ethics, 2004', <www.ahima.org>.

Andersen, B. and Aranson, E., 'Iceland's database is ethically questionable', *British Medical Journal*, 318(7197), 1999, p. 1565.

Annas, G. J., 'Baby Fae: The "anything goes" school of human experimentation', *Hastings Center Report*, 15(1), 1985, pp. 15–16.

——, 'The changing landscape of human experimentation: From Nuremberg and Helsinki to AIDS and cancer', talk given at Grand Rounds, Royal Prince Alfred Hospital, Sydney, 7 August 1992.

——, *Judging medicine*, Humana Press, Clifton, NJ, 1988.

Antiel, R. M., Curlin, F. A., Hook, C. C., and Tilburt, J. C., 'The impact of medical school oaths and other professional codes of ethics: Results of a national physician survey', *Archives of Internal Medicine*, 171(5), 2011, pp. 469–71.

Appelbaum, P. S. and Grisso, T., 'Capacities of hospitalized, medically ill patients to consent to treatment', *Psychosomatics*, 38(2), 1997, pp. 119–25.

Asch, D. A. and Ubel, P. A., 'Rationing by any other name', *New England Journal of Medicine*, 336(23), 1997, pp. 1668–71.

Associated Press, 'Baboon man out of hospital', *Weekend Australian*, 6–7 January, 1996, p. 11.

Australian Bureau of Statistics, *Hospitals Australia 1991–92*, Cat. no. 4391.10, Australian Bureau of Statistics, Canberra, 1993.

——, *Private hospitals 1994–95*, Cat. no. 4390.0, Australian Bureau of Statistics, Canberra, 1996.

Australian Federation of AIDS Organisations (AFAO), *Submission to the Baume Review of the Drug Evaluation and Access Process in Australia*, Sydney, 1991.

Australian Health Ethics Committee and Office of the Federal Privacy
    Commissioner, *Review of guidelines under Section 95 of the Privacy Act 1988*, AGPS,
    Canberra, 2003.

Australian Law Reform Commission, 'Background report no. 22', in *Australian Law
    Reform Commission, Privacy*, vol. 1, AGPS, Canberra, 1983.

Australian Medical Association, *AMA Code of Ethics*, AMA, Canberra, 2004.

Australian Research Council, Australian Vice-Chancellors' Committee, and National
    Health and Medical Research Council, *National statement on ethical conduct in
    human research*, Canberra, 2007, and as amended 2009.

Bacchetti, P. and Moss, A. R., 'Incubation period of AIDS in San Francisco', *Nature*,
    338, 1989, pp. 251–3.

Baker, S. M., Brawley, O. W., and Marks, L. S. 'Effects of untreated syphilis in the
    negro male, 1932–1972: A closure comes to the Tuskegee study, 2004', *Urology*,
    65(6), 2005, pp. 1259–62.

Barker, S. F., 'What is a profession?', *Professional Ethics: A Multidisciplinary Journal*,
    1(1/2), 1992, pp. 73–99.

Baume, P., 'Voluntary euthanasia and law reform', *Australian Quarterly*, 68(3), 1996,
    pp. 17–23.

Beauchamp, D. E., 'Community: The neglected tradition of public health', in
    Beauchamp, D. E. and Steinbock, B. (eds), *New ethics for the public's health*,
    Oxford University Press, Sydney, 1999, pp. 57–67.

Beauchamp, T. L. and Childress J. F., *Principles of biomedical ethics*, 2nd edn, Oxford
    University Press, New York, 1983.

——, *Principles of biomedical ethics*, 3rd edn, Oxford University Press, New York, 1989.

——, *Principles of biomedical ethics*, 4th edn, Oxford University Press, New York, 1994.

——, *Principles of biomedical ethics*, 5th edn, Oxford University Press, New York, 2001.

Benko, L. B. and Bellandi, D., 'The rough and tumble of it', *Modern Healthcare*, 31(12),
    2001, pp. 53–4.

Berg, K., 'Ethical aspects of early diagnosis of genetic diseases', *World Health*, 5, 1996,
    pp. 20–1.

Berglund, C. A., 'Australian standards for privacy and confidentiality of health
    records in research: Implications of the Commonwealth Privacy Act', *Medical
    Journal of Australia*, 152, 1990, pp. 664–9.

——, 'A survey of Sydney adults about the conduct of medical research', *Australian
    Health Review*, 17(1), 1994, pp. 135–44.

——, 'Children in medical research: Australian ethical standards', *Child: Care, Health
    and Development*, 21(2), 1995, pp. 149–59.

——, 'Mandatory HIV testing of patients and professionals: Bringing ethics into
    practice', *Medical Education*, 29, 1995, pp. 360–3.

——, 'Bioethics: A balancing of concerns in context', *Australian Health Review*, 20(1),
    1997, pp. 43–52.

——, 'Thoughts before whistling', *Australian Health Review*, 20(4), 1997, pp. 5–12.

Berglund, C. A. (ed.), *Health research*, Oxford University Press, Melbourne, 2001.

Berglund, C. and Devereux, J., 'Consent to medical treatment: Children making medical decisions for others', *Australian Journal of Forensic Sciences*, 32, 2000, pp. 25–6.

Berglund, C. A. and McNeill, P. M., 'Guidelines for research practice in Australia: NHMRC statement and professional codes', *Community Health Studies*, 13(2), 1989, 121–129.

Berglund, C. A., Mitchell, K., and Cox, K., *Exploring clinical ethics: Distance module in Masters of Clinical Education course*, 2nd edn, University of New South Wales, Sydney, 1993.

Berglund, C. A., Pond, C. D., Harris, M. F., McNeill, P. M., Gietzelt, D., Comino, E., Traynor, V., Meldrum, E., and Boland, C., 'The formation of professional and consumer solutions: Ethics in the general practice setting', *Health Care Analysis*, 5(2), 1997, pp. 164–7.

Berglund, C. A., Pond, D. C., Traynor, V., Gietzelt, D., McNeill, P. M., Harris, M. F., and Comino, E., 'General practice and ethics: Listening and understanding concerns raised by general practitioners and consumers', paper presented at the Fifth National Conference of the Australian Bioethics Association, Melbourne, 3–6 April 1997.

Berlant, J. L., *Profession and monopoly: A study of medicine in the United States and Great Britain*, University of California Press, Berkeley, CA, 1975.

Bernat, J. L. and Peterson, L. M., 'Patient-centered informed consent in surgical practice', *Archives of Surgery*, 141(1), 2006, pp. 86–92.

Berryman, J., 'Discussing the ethics of research on young children', in J. van Eys (ed.), *Research on children: Medical imperatives, ethical quandaries, and legal constraints*, University Park Press, Baltimore, MY, 1978, pp. 85–104.

Blackmer, J. and Haddad, H., 'The Declaration of Helsinki: An update on paragraph 30', *Canadian Medical Association Journal*, 173(9), 2005, pp. 1052–3.

Blonder, I., 'Blowing the whistle', in M. Coady and S. Bloch (eds), *Codes of ethics and the professions*, Melbourne University Press, Melbourne, 1996, pp. 166–90.

Bolsin, S., 'Professional misconduct: The Bristol case', *Medical Journal of Australia*, 169, 1998, pp. 369–72.

Brahams, D., 'Right to know in Japan' (letter), *Lancet*, 2, 1989, p. 173.

British Medical Association, 'Information revolution could mean patients have more access to records', 11 January 2011, <www.bma.org.uk>.

British Royal Infirmary Inquiry, *Learning from Bristol: the Report of the Public Inquiry into Children's Heart Surgery at the British Royal Infirmary*, Stationery Office, London, 2001.

Brody, H., 'The four principles and narrative ethics', in R. Gillon (ed.), *Principles of health care ethics*, John Wiley & Sons, Chichester, UK, 1994, pp. 207–15.

Brooks, M. J., 'Commentary: RU-486: Politics of abortion and science', *Journal of Pharmacy & Law*, 2, 1993, pp. 261–92.

Brown, N., 'The "harm" in euthanasia', *Australian Quarterly*, 68(3), 1996, pp. 26–35.

Burnard, P., *Counselling skills for health professionals*, 2nd edn, Chapman & Hall, London, 1994.

Callahan, D., 'Achievable goals', *World Health*, 5, 1996, pp. 6–8.

Campbell, A., Charlesworth, M., Gillett, G., and Jones, G., *Medical ethics*, 2nd edn, Oxford University Press, Auckland, 1997.

Cassarett, D. J., Karlawish, J. H. T., and Moreno, J. D., 'A taxonomy of value in clinical research', *IRB: Ethics & Human Research*, 24(6), 2002, pp. 1–6.

CCH, 'Death with dignity', *Australian Health and Medical Law Reporter*, CCH, Sydney, updated regularly, sections 22–268.

Centers for Disease Control, 'Revision of the CDC surveillance case definition for acquired immunodeficiency syndrome', *Morbidity and Mortality Weekly Report*, 36, supplement no. 1S, 1987 (inclusive page numbers).

——, 'Public Health Service statement on management of occupational exposure to human immunodeficiency virus, including considerations regarding zidovudine postexposure use', *Morbidity and Mortality Weekly Report*, 39, no. RR–1, 1990 (inclusive page numbers).

Chalmers, I. and Silverman, W. A., 'Professional and public double standards on clinical experimentation', *Controlled Clinical Trials*, 8(4), 1987, pp. 388–91.

Chant, K., Lowe, D., Rubin, G., Manning, W., O' Donoughue, R., Lyle, D., Levy, M., Morey, S., Kaldor, J., Garsia, R., Penny, R., Marriott, D., Cunningham, A., and Tracy, G. D., 'Patient-to-patient transmission of HIV in private surgical consulting rooms' (letter), *Medical Journal of Australia*, 342, 1993, pp. 1548–9.

Chapman, C., 'Swiss hospital lets terminally ill patients commit suicide in its beds', *British Medical Journal*, 332, 2006, p. 7.

Charlesworth, M., *Bioethics in a liberal society*, Cambridge University Press, Cambridge, 1993.

Chong, S. and Normile, D., 'How young Korean researchers helped unearth a scandal', *Science*, 311(5757), 2006, pp. 22–5.

Cica, N., *The euthanasia debate in Australia: Legal and political issues*, issues paper no. 2, Australian Institute of Health Law and Ethics, 1997.

Clarke, A., Devereux, J., and Werren, J., *Torts: A practical learning approach*, 2nd edn, LexisNexis, Sydney, 2011.

Collinson, D., *Fifty major philosophers: A reference guide*, Routledge, London, 1987.

Commission for Health Improvement, 'National patients survey programme: 2003 results', NHS, London, 2003, <www.chi.nhs.uk/eng/surveys/nps2003>.

Commonwealth Department of Foreign Affairs and Trade, 'Major step to protect rights of children', *Australian Foreign Affairs and Trade*, 61(12), 1990, p. 893.

Commonwealth Department of Health and Family Services, *Supplement to Medicare benefits schedule book*, 1 November 1996 (effective 1 May 1997), AGPS, Canberra, 1997.

Coney, S., *The unfortunate experiment: The full story behind the inquiry into cervical cancer treatment,* Penguin, Auckland, 1988.

Connell, J., 'Doctors seek powers to test for HIV', *Sydney Morning Herald,* 5 April 1994, p. 3.

Coombes, R., '"Paternalism" at the root of body parts nightmare', *Nursing Times,* 97(6), pp. 10–11.

Corsino, B. V., 'Bioethics committees and JCAHO patients' rights standards: A question of balance', *Journal of Clinical Ethics,* 7(2), 1996, pp. 177–81.

Coverdale, J., 'Ethics in forensic psychiatry', in W. Brookbanks (ed.), *Psychiatry and the law: Clinical and legal issues,* Brookers, Wellington, 1996, pp. 59–70.

Cox, K., 'Stories as case knowledge: Case knowledge as stories', *Medical Education,* 35, 2001, pp. 862–6.

Czecowoski, B. J. A., *Privacy and confidentiality of health care information,* American Hospital Association, Chicago, IL, 1984.

Davies, B. J. and Macfarlane, J., 'Clinical decision making by dentists working in the NHS General Dental Services since April 2006', *British Dental Journal,* 209(10), 2010, p. E17.

Dawson, R. T., 'Drugs in sport: The role of the physician', *Journal of Endocrinology,* 170(1), 2001, pp. 55–61.

Deber, R. B., Kraetschmer, N., and Irvine, J., 'What role do patients wish to play in treatment decision making?', *Archives of Internal Medicine,* 156, 1996, pp. 1414–20.

Deckers, J., 'Why current UK legislation on embryo research is immoral: How the argument from lack of qualities and the argument for potentiality have been applied and why they should be rejected', *Bioethics,* 19(3), 2005, pp. 251–71.

De Grazia, D., 'Moving forward in bioethical theory: Theories, cases, and specified principlism', *Journal of Medicine and Philosophy,* 17, 1992, pp. 511–39.

Department of Health (UK), *Governance arrangements for research ethics committees: A harmonised edition,* 2011, <www.dh.gov.uk>.

Department of Health and Human Services (US), 'Protections for children involved as subjects in research', *Federal Register,* 48, 1983, pp. 9814–20; revised *Federal Register,* 56, 1991, p. 28032, 45 CFR Part 46, Subpart D.

——, Food and Drug Administration, 'Additional safeguards for children in clinical investigations of FDA-regulated products', *Federal Register,* 66, 2001, pp. 20589–600, 21 CFR Parts 50 and 56.

——, Office for Human Research Subject Protections, 'Protecting human research subjects: Institutional Review Board Guidebook, 1993', <www.hhs.gov/ohrp>.

——, Office of Research Integrity, 'Sample policy and procedures for responding to allegations of research misconduct', <www.ori.dhhs.gov>.

——, 'HIPAA Administrative simplification statute and rules', <www.hhs.gov/ocr/privacy>.

de Ridder, D., Depla, M., Severens, P., and Malsch, M., 'Beliefs on coping with illness: A consumer's perspective', *Social Science & Medicine*, 44(5), 1997, pp. 553–9.

Devereux, J., *Medical law: Text, cases and materials*, 1st edn, Cavendish, Sydney, 1997.

——, *Medical law: Text, cases and materials*, 2nd edn, Cavendish, Sydney, 2002.

——, *Medical law: Text, cases and materials*, 3rd edn, Cavendish, Sydney, 2007.

de Vries, B. and Cossart, Y. E., 'Needlestick injury in medical students', *Medical Journal of Australia*, 160, 1994, pp. 398–400.

Di Angelis, A. J., Born, D. O., and Hill, A. J., 'State dental boards and mandatory HIV testing', *Northwest Dentistry*, 71(5), 1992, pp. 33–5.

Dickens, B. M., 'Issues in preparing ethical guidelines for epidemiological studies', *Law, Medicine & Health Care*, 19(3–4), 1991, pp. 175–83.

——, 'Legal approaches to health care ethics and the four principles', in R. Gillon (ed.), *Principles of health care ethics*, John Wiley & Sons, Chichester, UK, 1994, pp. 305–17.

Dickenson, D. L., 'Consent in children', in M. Parker and D. Dickenson (eds), *The Cambridge medical ethics workbook: Case studies, commentaries and activities*, Cambridge University Press, Cambridge, 2001, pp. 209–13.

Dickinson, G. M., Morhart, R. E., Klimas, N. G., Bandea, C. I., Laracuente, J. M., and Bisno, A. L., 'Absence of HIV transmission from an infected dentist to his patients: An epidemiologic and DNA sequence analysis', *Journal of the American Medical Association*, 269(14), 1993, pp. 1802–6.

'Doctor helped woman commit suicide', *Sydney Morning Herald* (reprinted from *New York Times*), 7 June 1990, p. 12.

'Dolly's cloners say no to families', *Australian*, 27 June 1997, p. 7.

Dorr-Goold, S. and Klipp, G., 'Managed care members talk about trust', *Social Science & Medicine*, 54(6), 2002, pp. 879–88.

Douglas, M., 'Risk acceptability according to the social sciences', *Social Research Perspectives—Occasional Reports on Current Topics*, Russell Sage Foundation, New York, 1985.

Dow, S., 'Trials and terror: Medical ethics under the microscope', *Sydney Morning Herald*, 14 June 1997, p. 35.

Doyal, L., 'Clinical ethics committees and the formulation of health care policy', *Journal of Medical Ethics*, 27, Supplement 1, 2001, pp. 144–9.

Dunne, E., 'Consultation, rapport, and collaboration: Essential preliminary stages in research with urban Aboriginal groups', *Australian Journal of Primary Health Interchange*, 6(1), 2000, pp. 6–14.

Dutch Pediatric Association, *To treat or not to treat? Limits for life-sustaining treatment in neonatology* (in Dutch), Utrecht, Netherlands, 1992, cited in F. J. Walther, 'Withholding treatment, withdrawing treatment, and palliative care in the neonatal intensive care unit', *Early Human Development*, 81(12), 2005, pp. 965–72.

Dworkin, G., 'Law and medical experimentation: Of embryos, children and others with limited capacity', *Monash University Law Review*, 13, 1987, pp. 189–206.

Economic and Social Research Council, *Revised framework for research ethics*, 2010, <www.esrc.ac.uk>.

Edgar A., 'A discourse approach to quality of life measurement', in A. Surbone and M. Zwitter (eds), 'Communication with the cancer patient: Information and truth', *Annals of the New York Academy of Sciences*, 809, 1997, pp. 30–9.

Emanuel, E. J., Wood, A., Fleischman, A., Bowen, A., Getz, K. A., Grady, C., Levine, C., Hammerschmidt, D. E., Faden, R., Eckenweiler, L., Tucker, C., and Sugarman, J., 'Oversight of human participants research: Identifying problems to evaluate reform proposals', *Annals of Internal Medicine*, 141, 2004, pp. 282–91.

English, V., Roman-Critchley, G., Sheather, J., Sommerville, A., and Dehn, G., 'Would you "blow the whistle"?', *British Medical Journal*, 325, 2002, p. 541.

Epstein, J. A. and Parmacek, M. S., 'Recent advances in cardiac development with therapeutic implications for adult cardiovascular disease', *Circulation*, 112, 2005, pp. 592–7.

Evans, B. T. and Pritchard, C., 'Cancer survival rates and GDP expenditure on health: A comparison of England and Wales and the USA, Denmark, Netherlands, Finland, France, Germany, Italy, Spain and Switzerland in the 1990s', *Public Health*, 114(5), 2000, pp. 336–9.

Faroque, F., 'Impolite doctors top list of complaints', *Age*, 7 December 1996, p. A8.

Ferngren, G. B., 'Roman lay attitudes towards medical experimentation', *Bulletin of the History of Medicine*, 59(4), 1985, pp. 495–505.

Finnis, J., 'The rights and wrongs of abortion', in M. Cohen (ed.), *The rights and wrongs of abortion*, Princeton University Press, Princeton, NJ, 1974, pp. 85–113.

Finucane, P., Myser, C., and Ticehurst, S., '"Is she fit to sign, doctor?": Practical ethical issues in assessing the competence of elderly patients', *Medical Journal of Australia*, 159, 1993, pp. 400–3.

Flaherty, D. H., *Protecting privacy in surveillance societies*, University of North Carolina Press, Chapel Hill, NC, 1989.

Flew, A., 'The principle of euthanasia', in A. B. Downing (ed.), *Euthanasia and the right to death*, Nash Publishing, Los Angeles, 1970, pp. 30–48.

Flores, J. A. and Dodier, A., 'HIPAA: Past, present and future implications for nurses', *Online Journal of Issues in Nursing*, 10(2), 2005.

Flynn, G., 'The NIH ethics crackdown: A message to the research community', *Annals of Emergency Medicine*, 47(1), 2006, pp. 57–60.

Foot, P., 'Killing and letting die', in J. L. Garfield and P. Henessey (eds), *Abortion: Moral and legal perspectives*, University of Massachusetts Press, Amherst, MA, 1985, pp. 177–85.

Forrester, K. and Griffiths, D., *Essentials of law for health professionals*, Harcourt, Sydney, 2001.

Foster, P., 'Girl, 15, forced to have new heart', *Sydney Morning Herald*, 17 July, 1999, p. 19.

Frankel, M. S., 'The development of policy guidelines governing human experimentation in the United States: A case study of public policy-making for science and technology', *Ethics in Science & Medicine*, 2, 1975, pp. 43–59.

Freckelton, I., 'Enforcement of ethics', in M. Coady and S. Bloch (eds), *Codes of ethics and the professions*, Melbourne University Press, Melbourne, 1996, pp. 130–65.

'Frozen embryos in legal limbo', *Sydney Morning Herald* (reprinted from *New York Times*), 3 June 1992, p. 15.

Fryback, D. G. and Lawrence, W. F., 'Dollars may not buy as many QALYs as we think: A problem with defining quality-of-life adjustments', *Medical Decision Making*, 17(3), 1997, pp. 277–84.

Gallagher, A., 'Ethical issues in patient restraint', *Nursing Times*, 107(9), 2011, pp. 18–20.

Gert, B., 'Morality, moral theory, and applied and professional ethics', *Professional Ethics: A Multidisciplinary Journal*, 1(1/2), 1992, pp. 5–24.

Gietzelt, D. and Jones, G., 'What language?', in C. Berglund and D. Saltman (eds), *Communication for health care*, Oxford University Press, Melbourne, 2002, pp. 15–32.

Gillett, G., 'The new ethical committees: Their nature and role', *New Zealand Medical Journal*, 102, 1989, pp. 314–15.

Gillon, R., *Philosophical medical ethics*, John Wiley & Sons, Chichester, UK, 1986.

—— (ed.), *Principles of health care ethics*, John Wiley & Sons, Chichester, UK, 1994.

Gilmore, N., 'The impact of AIDS on drug availability and accessibility', *AIDS*, 5, supplement no. 2, 1992, pp. S253–62.

Gomez, A. G., Grimm, C. T., Yee, E. F. T., and Skootsky, S. A., 'Preparing residents for managed care practice using an experience-based curriculum', *Academic Medicine*, 72(11), 1997, pp. 959–65.

Gong, Z. and Niklason, L. E., 'Use of human mesenchymal stem cells as alternative source of smooth muscle cells in vessel engineering', *Methods in Molecular Biology*, 698, 2011, pp. 279–94.

Gostin, L. O., 'Medical countermeasures for pandemic influenza: Ethics and the law', *Journal of the American Medical Association*, 295(5), 2006, pp. 554–6.

Grace, D. and Cohen, S., *Business ethics*, 3rd edn, Oxford University Press, Melbourne, 1995.

Grisso, T. and Vierling, L., 'Minors' consent to treatment: A developmental perspective', *Professional Psychology*, 9, 1978, pp. 412–27.

Hall, M., 'Bush OKs limited stem-cell funding', *USA Today*, 10 August 2001, p. 1.

Haimes, E. and Taylor, K., 'Fresh embryo donation for human embryonic stem cell (HESC) research: The experiences and values of IVF couples asked to be embryo donor', *Human Reproduction*, 24(9), 2009, pp. 2142–50.

Harman, G., 'Moral relativism defended', *Philosophical Review*, 84, 1975, pp. 3–22.

Harrison, C. and Laxer, R. M., 'A bioethics program in pediatric rheumatology', *Journal of Rheumatology*, 27(7), 2000, pp. 1780–2.

Hawkes, N., 'Arthritic Dolly is mutton dressed as lamb', *Times*, 5 January 2002, p. 22.

Hawkes, N. and Rhodes, T., 'Human clones within two years', *Weekend Australian*, 8–9 March 1997, p. 15.

'Health inequality: The UK's biggest issue', editorial, *Lancet*, 349, 1997, p. 1185.

Health Research Council of New Zealand, *HRC guidelines for ethics committee accreditation*, 2008, <www.hrc.govt.nz>.

Heard, S. E., 'Multidisciplinary response of San Francisco General Hospital to the AIDS epidemic', *American Journal of Hospital Pharmacy*, 46, 1989, pp. S7–10.

Henry, D., Keys, C., Balcazar, F., and Jopp, D., 'Attitudes of community-living staff members towards persons with mental retardation, mental illness, and dual diagnosis', *Mental Retardation*, 34(6), 1996, pp. 367–79.

Henry, D. and Lexchin, J., 'The pharmaceutical industry as a medicines provider', *Lancet*, 360(9345), 2002, pp. 1590–2.

Honderich, T. (ed.), *The Oxford companion to philosophy*, Oxford University Press, Oxford, 1995.

Hope, T. and Slowther, A., 'Clinical ethics committee in the UK', *Bulletin of Medical Ethics*, 178, 2002, pp. 13–15.

Horton, R., 'The real lessons from Harold Frederick Shipman', *Lancet*, 357, 2001, pp. 82–3.

Hoshino, K., 'Information and self-determination', *World Health*, 5, 1996, p. 12.

'Hospital faker ends in doc', *Sydney Morning Herald* (reprinted from Reuters), 30 December 1995, p. 10.

Hubert, E. M., Douglas-Stelle, D., and Bickel, J., 'Context in medical education: The informal ethics curriculum', *Medical Education*, 30, 1996, pp. 353–64.

Institute of Medicine (USA), *The AIDS Research Program of the National Institutes of Health*, National Academy Press, Washington DC, 1991.

International Committee of Medical Journal Editors, *Uniform requirements for manuscripts submitted to biomedical journals*, ICMJE, Philadelphia, PA, 2010.

Jagger, J., Hunt, E. H., Brand-Elnaggar, J., and Pearson, R. D., 'Rates of needle-stick injury caused by various devices in a university hospital', *New England Journal of Medicine*, 319(5), 1988, pp. 284–8.

James, P. D., *Devices and desires*, Penguin, London, 1989.

Jasny, B. R. and Zahn, L. M., 'A celebration of the genome', Part IV Essay—Genome Sequencing Anniversary, *Science*, 331, 2011, pp. 1024–7.

Jennett, B., 'Quality of care and cost containment in the U.S. and the U.K.', *Theoretical Medicine*, 10(3), 1989, pp. 207–15.

Joel, A., 'The man who cares for kids', *Good Weekend*, 4 January 1997, pp. 23–5.

Johnston, J., 'Stem cell protocols: The NAS Guidelines are a useful start', *Hastings Center Report*, 35(6), 2005, pp. 16–17.

Jonas, H., 'Philosophical reflections on experimenting with human subjects', *Daedalus*, 98(2), 1969, pp. 219–47.

——, *The imperative of responsibility: In search of an ethics for the technological age*, University of Chicago Press, Chicago, 1984.

Jones, J. H., *Bad blood: The Tuskegee syphilis experiment*, Free Press, New York, 1981.

Jonsen, A. R., Siegler, M., and Winslade, W. J., *Clinical ethics: A practical approach to ethical decisions in clinical medicine*, 4th edn, McGraw-Hill, New York, 1998.

Kerrison, S. and Pollock, A. M., 'The reform of UK research ethics committees: Throwing the baby out with the bath water?', *Journal of Medical Ethics*, 31(8), 2005, pp. 487–9.

Kitzhaber, J. and Kemmy, A. M., 'On the Oregon trail', *British Medical Bulletin*, 51(4), 1995, pp. 808–18.

Knultgen, J., *Ethics and professionalism*, University of Pennsylvania Press, Philadelphia, PA, 1988.

Krugman, S. and Giles, J. P., 'Viral hepatitis: New light on old disease', *Journal of the American Medical Association*, 212(6), 1970, pp. 1019–29.

Kuhse, H., 'Caution, not panic, on cloning', *Australian*, 12 June 1997, p. 11.

Larriera, A., 'Doctors' HIV: Patients will ask', *Sydney Morning Herald*, 3 August 1994, p. 5.

Lederberg, M. S., 'The psychological repercussions of New York State's do-not-resuscitate law', in A. Surbone and M. Zwitter (eds), 'Communication with the cancer patient: Information and truth', *Annals of the New York Academy of Sciences*, 809, 1997, pp. 223–36.

Lee, J. J., 'Comment: What is past is prologue: The International Conference on harmonization and lessons learned from European drug regulations harmonization', *University of Pennsylvania Journal of International Economic Law*, 26, 2005, p. 151.

Lee, J. W., 'Director-General Elect, speech to the Fifty-sixth World Health Assembly', 21 May 2003, Geneva, Switzerland, <www.who.int/dg_elect/wha56_jwlspeech/en/print.html>.

Leiken, S., 'A proposal concerning decisions to forgo life-sustaining treatment for young people', *Journal of Pediatrics*, 115(1), 1989, pp. 17–22.

Le Moncheck, L., 'Philosophy, gender politics, and in vitro fertilization: A feminist ethics of reproductive healthcare', *Journal of Clinical Ethics*, 7(2), 1996, pp. 160–81.

Lennane, K. J., 'Whistleblowing: A health issue', *British Medical Journal*, 307, 1993, pp. 667–70.

Levine C., Dubler, N. N, and Levine, R. J., 'Building a new consensus: Ethical principles and policies for clinical research on HIV/AIDS', *IRB: A Review of Human Subjects Research*, 13(1/2), 1991, pp. 1–17.

Levine, R. J., *Ethics and regulation of clinical research*, Urban & Schwarzenberg, Baltimore and Munich, 1986.

Levit, K., Smith, C., Cowan, C., Lazenby, H., Sensenig, A., and Catlin, A., 'Trends in U.S. health care spending, 2001', *Health Affairs*, 22(1), 2003, pp. 154–64.

Levitt, M., 'Let the consumer decide? The regulation of commercial genetic testing', *Journal of Medical Ethics*, 27(6), 2001, pp. 398–404.

Lewis, R. and Appleby, J., 'Can the English NHS meet the 18-week waiting list target?', *Journal of the Royal Society of Medicine*, 99(1), 2006, pp. 10–13.

Liang, B. A., 'The adverse event of unaddressed medical error: Identifying and filling the holes in the health-care and legal systems', *Journal of Law, Medicine & Ethics*, 29, 2001, pp. 346–68.

Lockwood, M., 'When does a life begin?', in M. Lockwood (ed.), *Moral dilemmas in modern medicine*, Oxford University Press, London, 1985, pp. 9–31.

Lovell, R., 'Ethics at the growing edge of medicine: The regulatory side of medical research', *Australian Health Review*, 9(3), 1986, pp. 234–50.

Lovett, K. M. and Liang, B. A., 'Direct-to-consumer cardiac screening and suspect risk evaluation', *JAMA*, 305(24), 2011, pp. 2567–8.

Lustig, B. A., 'The method of "principlism": A critique of the critique', *Journal of Medicine and Philosophy*, 17, 1992, pp. 487–510.

Lyall, K., '30-baht health care a fatal prescription', *Australian*, 24 April 2002, p. 8.

McBride, G., 'Living liver donor', *British Medical Journal*, 299, 1989, pp. 1417–18.

McCombs, J. S. (letter) *New England Journal of Medicine*, 335(19), 1996, p. 1465.

McDowell, B., 'The excuses that make professional ethics irrelevant', *Professional Ethics: A Multidisciplinary Journal*, 3(3/4), 1994, pp. 157–70.

MacLeod, P. and Clarke, F. F., 'Forget cloning and pay attention to China', *Canadian Medical Association Journal*, 159(2), 1998, pp. 153–5.

McNeill, P. M., 'The implications for Australia of the New Zealand Report of the Cervical Cancer Inquiry: No cause for complacency', *Medical Journal of Australia*, 150, 1989, pp. 264–96.

McNeill, P. M., Walters, J. D., and Webster, I. W., 'Ethical issues in Australian hospitals', *Medical Journal of Australia*, 160, 1994, pp. 63–5.

McPherson, K. M., Harwood, M., McNaughton, H. K., 'Ethnicity, equity, and quality: Lessons from New Zealand', *British Medical Journal*, 327(7412), pp. 443–4.

McVeigh, A., 'Violet Townsend Inquiry reaction', *Citizen*, 22 July 2003, pp. 12–13.

— 'We're improving our care services', *Gloucestershire Echo*, 29 July 2003, p. 9.

Magney, A. G. and Berglund, C. A., 'Co-ordinated care: Ethics debate as part of the trial process', *Evaluation*, 6(4), 2000, pp. 455–69.

Malley, B., 'Professionalism and professional ethics', in D. E. Edgar (ed.), *Social change in Australia*, Cheshire, Melbourne, 1974, pp. 391–408.

Mallon, D. F. J., Shearwood, W., Malla, S. A., French, M. A. H., and Dawkins, R. L., 'Exposure to blood borne infections in health care workers', *Medical Journal of Australia*, 157, 1992, pp. 592–5.

Mannion, R., 'General practitioner-led commissioning in the NHS: Progress, prospects and pitfalls (Review)', *British Medical Journal*, 97(1), 2011, pp. 7–15.

Marcus, R., 'Surveillance of health care workers exposed to blood from patients infected with human immunodeficiency virus', *New England Journal of Medicine*, 319, 1988, pp. 1118–23.

Marino, K., *Resumes for the health care professional*, John Wiley & Sons, New York, 1993.

Mill, J. S., 'On liberty', in *Three essays*, Oxford University Press, London, 1975, pp. 92–114.

Mitchell, K. R. and Lovat, T. J., *Bioethics for medical and health professionals*, Social Sciences Press, Wentworth Falls, NSW, 1991.

Momber, J. M. and Rueda, R. M., 'Bioethics and medical practice', *World Health*, 5, 1996, pp. 29–31.

Moodie, A-M., 'A code of ethics doesn't ensure business ethics', *Australian Financial Review*, 18 July 1997, p. 61, quoted in D. Grace and S. Cohen, *Business ethics*, Oxford University Press, Melbourne, 1995.

Mooney, G. H., Russell, E. M, and Weir, R. D, *Choices for health care: A practical introduction to the economics of health provision*, 2nd edn, Macmillan, London, 1986.

Morris, P., 'County dental care is in crisis', *Gloucestershire Echo*, 18 July 2003, pp. 1–2.

——, 'Queuing for NHS dentists: Is it Prestbury next?', *Gloucestershire Echo*, 30 July 2003, p. 3.

Morrow, L., 'When one body can save another', *Time*, 17 June 1991, pp. 46–50.

Motor Accidents Authority, *New South Wales Health bulk billing handbook*, State Health Publications No. (FB) 960105, Motor Accidents Authority, Sydney, May 1996.

Mulhall A., 'Anthropology, nursing and midwifery: A natural alliance?', *International Journal of Nursing Studies*, 33(6), 1996, pp. 629–37.

Murphy, T. F., 'Physician-assisted suicide and the slippery slope', *Department of Medical Education Bulletin*, 3(2), 1996, p. 1.

Naik, G., 'Patent ruling sets back EU stem-cell scientists', *Wall Street Journal*, 19 October 2011, <online.wsj.com>.

Nakajima, H., 'Health, ethics and human rights', *World Health*, 5, September–October, 1996, p. 3.

National Commission for the Protection of Subjects of Biomedical and Behavioral Research, *Report and recommendations: Institutional Review Boards*, Department of Health, Education and Welfare publication no. (OS) 78-0008, US Government Printer, Washington DC, 1978.

National Health and Medical Research Council, *The media and public health: A discussion of the role of the media in promoting the health of the public* (Standing Subcommittee on Health Promotion and Education, and Subcommittee on the Media and Health Promotion), NHMRC, Canberra, 1984.

——, 'General guidelines for medical practitioners on providing information to patients', 2004.

——, *National statement on ethical conduct in research involving humans*, Canberra, AGPS, 1999.

——, Australian Research Council, and Australian Vice-Chancellors' Committee, *National statement on ethical conduct in research involving humans*, 2009.

Nelson, R. M. and Ross, L. F., 'In defense of a single standard of research risk for all children', *Journal of Pediatrics*, 147(5), 2005, pp. 565–6.

New Zealand Medical Association Newsletter, 108, 1994, p. 3.

New Zealand Ministry of Health and National Ethics Advisory Committee, *Operational standard for ethics committees* (last updated 2002), <www.moh.govt.nz>.

Newton, J. S., Ard, W. R., Horner, R. H., and Toews, J. D., 'Focusing on values and lifestyle outcomes in an effort to improve the quality of residential services in Oregon', *Mental Retardation*, 34(1), 1996, pp. 1–12.

Nicholson, R. H., *Medical research with children: Ethics, law, and practice*, Oxford University Press, Oxford, 1986.

——, 'Bioethics attacked in Germany' (editorial review), *Bulletin of Medical Ethics*, 61, 1990, pp. 19–23.

Noonan, J. T., 'An almost absolute value in history', in J. Feinberg (ed.), *The problem of abortion*, Wadsworth, Belmont, CA, 1973, pp. 10–17.

NSW Department of Health, 'Waiting time and elective patient management policy (PD 2009_018), < www.health.nsw.gov.au/policies>.

——, 'Health records and information', Ch. 9 in *Patient matters: Manual for area health services and public hospitals*, NSW Department of Health, Sydney (updated regularly and current as at 2011), PD2005-004, PD2005-406, IB2005-054, <www.health.nsw.gov.au>.

NSW Medical Board, *2004 Annual Report*, NSW Medical Board, Sydney, 2004.

O'Brien, E., 'Making a note and handover', in C. Berglund and D. Saltman, *Communication for health care*, Oxford University Press, Melbourne, 2002, pp. 113–34.

Oliver, J. and Webb, D. J., 'Sildenafil for "blue babies": Such unlicensed drug use might be justified as last resort', *British Medical Journal*, 325(7373), 2002, p. 1174.

Olsen, D. P., 'Populations vulnerable to the ethics of caring', *Journal of Advanced Nursing*, 18, 1993, pp. 1696–700.

Oosterhof, J. E. J., Scholten-Linde, J. L. J., Houtepen, R., and Berglund, C. A., The interpretation of morality: Cross-purposes in the Australian euthanasia debate. Unpublished paper.

Organization for Economic Co-operation and Development, *OECD Health Data 2009*, OECD, Paris, <www.oecd.org>.

Otlowski, M., *Implications of genetic testing for Australian insurance law and practice*, Occasional Paper No. 1, Centre for Law and Genetics, University of Tasmania Law School, University of Melbourne Faculty of Law, Hobart and Melbourne, 2001.

Parker, M. and Dickenson, D., *The Cambridge medical ethics workbook: Case studies, commentaries and activities*, Cambridge University Press, Cambridge, 2001.

Parliament of New South Wales, 'Budget Paper No. 3', Budget estimates 2011–12, New South Wales Budget Tabled on 6 September 2011, Parliamentary Paper No. 107, in Session 551, <www.budget.nsw.gov.au>.

Parry, J., 'Funding of bird flu initiative exceeds expectations', *British Medical Journal*, 332(7535), 2006, p. 198.

Patterson, K., 'A fairer Medicare: Better access, more affordable', Media Release, 28 April 2003.

Peabody, J. W., Bickel, S. R., and Lawson, J. S., 'The Australian health care system: Are the incentives Down Under or right side up?', *Journal of the American Medical Association*, 276(24), 1996, pp. 1944–50.

Pearson, S. D., Sabin, J. E., and Hyams, T., 'Caring for patients within a budget: Physicians' tales from the front lines of managed care', *Journal of Clinical Ethics*, 13(2), 2002, pp. 115–23.

Peel, P., 'Community participation in decision-making and service delivery', *Canberra Bulletin of Public Administration*, 94, 1999, pp. 34–51.

Pellegrino, E., 'The metamorphosis of medical ethics: A 30 year retrospective', *Journal of the American Medical Association*, 269(9), 1993, pp. 1158–62.

Pellegrino, E. D. 'Character, virtue and self-interest in the ethics of the professions', *Journal of Contemporary Health Law and Policy*, 5, 1989, pp. 53–73.

Pellegrino, E. D. and Thomasma, D. C., *For the patient's good: The restoration of beneficence in health care*, Oxford University Press, New York, 1988.

Pennisi, E. and Williams, N., 'Will Dolly send in the clones?', *Science*, 275, 1997, pp. 1415–16.

Pharmacy Board of Australia, *Pharmacy Code of Conduct for registered health practitioners*, <www.ahpra.gov.au>.

Plomer, A., 'Beyond the HFE Act 1990: The regulation of stem cell research in the UK', *Medical Law Review*, 10, 2002, pp. 132–64.

Price, V. and Roberts, D. F., 'Public opinion processes', in C. R. Berger and S. H. Chaffee (eds), *Handbook of Communication Science*, Sage, Newbury Park, CA, 1987, pp. 781–816.

Powell, I., 'Providing quality healthcare under funding constraints', *New Zealand Medical Journal*, 118(1215), 2005, U1471.

Qiu, R-Z., 'Bioethics in an Asian context', *World Health*, 5, 1996, pp. 13–15.

Queensland Law Reform Commission, *Assisted and substituted decisions: Decision-making by and for people with a decision-making disability*, report no. 49, vol. 1, Queensland Law Reform Commission, Brisbane, 1996.

Quill, T. E. and Brody, H., 'Physician recommendations and patient autonomy: Finding a balance between physician power and patient choice', *Annals of Internal Medicine*, 125(9), 1996, pp. 763–9.

Rachels, J. A., 'Active and passive euthanasia', *New England Journal of Medicine*, 5, 1975, pp. 39–45.

Ramsay, S., 'Audit further exposes UK's worst serial killer', (news) *Lancet*, 357, 2001, pp. 123–5.

Ramsey, P., 'The enforcement of morals: Non-therapeutic research on children', *Hastings Center Report*, 6(4), 1976, pp. 21–30.

Rawls, J., *A theory of justice*, Belknap Press, Cambridge, MA, 1971.

Redfern, M., Keeling, J. W., and Powell, E., *The Royal Liverpool Children's Inquiry, Summary and Recommendations*, The Stationery Office, London, 30 January 2001.

Richardson, J., 'The importance of perspective in the measurement of quality-adjusted life years', *Medical Decision Making*, 17(1), 1997, pp. 33–41.

Robertson, J. A., 'Embryo stem cell research: Ten years of controversy', *Journal of Law, Medicine & Ethics*, 38(2), 2010, pp. 191–203.

Robotham, J., 'Thigh gives heart a leg-up and offers alternative to stem cells', *Sydney Morning Herald*, 9 May 2002, p. 3.

——, 'High-dose bird flu vaccine trial fails', *Sydney Morning Herald*, 18–19 February 2006, p. 3.

Rocker, G. M., Cook, D. J., Martin D. K., and Singer, P. A., 'Seasonal bed closures in an intensive care unit: A qualitative study', *Journal of Critical Care*, 18(1), 2003, pp. 25–30.

Royal College of Surgeons of England, 'Working party report, facial transplantation', 2003.

Salmon, D. A., Teret, S. P., MacIntyre, C. R., Salisbury, D., Burgers, M. A., and Halsey, N. A., 'Compulsory vaccination and conscientious or philosophical exemptions: Past, present, and future', *Lancet*, 367, 2006, pp. 436–42.

St Vincent's Bioethics Newsletter, 1(3), 1983, p. 12.

Schlink, L., 'Dolly dies of lung disease', *Sunday Telegraph*, 16 February 2003, p. 40.

——, 'New baby from dead husband', *Sunday Telegraph*, 10 February 2002, p. 46.

Schneider, G. W. and Snell, L., 'C.A.R.E.: An approach for teaching ethics in medicine', *Social Science & Medicine*, 51(10), 2000, pp. 1563–7.

Schroeder, S., 'Ethical issues for parents of extremely premature infants', *Journal of Paediatrics and Child Health*, 44(5), 2008, pp. 302–4.

Scott, J., 'Syringe may have held virus: QC', *Australian*, 30 August 1994, p. 3.

Seal, M., 'Patient advocacy and advance care planning in the acute hospital setting', *Australian Journal of Advanced Nursing*, 24(4), 2007, pp. 29–36.

Secretary of Health and Human Services, Presidential Commission for the Study of Bioethical Issues, *Charter*, Washington, DC 20201, 10 March 2010.

Shapiro, J., Rucker, L., and Robitshek, D., 'Teaching the art of doctoring: An innovative medical student elective', *Medical Teacher*, 28(1), 2006, pp. 30–5.

Shawndra, S., 'State intervention in the family: Child protective proceedings and termination of parental rights', *Columbia Journal of Law and Social Problems*, 40(4), 2007, pp. 485–93.

Shooner, C., 'The ethics of learning from patients', *Canadian Medical Association Journal*, 156(4), 1997, pp. 535–8.

Singer, P., *Practical ethics*, Cambridge University Press, Cambridge, 1979.

Singh, K. and Gan, G. L., 'An Asian perspective on euthanasia', *Australian Quarterly*, 68(3), 1996, pp. 36–45.

Skene, L., 'What should doctors tell patients?', *Medical Journal of Australia*, 159, 1993, pp. 367–8.

Slaytor, E. and Lesjak, M., 'Euthanasia seminar', in *News* (Newsletter of the NSW Branch of the Public Health Association), 11(2), 1997, p. 7.

Smets, T., Bilsen, J., Cohen, J., Rurup, M. L., Dekeyser, E., and Deliens, L., 'The medical practice of euthanasia in Belgium and the Netherlands: Legal notification, control and evaluation procedures', *Health Policy*, 90(2–3), 2009, pp. 181–7.

Smith & Nephew Surgical, *Hospital and health services year book 1995/96*, 20th edn, Peter Isaacson Publications Pty Ltd, Melbourne, 1996.

Smith, D., 'Cloning study points to early end for Dolly', *Sydney Morning Herald*, 11 February 2002, p. 6.

Smith, J., *The Shipman Inquiry. Third Report: Death certification and investigation of deaths by coroners*, presented to Parliament by the Secretary of State for the Home Department and the Secretary of State for Health by Command of Her Majesty July 2003. Cm5854. Whitehall, London, July 2003.

Smith, S., Newhouse, J. P. and Freeland, M. S., 'Income, insurance, and technology: Why does health spending outpace economic growth?', *Health Affairs*, 28(5), 2009, pp. 1276–84.

Solomon, W. D., 'Rules and principles', in W. T. Reich (ed.), *Encyclopedia of bioethics*, vol. 1, Free Press, New York, 1978, pp. 407–13.

Sorlier, V., Forde, R., Lindseth, A., and Norberg, A., 'Male physicians' narratives about being in ethically difficult care situations in paediatrics', *Social Science & Medicine*, 53(5), 2001, pp. 657–67.

Spark, M., *Memento mori*, Penguin, Middlesex, 1959.

Spicker, S. F., Alon, I., de Vries, A., and Engelhardt, H. T. Jr, *The use of human beings in research*, Philosophy and Medicine no. 28, Kluwer Academic Publishers, Dordrecht, 1988.

Spurgeon, B., 'Surgeons pleased with patient's progress after face transplant', *British Medical Journal*, 331(7529), p. 1359.

Stacey, G. and Hunt, C. J., 'The UK stem cell bank: A UK government-funded, international resource center for stem cell research', *Regenerative Medicine*, 1(1), 2006, pp. 139–42.

Stecher, J., 'Ethics at the end of life in transplant recipients', *Progress in Transplantation*, 21(1), 2011, pp. 83–7.

Sullivan, R. J., *Immanuel Kant's moral theory*, Cambridge University Press, Cambridge, 1989.

Surbone, A., 'Truth-telling, risk, and hope', in A. Surbone and M. Zwitter, 'Communication with the cancer patient: Information and truth', *Annals of the New York Academy of Sciences*, vol. 809, New York Academy of Sciences, New York, 1997, pp. 72–9.

Suzuki, D. and Knudtson, P., *Genethics: The ethics of engineering life*, Allen & Unwin, Sydney, 1989, pp. 345–6.

Taerk, G., Gallop, R. M., Lancee, W. J., Coates, R. A., and Fanning, M., 'Recurrent themes of concern in groups for health care professionals', *AIDS Care*, 5(2), 1993, pp. 215–22.

Tanne, J., 'South Dakota abortion ban encourages other states', *British Medical Journal*, 332(7542), 2006, p. 626.

Taylor, H. A. and Kass, N. E., 'Attending to local justice: Lessons from pediatric HIV', *IRB: Ethics & Human Research*, 24(6), 2002, pp. 9–17.

Tegtmeier, J. W., 'Ethics and AIDS: A summary of the law and critical analysis of the individual physician's ethical duty to treat', *American Journal of Law & Medicine*, 16(1–2), 1990, pp. 249–65.

The President's Council on Bioethics, *Alternative sources of pluripotent stem cells*, Washington, DC, 2005.

Thomson, C., 'Personnel', in *CCH Australian Health & Medical Law Reporter*, (looseleaf service), updated regularly, pp. 6–400.

Thomson, J. J., 'A defense of abortion', *Philosophy and Public Affairs*, 1(1), 1971, pp. 47–66.

Todd, A. M., Lacey, E. A., and McNeill, F., '"I'm still waiting . . .": Barriers to accessing cardiac rehabilitation services', *Journal of Advanced Nursing*, 40(4), 2002, pp. 413–20.

Tomaszewski, T., 'Ethical issues from an international perspective', *International Journal of Psychology*, 124, 1979, pp. 131–5.

Tooley, M., 'Abortion and infanticide', in J. Feinberg (ed.), *The problem of abortion*, Wadsworth, Belmont, CA, 1973, pp. 51–91.

'Troubled transplant man throws in bad hand', *Australian*, 5 February 2001, p. 5.

Ubel, P. A., DeKay, M. L., Baron, J., and Asch, D. A., 'Cost-effectiveness analysis in a setting of budget constraints', *New England Journal of Medicine*, 334(18), 1996, pp. 1174–7.

United Nations, 'Convention on the Rights of the Child', entry into force 2 September 1990, in accordance with article 28, <www.un.org>.

——, 'International Covenant on Civil and Political Rights', entry into force 23 March 1976.

United Nations Educational, Scientific and Cultural Organization, 'Universal Declaration on the Human Genome and Human Rights', adopted 11 November 1997, UNESCO's 29th General Conference, Endorsed UN General Assembly 1998.

——, 'Universal Declaration on Bioethics and Human Rights', adopted by acclamation on 19 October 2005 by the 33rd Session of the General Conference of UNESCO.

United States Department of Health, Education, and Welfare, *Ethical principles and guidelines for the protection of human subjects of research* (the Belmont Report), publication no. OS 78–0012, US Department of Health, Education, and Welfare, Washington DC, 1978.

—, Privacy Rule, *Federal Regulations*, 67(157), 14 August 2002, pp. 53181–273.

—, revised *Federal Register*, 56, 1991, p. 28032, 45 CFR Part 46, Subpart D.

Urbina, C., Kaufman, A., and Derksen, D., 'The managed health care scenario: Challenges to future medical training', *Education for Health*, 10(1), 1997, pp. 25–33.

'Urgent changes needed for authorisation of phase I trials', editorial, *Lancet*, 367(9518), 2006, p. 1214.

Veatch, R. M., *Cross cultural perspectives in medical ethics*, Jones & Bartlett Publishers, Boston, 1989.

—, 'Justice in health care: The contribution of Pellegrino', *Journal of Medicine and Philosophy*, 15, 1990, pp. 269–87.

Vinten, G., 'Whistle while you work in the health related professions?', *Journal of the Royal Society of Health*, 114(5), 1994, pp. 256–62.

Walker, J., Lyall, K., and Hawes, R., 'Wooldridge backs inquiry on guinea-pig babies', *Australian*, 11 June 1997, pp. 1, 2.

Wall, S. D., Olcott, E. W., and Gerberding, J. L., 'AIDS risk and risk reduction in the radiology department', *American Journal of Roentology*, 157(5), 1991, pp. 911–17.

Walsh, M., *The National Childhood Immunisation Campaign—ethical issues: Topics for attention*, Issues Paper No. 3 (Autumn 1997), Australian Institute of Health Law & Ethics, 1997.

Walther, F. J., 'Withholding treatment, withdrawing treatment, and palliative care in the neonatal intensive care unit', *Early Human Development*, 81(12), 2005, pp. 965–72.

Warnock, M., 'Do human cells have rights?', *Bioethics*, 1(1), 1987, pp. 1–14.

Warnock, M., *Making babies: Is there a right to have children?*, Oxford University Press, Oxford, 2002.

Weed, M., 'Ethics, regulation, and biomedical research', *Kennedy Institute of Ethics Journal*, 14(4), 2004, pp. 361–8.

Weeramantry, C. G. and Giantomasso, D. F., *Consent to the medical treatment of minors and intellectually handicapped persons*, Faculty of Law, Monash University, Melbourne, 1983.

Westin, A. F., *Privacy and freedom*, Atheneum, New York, 1970.

Whitney, S. N., Ethier, A. M., Frugé, E., Berg, S., McCullough, L. B., and Hockenberry, M., 'Decision-making in pediatric oncology: Who should take the lead? The decisional priority in pediatric oncology model', *Journal of Clinical Oncology*, 24(1), 2006, pp. 160–5.

Williams, M. V., Parker, R. M., Baker, D. W., Parik, N. S., Pitkin, K., Coates, W. C., and Nurss, J. R., 'Inadequate functional literacy among patients at two public hospitals', *Journal of the American Medical Association*, 274(21), 1995, pp. 1677–82.

World Health Organization, *Basic Documents*, 26th edn, WHO, Geneva, 1976.

——, 'Preamble to the constitution of the World Health Organization', in WHO *Basic Documents*, 26th edn, WHO, Geneva, 1976, p. 1.

——, 'Alert, verification and public health management of SARS in the post-outbreak period', 14 August 2003 <www.who.int/csr/sars>.

——, 'WHO News: Pandemic flu: Communicating the risks', *Bulletin of the World Health Organization*, 84(1), 2006, pp. 9-11.

—— 'Projected supply of pandemic influenza vaccine sharply increases', 23 October 2007, <www.who.int>.

World Medical Association, 'Declaration of Helsinki', as amended in 2000 with note of clarification on paragraph 29, 2002, and paragraph 30, 2004, <www.wma.net>.

——, 'Ethical principles for medical research involving human subjects, Declaration of Helsinki'. Adopted 1964, as amended 2008, <www.wma.net>.

——, 'WMA to continue discussion on Declaration of Helsinki', Press release, 14 September 2003, <www.wma.net>.

Wueste, D., 'A philosophical yet user-friendly framework for ethical decision making in critical care nursing', *Dimensions of Critical Care Nursing*, 24(2), 2005, pp. 70-9.

Yarborough, M., Jones, T., Cyr, T. A., Phillips S., and Stelzner, D., 'Interprofessional education in ethics at an academic health sciences center', *Academic Medicine*, 75(8), 2000, pp. 793-800, at p. 794.

Young, T., 'Teaching medical students to lie', *Canadian Medical Association Journal*, 156(2), 1997, pp. 219-22.

Zeleznik, D., Habjanic, A., and Micetic Turk, D. M., 'Teaching ethics to students in the University College of Nursing Studies in Maribor', *Medicine and Law*, 19(3), 2000, pp. 433-9.

Zwart, H., 'Rationing in the Netherlands: The liberal and communitarian perspective', *Health Care Analysis*, 1(1), 1993, pp. 53-6.

INDEX

abortion 136–40
  Catholic health institutions 194
  China 137
  Islamist views 192
  United States 138–9, 145
absolutism 6–7, 31
acceptance of health status 155
access to information 108
accountability 28
advance directives 171
aged care 169–72
  assessing competence 169
  degenerative conditions 174–5
  dementia 171–2
  resuscitation 170
  use of restraints 170
AIDS Clinical Trials Group (ACTG) [USA] 185
AIDS education, Catholic views 195
American Medical Association 113
Ancliffe, Jacqui 159, 162
Andrews Bill (Cth) 176, 178
Appelbaum, Paul 157
Aristotle 5, 26
Asch, D.A. 64, 66
Association of Salaried Medical Professionals [NZ] 62
Australia
  health care system 65
  health spending 53
  Medicare 57–8
Australian Health Practitioner Regulation Agency (AHPRA) 37, 199
Australian Research Council 203
Australian Vice-Chancellors' Committee 203
autonomy
  within beneficence 87
  children 144–52
  competence 147–8, 157
  comprehension 148–9
  developmentally disabled clients 158
  end-of-life decisions 171–80
  enhanced 87
  ethically robust decisions 146–7
  ethics principle 14, 29–33, 72, 131
  euthanasia 176–8
  libertarianism 48
  life support decisions 87
  limiting 77–9
  promoting 77–9
  suicide 175
  treatment responsibility 86–9, 91–6
  voluntariness 149–50
  vs social responsibility 156–7
avian influenza (H5N1 strain) 111–12, 187

Baron, J. 66
Beauchamp, T.L. 14–15, 29–32, 87, 89–90, 134, 170
Belmont principles 30–1, 214–218
beneficence
  Belmont principles 30–1, 214
  end-of-life decisions 171
  ethics principle 14, 29–33, 52, 80
  treatment responsibility 81–3, 85–9
benefit 76
Bentham, Jeremy 206
Berg, Kare 136
Bernat, J.L. 158
best interests 145–6, 149, 171
bioethics 3
bird flu (H5N1 strain) 111–12, 187
Blonder, Irene 200
blood donors
  confidentiality 110
  harm minimisation 121
Boase, Leanne 76, 84, 115, 155
bone marrow donation 146
Bristol Inquiry 201
British Medical Association 114
Brown, Neil 180
Bush, George W. 128–9

Callahan, Daniel 52
cardiopulmonary resuscitation (CPR) 170

'CARE'   187
carer-client relationship
    risks   120
    terminating   121-2
    trust   115-16, 155
Cartwright, Jade   174, 193
casuistry   13-14, 94-5
Chalmers, I.   190
Charlesworth, Max   91
children
    autonomy   144-52
    best interests   145
    competence   147-8
    immunisation   156-7
    quality of life decisions   161
    research participation   150-2, 186
    tattooing   145
Childress, J.F.   14-15, 29-32, 87, 89-90,
    134, 171
Cica, N.   178
claim right   140
claims on health resources   47
client-carer relationship
    risks   120
    terminating   121-2
    trust   115-16, 155
clients   39
    as consumers   154-7
    injured or 'wronged'   207
    negotiating treatment with   89-96
    non-compliant   161-3
    passive   156
clinical ethics committees   202-3
Clinical Ethics Network [UK]   191
clinical trials   166
Clinton, Bill   135
cloning   135
codes of ethics   34-7, 198
    American Health Information
        Management Association   104
    American Medical Association   113-14
Cohen, Stephen   36
communitarianism   8, 12, 79, 183
community consultation   182-90
community limits   183
competence

aged care   169-70
    autonomy   147-8, 157
    children   147-8
    consent   157-8, 169
complaints against practitioners
    199-200
comprehension   148-9, 158
compulsory actions   118
'concept mapping'   155
confidentiality   100-10, 121, 216
conflict of interest   205
consent   86
    acutely ill patients   157-8
    balance of power   155
    competence   147-8, 157-8, 169
    comprehension   148-9, 158
    informed   88, 90-6, 146-7, 157-8
    limiting what is asked   150-2
    surrogate decision makers   145-6, 158
    use of organs   151
    voluntariness   149-50
    waiving   109
consequentialism   7, 31, 136
consumer perspectives
    on health care system   155-6
    on illness   155
Consumer Reports   185
Consumers Union [USA]   185
Convention on the Rights of the Child
    (United Nations)   50, 147
convictions   193-4
cost-benefit analysis   66-7
cost-effectiveness analysis   66
counselling relationships   73
Covenant on Civil and Political Rights
    (United Nations)   216
Cox, Ken   22
cultural beliefs and practices   183-4, 188,
    192-3
cultural safety   62
culture   187

de Ridder, D.   155
Declaration of Helsinki (World Medical
    Association)   215, 219-20
degenerative conditions   174-5

DeKay, M.L.   66
dementia   171–2
deontology   6–7, 11, 31–2, 87, 131, 136, 140, 180, 183
Department of Health and Human Services [USA], Privacy Rules and Security Rule   106–7
Depla, M.   155
Devereux, John   148
Dickenson, Donna   145
dignity   72
disclosure of information
    about dangerous practices   79
    by clients/patients   100
    to clients/patients   11, 89–92, 94–5, 114–15
    public interest   108–10, 121
    see also confidentiality
'do no harm'   11, 30, 214–15
'Do Not Resuscitate' (DNR)   170
doctrine   84
Dolly [cloned sheep]   135
'double effect,' doctrine of   84–5
Douglas, M.   188–9
drug development   164–6, 211
duties   26
duty of care   82–3, 158

Edwards, Tracy   171
embryos, treatment of   127–9, 188
entitlement   50
ethics committees
    clinical   202–3
    lay members   205
    research   165, 184–5, 190, 202–5, 215, 218–23
ethics, definition   3
eugenics   188
European Court of Justice   130
euthanasia   176–80
    assistance devices   179
    Northern Territory Act   176–8
    'slippery-slope' argument   178
Euthanasia Laws Act 1997 (Cth)   176

female circumcision   145
feminist research   184

Finnis, John   139–40
Flew, Anthony   178
Food and Drug Administration (FDA) [USA]   139
Foot, Philippa   85
Foottit, Jenneke   29, 51, 55, 105, 113, 184, 202
Frankel, M.S.   189

Gallagher, Ann   170
generic drugs   165
genetic testing   133–6
genetics and ethics   132–6
Gillon, R.   30, 52, 179
goals   26
Godecke, Erin   159, 162
Goh Lee Gan   192
good   46–7, 50, 52–3, 66, 131, 151
    definition   5
    utilitarianism   7
good Samaritan principle   82, 139, 158
Grace, Damian   36
Granger, Andrew   159, 162
Greenpeace   130
Grisso, Thomas   157
guardianship   145–6, 156–7

harm minimisation   79
Harman, G.   39
health and disability ethics committees (HDECs) [NZ]   205
health care   22
health care professionals   22
health records   74
health spending
    Australia   53
    international comparisons   53
health, WHO definition   52–3
hepatitis C   120
HIV transmission   117–20, 166
HIV/AIDS treatments research   165–6, 185, 211
Hohfeld, W.N.   52, 140
Human Genome Organisation   132
Human Genome Project   132
human rights   132

Hume, David   99

ideals   5
immunisation   156–7
    trials on orphans   152, 186
in vitro fertilisation (IVF)   126–9
    after husband's death   173
infants
    care of disabled   179
    'non-viable'   173
    pre-term   173
infection control standards   118
information disclosure   89–96, 100,
    108–10, 114–15, 121
    standards   90
informed consent   88, 90–6, 146–7, 157–8
informed decision making   94
Inquiry into Human Fertilisation and
    Embryology [UK]   126
insight   200
institutional ethics committees (IECs)
    [NZ]   205
institutional review boards (IRBs) [USA]
    185, 204–5
institutions
    institutional cultures   190–1
    operating guidelines   191
    standards   202–5
interests   47–8, 50–2

Japanese health practices   88
Jehovah's Witnesses   194
Jennett, B.   15, 85
Jonas, Hans   35, 188
Jonsen, A.R.   15, 74, 160, 170
justice
    Belmont principles   30–1, 214, 217–18
    comparative   54
    distributive   54–5
    ethics principle   14, 29–33, 52
    as fairness   53
    models of   53–6

Kant, Immanuel   32, 34, 183
Kemmy, A.M.   67
Kitzhaber, J.   67
Knultgen, J.   35

law   41–2, 52, 206–7
    see also abortion; euthanasia
legal standards   206–7
Leontini, Rose   25
libertarianism   7, 10, 12, 47, 78, 91, 183
    autonomy   48
liberty   47, 77–8, 89, 140
life support decisions   87
limiting what is asked   150–2
'living wills'   171

Magney, Alix G.   12
Making babies (Warnock)   126
Malsch, M.   155
managed care   61–5
mandatory actions   118, 157
mass media   186
McCorvey, Norma   138
Medical Education   117
medical ethics   3
medical records   74
    client access   114–15
Medical Research Council [UK]   130
Medicare   57–8
Mill, John Stuart   7, 32, 47–8, 77–8, 109, 119
moral
    definition   3
    ideals   34
    rules   34
'moral perfection'   32
morality
    character   199
    personal   77–8, 195
    social   77–9
morals, definition   2
Moreno, J.D.   39
morning-after pill   139

narrative approach to ethics   160
National Academy of Sciences [USA]   129
National Ethics Advisory Committee and the
    Ministry of Health [NZ]   205
National Health and Medical Research
    Council   203
National Health Service (NHS) [UK]   62,
    114, 157
        consumer representation   185

National Institute of Health [USA]   129
National Institutes of Health (NIH)
    [USA]   210
*National statement on ethical conduct in research
    involving humans* (NHMRC et al)   203
need   54
needlestick injuries   118
negligence law   207
negotiating treatment with clients   89–96
Nelson, R.M.   151
New Zealand cervical cancer experiments
    201, 210
New Zealand health system   62
no-fault compensation scheme [NZ]   207
non-compliant patients   161–3
non-maleficence   14, 29–33
    ethics principle   29–33
non-therapeutic research   151, 215
norms   4
notifiable conditions   110–11
Nuffield Council on Bioethics   191
Nuremberg Code   219
nursing, tasks   27

Obama, Barack   129
obligations   26, 52
occupational health and safety   120
    HIV transmission   117–20
occupational therapy   27
Office of Research Integrity [USA]   191, 221
Olsen, D.P.   195
On Liberty (Mill)   7
Oregon experiment   67–8
Organization for Economic Co-operation and
    Development (OECD)   53
organs, post death use   151

palliative pain relief   84–5
pandemics   110–12
parental decision-making   144–52, 156–7
paternalism   11, 31, 78, 86–7, 91, 96,
    112, 121
patients   39
    as consumers   154–7
    negotiating treatment with   89–96
    non-compliant   161–3
    passive   156

peer review   190, 200
peer standards   197–9
Pellegrino, E.   23, 33, 87, 91
performance enhancing drugs
    use   79
person   126
personhood   126, 128, 130, 140
Peterson, L.M.   158
pharmaceuticals   164–6
Pharmacy Board of Australia, Code of
    Conduct   109
Philosophical medical ethics (Gillon)   179
Plato   5
potentiality   128
premature births   173
Presidential Commission for the Study of
    Bioethical Issues   129
President's Council on Bioethics   129
Principle Approach   12–13
principlist frameworks   11–12, 14–15
privacy   72–3, 100–10
private interests   108–9, 121
professional caring   176
professional standards
    breaches   27–8, 116, 201
    character   199
    community trust   35–6
    disciplinary records   199–200
    law   206
    maintaining   197–9
    registration board inquiries
        199–200
    see also codes of ethics
professions   34
proportionism   8, 189
public health   112, 120–1
public interests   108–9, 120–1

Qiu, R-Z.   79
quality assurance   190, 202
quality-adjusted life years (QALY)   160–1
quality-of-life dilemmas   160–1
quarantine   121

Rawls, John   37–8, 53, 55
reflection   2
registration   27, 198

Australian Health Practitioner Regulation
     Agency (AHPRA)   37, 199
   English proficiency   199
registration board inquiries   199
relativism   7, 13, 16, 39
relaying bad news   112–13
religion and health care   191–5
   Catholic church   194–5
   Chinese views   191–2
   Islamic views   192–3
   Jehovah's Witnesses   194
   Singaporean views   192
reproductive technology   125–36
research
   Belmont principles   214–18
   carers as researchers   209–10
   community consultation   189
   culturally informed   184
   dissemination of information   217–18
   drug development   164–6
   ethics committees   165, 184–5, 190,
     202–5, 215, 218–23
   ethics concerns   211–14, 218
   feminist   184
   funding by pharmaceutical companies
     210
   HRECs   203–4, 218–23
   non-therapeutic   151, 215
   payment of participants   216–17
   placebo groups   219–20
   proposals   220–3
   therapeutic   150, 152, 215
   transparency   223
   unethical, cervical cancer   201, 210
   unethical, syphilis   190, 210
research ethics committees (RECs) [UK]   204
research participants
   children   145, 150–2, 186
   community perceptions   190
   developing countries   165
   patients   211
resource allocation   57–69
respect for persons   30–1, 72
   Belmont principles   30–1, 214–17
responsibility   28, 156–7
Revay, Beah   137

'right to life'   126
rights   49–52, 140, 157
Rights of the Terminally Ill Act 1995 [NT]   176
risk
   acceptable   86, 150–1, 166, 190
   to carers   117–20
   to clients   117–20
   liberty and   77
   to others   120–1
Roe v. Wade   138
Ross, L.F.   151
Royal College of Surgeons [UK]   187
RU486 (morning-after pill)   139
rules   34

'scrupulous parent' standard   151
self-care   25, 27
severe acute respiratory syndrome
   (SARS)   110–11
Severens, P.   155
Shapiro, J.   161
Shipman, Harold   28
Shipman Inquiry   28
Shooner, Caroline   116
Siegler, M.   15, 74, 160
Silverman, W.A.   190
Singer, Peter   81–2, 188
Singh, Kamaljit   192
skill   23
Smith, Janet (Dame)   28
Socrates   4–5
St Thomas Aquinas   126
St Vincent's Bioethics Newsletter   195
stem cell research   125, 127–30, 135
suicide   175–6
surrogate decision makers   145–6, 158
Suzuki, David   134

Tarasoff v. Regents of University of California
   121
Thailand health system   65
thalidomide   164–5
Therapeutic Goods Administration (TGA)
   139
therapeutic research   150, 152, 215
Thomasma, D.C.   87, 91
Thomson, J.J.   139–40

transparency   223

transplants
  bone marrow   131, 146
  cells   130
  facial   187–8
  hands   187
  inter-species   211
  organs   51, 149, 151

treatment responsibility
  autonomy   87–9, 91, 157–60
  beneficence   81–3, 85–9
  negotiation with clients   89–96
  non-compliant patients   161–3
  quality-of-life dilemmas   160–1
  surrogate decision-makers   159–60

triage system of health care delivery   54

trust   76, 99–100, 115–16

truth   113–14

Tuskegee Study of Untreated Syphilis
  190, 210

Ubel, P.A.   64, 66

United Kingdom health system   61–2, 80–1

United Nations Educational, Scientific and
  Cultural Organization (UNESCO)   38

United States health system   62–4

Universal Declaration on Bioethics and
  Human Rights (UNESCO)   38, 216

Universal Declaration on the Human
  Genome and Human Rights (UNESCO)
  132

'Universal Precautions'   118

utilitarianism   7, 31–2, 66, 87, 131, 140,
  180, 206

utility   66

vaccine research   152

values, definition   4

Veatch, Robert   191

veracity   113–14

Vinten, G.   200

virtue   99

voluntariness   149–50

Walsh, Michael   156

Warnock, Mary   126

whistleblowing   200–2

Willowbrook experiments   152

Winslade, W.J.   15, 74, 160

wishes   72

World Health Organization
  110–12, 165

World Medical Association (WMA)
  215, 219

Wueste, Daniel   189

Young, Tara   113